Building Health and Wellbeing

This book focuses on the relationship between buildings and our health and wellbeing, and by extension our quality of life. Expanding on the 50th anniversary Special Issue of *Building Research & Information* (BRI), which was dedicated to health and wellbeing, articles have been extended and updated to complement contributions from new authors. *Building Health and Wellbeing* covers design for ageing, energy poverty and health, productivity and thermal comfort in offices, housing space and occupancy standards, and much more. The aim is to explore the inter-relationship between people and our buildings. Chapters are supported with new case studies to illustrate global approaches to a common challenge, while demonstrating local strategies to suit different climates. The content covers housing, offices, and healthcare facilities and the unique aspect of the book is the people perspective, providing outlooks from different age groups and users of buildings. It will act as an important reference for academics in the built environment and healthcare sectors.

Stephen Emmitt is an architect and Professor of Architectural Practice at the Department of Architecture and Civil Engineering, University of Bath. He has also held professorial posts at Loughborough University and the Technical University of Denmark as well as a visiting professor position at Halmstad University, Sweden. He is an established author and Editor-in-Chief of *Building Research & Information* (BRI). Stephen's research interests range from the management of design and design offices, architectural technologies and the performance of buildings, to how people interact with buildings.

BRI Research Series

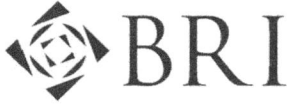

❖BRI

This book series shares similar aims and scope to the journal, *Building Research & Information*, but allows for a more focused and deeper investigation of interdisciplinary topics and issues.

This book series focuses on the entire life cycle of buissldings, from inception to designing, engineering, and making, through the building in use phase, to disassembly and recovery. Unique to this series is a holistic and interdisciplinary approach to a sustainable built environment, centred on the building and its context. The journal scope includes research on a wide range of topics relating to buildings, embracing the what, why, how, and when questions relating to:

- **People:** Motivations and actions of designers, engineers, makers, managers and users of buildings; user satisfaction; universal and inclusive design; education of stakeholders; supply chain capabilities; stakeholder needs; stewardship; sustainable communities; culture.
- **Performance:** The performance and impact of buildings in relation to design, engineering, environmental, economic, social, organiational, structural, and technical factors; impact assessment and performance monitoring; thermal comfort and indoor climate; resource use.
- **Policy:** Innovation; legislation, standards and codes; ethics and ethical sourcing; health, wellbeing and quality of life; building values; value of buildings; public policy; space standards; societal interests and sustainable building; engagement with buildings; security.
- **Product:** De-carbonised buildings; regenerative and restorative building design and development; mitigation, resilience, and adaption to climate change; active building technologies and smart buildings; innovative and non-conventional building materials; healing environments; adaptive re-use, retrofit, disassembly, and resource recovery; quality.
- **Process:** Integrated and creative processes and systems; automation and craft; creation and making of buildings; management and use of built assets within a digital, creative, and circular economy; optimiation of design; innovative solutions to complex challenges; interfaces.

Building Health and Wellbeing

Edited by Stephen Emmitt

Routledge
Taylor & Francis Group

LONDON AND NEW YORK

First published 2024
by Routledge
4 Park Square, Milton Park, Abingdon, Oxon OX14 4RN

and by Routledge
605 Third Avenue, New York, NY 10158

Routledge is an imprint of the Taylor & Francis Group, an informa business

British Library Cataloguing-in-Publication Data
A catalogue record for this book is available from the British Library

ISBN: 978-1-032-38021-6 (hbk)
ISBN: 978-1-032-38375-0 (pbk)
ISBN: 978-1-003-34471-1 (ebk)

DOI: 10.1201/9781003344711

Typeset in Times New Roman
by MPS Limited, Dehradun

Contents

Series Preface   *vii*

Introduction   1

1   Exploring the concept of a healthy office and
    healthy employees   5
    MELINA FOROORAGHI, ANTONIO COBALEDA-CORDERO,
    AND MARAL BABAPOUR CHAFI

2   The productivity of office occupants in relation
    to the indoor thermal environment   31
    JAIME SOTO MUÑOZ, MAUREEN TREBILCOCK KELLY,
    VICENTE FLORES-ALÉS, AND RAÚL RAMÍREZ-VIELMA

3   Use of portable air purifiers, occupant behaviour,
    and indoor air quality in homes in three
    European cities   60
    ELIZABETH COOPER, YAN WANG, SAMUEL STAMP,
    AND DEJAN MUMOVIC

4   Hospitalised patients' adaptation strategies and how
    they influence their indoor environmental comfort   88
    SARA WILLEMS, DIRK SAELENS, AND ANN HEYLIGHEN

5   Environmental qualities and features in mental
    and behavioural health environments   111
    MARDELLE MCCUSKEY SHEPLEY, KATI PEDITTO,
    NAOMI A. SACHS, Y PHAM, RUTH BARANKEVICH,
    GARY CROUPPEN, AND KARYN DRESSER

6   Mobility, independence, and spatial distance
    in rehabilitation centres for stroke   139
    MAJA KEVDZIJA AND GESINE MARQUARDT

7   Outdoor activity-friendly environments for older
    adults with disabilities: A case study in China
    from a functioning perspective   164
    QING XIE AND XIAOMEI YUAN

8   Healthy ageing and the relationship with the
    built environment and design   193
    LINA ENGELEN, MARGIE RAHMANN, AND ELLEN DE JONG

9   Energy poverty, poor housing, and the wellbeing
    of older Australians   221
    CAROLINE VALENTE, ALAN MORRIS, AND SARA WILKINSON

    Conclusion   248

    Index   *250*

Series Preface

Building Research & Information (BRI) is a leading international refereed journal focused on the entire life cycle of buildings, from inception to designing, engineering, construction and assembly, through the building in use phase, to disassembly and recovery. Unique to *BRI* is a holistic and interdisciplinary approach to a sustainable built environment, centred on the building and its context. This book series shares the journal's philosophy and commitment to high-quality research, providing the space for more detailed and nuanced exploration of a particular theme. Each book in the series aims to explore the complex and inter-related nature of our sustainable built environment, embracing what? why? how? and when? questions in relation to a specific research theme.

The content of the journal, except for Special Issues, is very much determined by what is submitted to the journal for consideration; and what gets through a rigorous anonymous peer review process. Thus, the content is wonderfully varied, and individual Issues are rarely themed in the way that an edited book can be. The journal content does, however, often suggest the need for further enquiry and exploration that lends itself a little better to a research book format. This research book series is a mechanism that allows the curation of chapters as a themed anthology and builds on the content of the journal. Like any edited collection, difficult decisions must be made about what to include and what to exclude to create books that are integrated around a specific topic. The rationale is to provide unbiased peer-reviewed content by expert authors, championed by the book editor and supported by the book series editor. In this way, the book series aims to be fresh and engaging, and by design, not formulaic. We believe that these books will be a valuable starting point for early career academics and readers wanting to discover more about a specific topic. With this book series, we hope to further inform and stimulate rapid advances in the performance of our buildings.

In this book, the focus is on the relationship between buildings and our health and wellbeing, and by extension our quality of life. The genius of this book is to be found in the 50th anniversary Special Issue of *Building Research & Information* (BRI), which was dedicated to health and wellbeing. The focus of the research presented in this book is on the how people interact with buildings and the mechanisms and stimuli that can make a positive impact to our comfort, health, and wellbeing.

Professor Stephen Emmitt
Department of Architecture and
Civil Engineering
University of Bath, UK

Introduction

Although we have known for a long time about the health benefits that well designed, constructed, and maintained buildings bring to building users, it is not always the most important factor when stakeholders are making decisions concerning our built environment. Priorities may lie elsewhere, and the raft of legislation and guidance documents can sometimes cloud our collective decision-making; unintentionally resulting in buildings that do little to promote a healthy lifestyle. For example, the move to highly insulated and airtight buildings has helped with the drive to reduce energy consumption; however, it has also led to issues with poor indoor air quality, condensation, and overheating in hot weather. Similarly, once in use, building owners and managers may not always have the occupants' health and wellbeing as their priority, making changes and maintenance decisions based on other criteria. Thus, as building users, we sometimes experience frustration because our buildings do not always perform as we would like. In some cases, this may result in minor inconvenience, while in others there may be more serious consequences for our comfort, health, and wellbeing.

There is a growing body of evidence that has explored the relationship between buildings and the physical and psychological health of building users. This interdependence has been brought into sharp focus by the recent global pandemic, alongside challenges associated with an ageing global population and the climate emergency facing our planet. Attention has been on internal air quality, energy conservation and reduction, thermal comfort, and the useability of internal spaces. This has resulted in many building owners and users questioning why so many of our buildings are not performing as well as they should. While many of these questions relate to energy performance and environmental performance, increasingly, attention is turning to the building users' health and wellbeing. In most cases, buildings are designed for people to live, work and play in, and putting people back at the centre of the debate is long overdue.

As a global society, we are developing a much better understanding of the influence of buildings and building materials on our health and wellbeing, but there is more to be done. As we adapt to a warming planet, the practical challenges relating to how we design resilient, adaptable, and healthy

DOI: 10.1201/9781003344711-1

buildings that are net zero carbon becomes ever more urgent. How we can best achieve this will no doubt feature in future issues of *Building Research & Information* and other leading peer-reviewed journals. What is clear is that we need to move rapidly to a more sensual, textile, beautiful, sustainable, and restorative built environment that is accessible to all. We need to design and maintain buildings that make a positive contribution to our health and wellbeing as well as to our planet. How people interact with buildings and how design can contribute to a healthier and better quality of life for all is clearly an important factor. This has led to efforts to improve our links to nature through biophilic design and is leading to a better understanding of what building users want from the buildings they interact with.

There are many definitions and understandings of "health" and "well-being" in the literature. As witnessed in this book, the interpretation and application is very much related to context and the viewpoint of the authors. The wide range of building users' age, physical and mental characteristics, combined with variety of building typologies, ages, and functions, makes it challenging to generalise. For example, we may have different expectations and experiences of office buildings, compared to healthcare buildings or our homes. Similarly, we may have different interpretations and understandings based on where we life and work. Expectations and experiences also vary with age and the various environmental, economic, and societal pressures that influence our behaviour and decision-making. Thus, buildings that worked well when we were younger may not be so functional or enjoyable as we age and become less independent. As an editor, it is encouraging to see differences in interpretation and approaches to the relationship between our buildings and our physical and mental wellbeing expressed in this book.

The chapters curated for this book provide a wide range of insights into how buildings and their immediate environs may contribute to our health and wellbeing, comfort, quality of life, and our productivity. The health and wellbeing theme is confronted from a variety of perspectives and geographical locations. It is, of course, not possible to include every aspect of buildings and health, and this collection has gravitated to themes around offices, healthcare buildings, and our homes. Chapters are based on articles published in the 50th anniversary Special Issue of *Building Research & Information*. It was challenging to decide what to include and what to exclude given that space in this book was at a premium. The rationale was to present chapters that linked in such a way as to carry a narrative through the chapters, while also covering a variety of age groups and physical and mental characteristics. The overall aim was to provide an engaging book that would also act as a primer for further investigations and interventions.

Building Research & Information has a long history of research into workplace environments and the relationship to performance and health. The first chapter of this book extends that tradition by exploring the concept of a healthy office environment and healthy employees. The focus of Forooraghi et al. is on employees' perception of their previous and new office environments, with a unique longitudinal study revealing a wealth of information relating to the work environment. The authors draw on the concept of coherence and an individual's ability to cope with various stressors. One could deduce that there is also a link to productivity, and the second chapter by Muñoz et al. provides a window on the relationship between productivity and the workplace thermal environment. Their work draws on office buildings based in two cities in Chile, helping to identify the occupants' perceived relationship between temperature and productivity. Both chapters provide insights for designers, employers, and building owners that could be taken forward to inform future office design.

Chapter 3 also explores the internal environment, with the context shifting to homes located in three major European cities. Indoor air quality has always been a determinant of healthy living, which has taken on even more prevalence with the global COVID-19 pandemic. The use of portable air purifiers is, therefore, highly topical. Cooper et al. provides evidence and insights into why these devices are used and the perceptions of the users in terms of their health. As the authors note, there is much more research required to fully understand the contribution of such devices to the residents' comfort and wellbeing. One could be forgiven for wondering why these buildings have not been better designed and constructed so that these devices are not necessary. It is, of course, a question that relates to psychological issues as much as it does the physical building fabric.

Healthcare buildings cover a wide variety of functions and patient needs, and the facilities covered in Chapters 4–6 include hospital rooms, mental and behavioural facilities and rehabilitation clinics for stroke patients. In Chapter 4, Willems et al. have provided unique glimpses into how patients perceive and respond to, and adapt, their immediate environment in hospital wards. Their mixed methods approach has created a comprehensive data set that provides evidence on patients' perceived control over their indoor climate. This concerns the degree of autonomy, or not, bestowed on patients while they are staying in hospital, and by extension their sense of comfort and wellbeing. Chapter 5 addresses environmental qualities and features in mental and behavioural health environments in the USA. Shepley et al. have researched the perceptions of clinical staff and resident patients. The research reveals differences between how the resident patients perceive their environment compared to the clinical staff, helping to shed light on the need for more supportive facilities.

Chapter 6 is focused on mobility and independence in rehabilitation centres. Kevdzija and Marquardt have used patient shadowing to observe the challenges facing stroke patients as they attempt to move around buildings. Their wayfinding research has highlighted some of the physical barriers facing stroke patients, and especially the difficulties of patients who are reliant on wheelchairs following a stroke. The findings clearly indicate a need for better designed clinics to facilitate ease of movement, and with it the potential for patients to be more active as they recuperate.

These chapters raise questions about the suitability of healthcare facilities and reinforce the need to include the needs of different building users in the design and maintenance of buildings.

Attention moves to elderly members of society for Chapters 7–9. External environments surrounding our buildings can affect our wellbeing in positive and negative ways. In Chapter 7, Xie and Yuan have investigated how activity-friendly environments contribute to the wellbeing of older disabled residents in a long-term care facility in China. Their research contributes to the understanding of stimuli and the relationship between residents and their immediate external environment. The message being that user experience, satisfaction, and wellbeing could be improved by paying more attention to the needs of the users of such facilities.

Chapters 8 and 9 both draw on research conducted in Australia, and both focus on elder members of our society. Chapter 8 explores healthy ageing and the relationship with the built environment and design. Engelen et al. have identified several themes in the literature that colour the quality of life and wellbeing of older people. Their conclusions point to the relationship between adults having the ability to exert control over their environment and their health and wellbeing. The review will provide evidence for designers striving to provide buildings that support and facilitate healthy ageing. In Chapter 9, Valente et al. have explored the three factors contributing to energy poverty; energy efficiency of dwellings, the cost of energy to heat and cool the buildings, and household income. Based on interviews with individuals experiencing energy poverty the findings highlight their vulnerability to quite small changes, leading to thermal discomfort and other issues, such as social exclusion. Although the focus is on Australia, energy poverty is a challenge for many countries around the world and one that appears to be complex and difficult to resolve.

1 Exploring the concept of a healthy office and healthy employees

Melina Forooraghi, Antonio Cobaleda-Cordero, and Maral Babapour Chafi

Introduction

Recent decades have seen increasing interest in studying the impact of office environment on health-related outcomes (cf. Clements-Croome, 2018; Jensen & van der Voordt, 2019). However, as revealed by recent literature reviews (Colenberg et al., 2021; Groen et al., 2018; Jensen & van der Voordt, 2019), most studies focus on alleviating the negative effects on employees while the health-promoting potential of office environments is overlooked. These include, for example, nature as a means of recovering from stress or space personalisation as a means of enhancing wellbeing (Colenberg et al., 2021). Moreover, the health and wellbeing agenda within the corporate real estate sector focuses on flexible office concepts, predominantly with respect to short-term effects of relocation to a new office (cf. Appel-Meulenbroek et al., 2018; Engelen et al., 2019). Therefore, we know little about what happens when we become habituated to the new office environment and the novelty begins to wear off. This leads to an important question: are the perceived health benefits of office environments permanent or do they eventually fade away? This chapter explores ways in which employees' perceptions of the office environment relate to their perceived health in the long term to provide a unique insight into an under-researched area.

Studies on the influence of office environment on employee health in the long term are rare and disparate. Some researchers have observed improvements in perceived health 15 months after relocation to an activity-based office (Meijer et al., 2009). Conversely, other studies have observed a decline in perceived health, wellbeing, and performance in the long term due to increased exposure to environmental stressors in open plan offices (Bergström et al., 2015; Brennan et al., 2002; Lamb & Kwok, 2016). Furthermore, most longitudinal studies focus on comparing employee perceptions pre-relocation and within the three to nine months post-relocation (Blok et al., 2009; Candido et al., 2019; Gerdenitsch et al., 2018; Rolfö et al., 2018) which may be enough time for employees to adjust to the new environment and capture novelties. According to Wijk et al. (2020), a follow-up after nine months may be too short, as they did not find any

DOI: 10.1201/9781003344711-2

changes in health after a move to an activity-based office from multiple office types. Short-term evaluations may not be sufficient to give in-depth knowledge on how novelties are appropriated over time. Exceptions are Wohlers and Hertel (2018) and Haapakangas et al. (2019) who investigated the long-term effects of relocation to activity-based offices and found decreased satisfaction with communication. Both studies emphasised that the long-term effects of relocations may vary depending on follow-up time, previous office layout and concept, and differences between cases. Hence, if the case-specific circumstances play an important role in explaining the observed discrepancies between studies, qualitative and in-depth research approaches appear to be particularly relevant to further understand:

- how and why initial perceptions evolve over time,
- how the new routines or coping strategies remain or change over time.

A recent systematic literature review that reported the influences of physical work environments on employee health and wellbeing evidenced that longitudinal studies with a qualitative approach are scarce (Berlin & Babapour Chafi, 2020). This chapter explores the concept of a healthy office and healthy employees via a case study, using salutogenesis and sense of coherence as the underpinning theory.

Salutogenesis and sense of coherence

This chapter uses the conceptualisation of health proposed by Huber et al. (2011), as "the ability to adapt and to self-manage in the face of social, physical and emotional challenges". This conceptualisation was adopted because it is dynamic, and it emphasises the resilience and capacity of people to cope with disease. Moreover, it considers the opportunities for individuals' health gains, rather than focusing only on their ill health. Huber's conceptualisation has received criticism as it is only applicable in circumstances wherein the individuals are in control, whereas some social conditions may prevent individuals and communities adapting to their circumstances (Jambroes et al., 2016). Nevertheless, health in this conceptualisation is regarded as a dynamic balance between opportunities and limitations influenced by social and environmental challenges (Huber et al., 2011). By effectively providing inclusive work environments, people who are less able to take care of their own health can work or participate in social activities and be part of society, despite limitations. Hence, this conceptualisation is preferred over the definition of health by the World Health Organisation (1948) as a state of "complete physical, mental and social wellbeing" which has been often taken as a reference point, but also criticised for being overly idealistic, especially due to the word "complete". The conceptualisation by Huber et al. fits with this chapter's perspective on health as a dynamic concept on a health-ease and dis-ease spectrum, i.e., a salutogenic approach.

Antonovsky (1979) coined the term "salutogenesis" to refer to a health approach that focuses on the factors promoting health, rather than on those causing illness. From this perspective, health and illness are not separate variables but the ends of a continuum; and movement towards the health end is facilitated or hindered by competing forces (Eriksson & Lindström, 2006). Antonovsky (1979) developed the construct of "sense of coherence" to explore what helped people stay healthy in stressful situations, consisting of three interrelated components: comprehensibility, manageability, and meaningfulness. This construct is framed in the salutogenic approach to health and refers to a person's, a community's, or a society's ability to overcome challenges by understanding the character of the problems (comprehensibility), identifying and deploying relevant resources (manageability) while finding the perceived problems as challenges worthy of investment and engagement (meaningfulness) (Antonovsky, 1987). Accordingly, the sense of coherence determines an individual's ability to cope effectively with stressors and subsequently their position on the "health-ease"–"dis-ease" continuum (Eriksson & Lindström, 2006).

Studies indicate that the components of sense of coherence are health-promoting resources that may protect individuals from stress and reduce health risks (Eriksson & Lindström, 2006, 2007). Thus, people with a stronger sense of coherence adopt healthier behaviour and are more motivated to cope with stressors, thereby becoming more resilient with better perceived health and quality of life (Braun-Lewensohn et al., 2016; Eriksson & Lindström, 2007; Idan et al., 2017; Koelen et al., 2016). Moreover, a resourceful working environment helps employees build up sense of coherence, thus leading to greater work engagement (Vogt et al., 2016).

Health is developed through the interaction between individuals, their individual health determinants, and their relevant living environments (Bauer & Jenny, 2016). Accordingly, organisations can be considered a living environment and thus a significant contributor to both pathogenic and salutogenic health development. In that sense, the organisational structure, strategy, and culture interact with individual competence, motivation, and identity to influence health (ibid). Hence, health in an office context becomes relevant when studying individual health developments.

Sense of coherence in the office context

This study focuses on the physical office environment which encompasses every material object and stimulus that people encounter in their work, such as building design, room size and layout, furnishings, material and equipment, plus indoor environmental quality such as noise, lighting, and air quality (Davis et al., 2011; Sander et al., 2019). The components of sense of coherence are further described and interpreted with respect to the office context (summarised in Figure 1.1).

Crowding, disorientation, sick building syndrome
(fatigue, allergic reactions, respiratory problems)

Pathogenic forces

Dis-ease ⟵⟶ Health-ease

Salutogenic forces

Sense of coherence

Comprehensibility Ease of wayfinding
Spatial readability
Behavioral rules
Information sharing

Manageability Control over environment
Participation & empowerment
Life management amenities

Meaningfulness Nature references
Personalization
Social relations and support

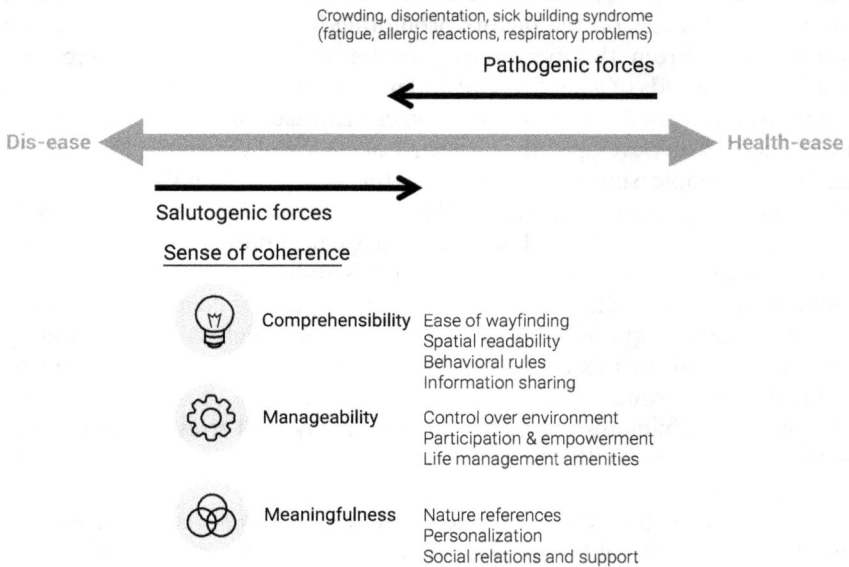

Figure 1.1 The sense of coherence framework in the context of physical office environment.

Comprehensibility

Comprehensibility in the work environment is the capacity to understand and negotiate the contexts in which we find ourselves (Golembiewski, 2016). Wayfinding is an architectural feature that has important implications for a person's stress and anxiety levels and effectiveness in coping (Danko et al., 1990). People tend to use landmarks, boundaries, nodes, and colours to understand and navigate in buildings (Oseland, 2009). Hence, a comprehensible space has cues and signs and is psychologically accessible. Moreover, comprehensibility relates to behavioural rules that are often necessary for structure and predictability. Involving users in the design process and making rules more explicit may result in increased acceptance and greater compliance (Rolfö, 2018). Comprehensibility also refers to environments that communicate their intended use and differences between different workspace types by, say, colour-coding or using different materials and furniture. Finally, when a relocation takes place, it is often unclear to employees what a change in the work environment will mean for them. Transparency and predictability are necessary during a change process, perhaps by giving early and ongoing information about the change and its anticipated results (Kämpf-Dern & Konkol, 2017; Lahtinen et al., 2015). Hence, office environment comprehensibility may be fostered through:

- ease of wayfinding,
- clear behavioural rules,
- easy-to-understand environments,
- transparent information sharing.

Manageability

Manageability reflects the feeling that a person is in control of their environment and work. A sense of control may refer to freedom of choice in perceiving visual and acoustic stimuli, plus isolation from unwanted observation and background noise (called "visual and acoustic privacy"; Kupritz, 1998; van der Voordt et al., 1997). Another form of control is empowerment by increasing employee opportunities to participate in the decision-making process (Vischer, 2008). It has also been suggested that the feeling of empowerment impacts the sense of belonging or ownership over the employee's workspace (ibid). Finally, resources that help employees manage work and home pressures represent important stress relief and mental relaxation outlets. These cover a wide array of services, such as childcare or work autonomy (Danko et al., 1990). Therefore, manageability in the context of an office environment may apply to:

- a sense of control over one's surroundings (such as tools, resources, and stimuli),
- participation and empowerment,
- life management amenities.

Meaningfulness

Meaningfulness in the work environment refers to the extent to which one feels that the stressors of that environment are worthy of investment and engagement (Antonovsky, 1993). Factors that evoke meaning in an office environment may include colours, materials, art, and elements of the natural environment, such as daylight, indoor plants, views and/or access to the natural landscape. It is suggested that humans have an innate tendency to seek connections with nature and other forms of life, and that nature contact is linked with health and wellbeing benefits (Wilson, 1984). Thus, nature references in office environments can be seen as a salutogenic resource that renders meaning to office environments by integrating other forms of life. Moreover, personalisation is another form of affording meaning to space. This may lead to "place attachment"; the emotional bonds between people and their physical environment, including personal space or valued items and facilities (Inalhan & Finch, 2004). Artefacts and symbols of cultural and group identity are examples of meaningful resources that may promote a collective sense of meaning (Heerwagen et al., 1995). Similarly, meaning is found in social relations. The physical layout of the office influences patterns of social interaction. It thereby shapes the social and relational aspects of work because it facilitates or restricts with whom and how often one interacts (Davis et al., 2011). In an office environment meaning may be fostered through:

- integration of the elements of the natural environment,
- personalisation,
- social relations.

The salutogenic approach has received scant attention in built environment research, specifically in the office context. A few studies have applied salutogenesis to healthcare building design (Golembiewski, 2010, 2016) and there is a growing interest in its application in the office context. From a salutogenic perspective, Roskams and Haynes (2019) proposed a conceptual framework in which environmental demands and resources such as behavioural rules, opportunities for personal identity expression, and biophilic design solutions were proposed as influencing a sense of coherence. Ruohomäki et al. (2015) related sense of coherence to office relocation, but no explicit relation was made to the physical environment. Similarly, a case study was used to investigate indicators of sense of coherence during relocation to an activity-based office, using a two-wave questionnaire and focus group interviews (Wijk et al., 2020). The study found that meaningfulness, manageability, and comprehensibility significantly increased from the baseline to nine months post-relocation. The implementation process facilitated a sense of coherence with support from managers, tools on how to work in an activity-based office, and clear communication.

However, there is a lack of research that identifies features of office environments important to employees' sense of coherence in the long term. Increased knowledge about the salutogenic aspects can help to provide evidence for designers, facility managers, and property owners in the drive for healthier offices and employees. To address this knowledge gap, this research aimed to investigate ways in which employees' perceptions of the office environment related to their sense of coherence in the long term. The research question was: what are the short-lived and long-lasting interrelations between employees' perceptions of the office environment and their sense of coherence?

Method

A case-study approach was adopted comprising two waves (six months and two years post-relocation) to investigate ways in which employees' perceptions of the office environment related to their sense of coherence over time.

Context

The case study concerns a division of employees at a Swedish university department that had relocated from cellular offices to a combi office.

The combi office was in a renovated five-storey building. The two middle floors were allocated to university staff, with the rest excluded from the study as it mostly served educational purposes. Employees had assigned desks on the fourth floor, in rooms shared by either two or eight employees. All office rooms had homogeneous conditions in terms of, e.g., type of furniture, technical equipment, glass partitions, daylight, and temperature. The only minor difference was the position of the workstations within the rooms. Back-up spaces included meeting rooms, phone booths, quiet rooms, flexible work rooms, breakout areas and balconies, most of which faced a central atrium (Figure 1.2). Employees had access to all shared facilities in the building. Some modifications had been applied to the office interior by facility management between the Wave 1 data collection phase and Wave 2, which are as follows:

i A quiet room with couches was turned into a shared office room due to a lack of workstations.
ii A windowless meeting room (rarely observed in use during Wave 1) was turned into a print room, following complaints about a lack of printers.
iii Curtains were added to rooms facing the staircases to enhance visual seclusion (privacy) following spontaneous interventions by employees who, for example, covered the glass walls with paper.
iv Couches in the dining room were moved to the other breakout areas and replaced with more dining tables and chairs to accommodate more employees during lunch.

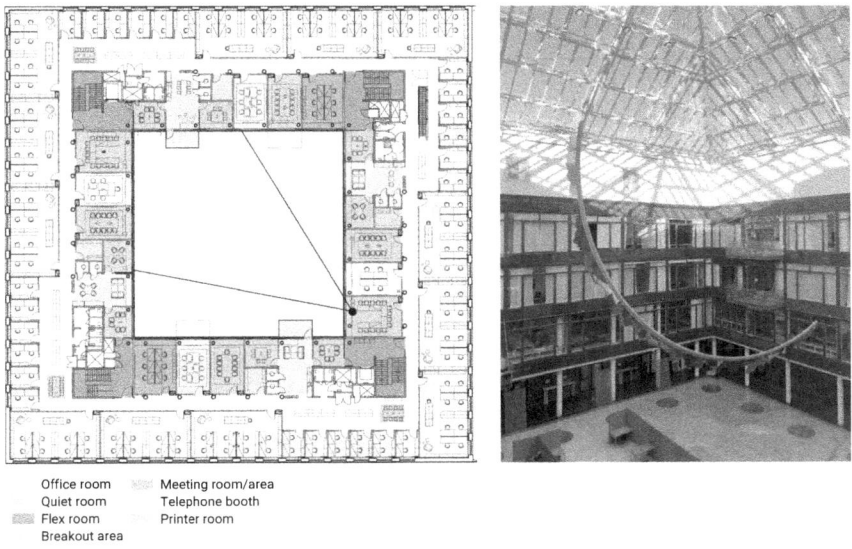

Office room   Meeting room/area
Quiet room   Telephone booth
Flex room   Printer room
Breakout area

Figure 1.2 Representative floorplan of the office and photograph of the office interior.

Data collection procedure

The data collection involved individual semi-structured interviews and structured observations, using the same data collection protocols in both waves. Invitations to participate in interviews went out to all division employees. In Wave 1, 16 employees volunteered to participate in the study, out of which 11 volunteered for Wave 2. Two employees had left the organisation at the time of the second study due to the ending of contract/research projects. The temporality of research contracts causes a moderate rotation of personnel in the organisation, thus, to preserve a sample that was representative of the population as it was in Wave 1, six additional employees who volunteered for Wave 2 were included in the study. Three had experienced the previous office and the other three had been working in the organisation for about or less than one year (Table 1.1).

Prior to the second study (Wave 2), the authors held several discussions among themselves to ensure that data collection was conducted in the same way as the first study. Discussions concerned information and techniques on how to guide the interviewees through the interviews, formulate the questions, introduce the mediation tools in the interviews, as well as how to plan the observations routes and avoid disrupting employees' routines. This was followed by a pilot interview and a test of the observation protocols. The questions addressing the relocation process in

Table 1.1 Interviewees' demographics and job positions

Relocation August 2017	Wave 1 Six months after	Wave 2 Two years after
No. of division employees	Total = 36 Female = 20.5% Male = 79.5%	Total = 35 Female = 22.8% Male = 77.1%
No. of interviewees	Total = 16 Female = 31.2% Male = 68.8%	Total = 17 Female = 29.4% Male = 70.5%
Researcher	11	9
Professor/lecturer	4	4
Project assistant	1	0
Other categories (e.g., project manager, admin)	0	4
Time working in the organisation	Total = 16 0–1 year = 18.7% 2–5 years =62.5% 6> years = 18.7%	Total = 17 0–1 year = 17.6% 2–5 years = 41.1% 6> years = 41.1%
Interviewees participating in both study waves	11	
Interviewees participating in one study wave only	5	6
Interviewees' median age	31.5 years	34 years

Wave 1 were adapted to Wave 2 to focus on employees' perceptions and involvement in decisions concerning modifications in the office over time. For instance, the question about degree of involvement in the relocation process was changed to the degree of involvement in the post-relocation modifications.

A card sorting exercise plus floorplan drawings, markers, and sticky notes were used as mediation tools during the interviews. The card sorting exercise consisted of a biaxial chart visualising levels of satisfaction and importance, and a set of cards relating to predefined themes to be sorted on the chart by employees. The themes covered office environment features such as daylight, personal storage or visual privacy, and contextual aspects such as job conditions, activities, etc. The participants were asked to sort the cards one by one while motivating their choice. Blank cards were also available at the end in case the participants wanted to contribute with new themes. The drawings, markers, and notes were used to help interviewees elaborate on their explanations, note the spaces used for their routines, or signal relevant aspects from these. Interviews averaged an hour in length and were audio recorded. Questions were designed to enable interviewees to share their insights on how they experienced the office, their activities and preferences, and contextual socio-organisational aspects. For instance, the question "are there any rules or agreements between colleagues on how to use the different office zones depending on your activity?" was asked to investigate structure and predictability in the office. Follow-up questions were asked depending on the answers, such as: (if yes) are those rules respected; (if no) do you wish to have them?

The observations in the office involved structured observations. Rounds were conducted according to a systematic plan and employees were aware of the observer. Nineteen rounds were conducted in Wave 1 and 18 rounds in Wave 2. In both waves, the rounds were scheduled over two weeks and across four intervals (8:00–10:00, 10:00–12:00, 13:00–15:00, and 15:00–17:00), according to the availability of the observer and avoiding events that were not part of the daily routine. The goal was to cover the equivalent of a regular Monday-to-Friday working week. Each round involved walking a pre-defined route covering all workstations, back-up spaces, and breakout areas, taking structured field notes and blueprint annotations as well as photographs. The field notes recorded details about workstations and back-up spaces in use, the number of employees per space, available facilities and equipment, activity patterns and flows of people between spaces, and whether different spaces were organised as they should have been.

Data handling complied with the General Data Protection Regulation, assuring interviewees of their right to request access to their notes. Interviewee names were coded, and their data aggregated. Preliminary findings from the analysis were presented during a seminar in the division to get feedback and confirmation that the data were an accurate reflection.

Data analysis procedure

Interview audio recordings were transcribed and coded using NVivo 12. An abductive approach was adopted to analyse the content that is defined as a "creative inferential process" combining an inductive and deductive approach, i.e., using empirical data and theoretical prepositions in a dialogical process for analysing qualitative data (Timmermans & Tavory, 2012). In step 1, the interview transcripts were analysed to identify recurring themes related to perceptions of the physical office environment and contextual aspects regarding organisation, activities, and individual preferences (see examples in Table 1.2). This led to identifying recurring positive and negative perceptions. For example, 17 interviewees in Wave 2 referred to a lack of cleanliness and individual responsibility in 27 instances. In a further round of coding in the second step, the codes (perceptions) were related to office environment features from the sense of coherence framework. For example, "too much transparency due to

Table 1.2 Examples of deductive coding process

Excerpt	Step 1: Perceptions of the environment	Step 2: Office environment feature	Step 3: Sense of coherence components
"*[I am] slightly dissatisfied with it [cleaning] maybe, but that's perhaps because we have colleagues who don't put things in the dishwasher and that's a problem*". (I07-W2)	• Cleanliness and visual clutter • Individual responsibilities	Behavioural rules	Comprehensibility
"*Since I don't go anywhere, I sit at my desk, so I just avoid seeing anyone who is going. I know people are going because … it's a 360-degree kind (at least 270 degree) view. So, you can't avoid knowing that someone is going*". (I20-W2)	• Too much transparency due to glass partitions	Exposure to visual stimuli and lack of control	Manageability
"*The social atmosphere is much, much better. … You see more people and friends and start talking with them.*" (I3-W1)	+ Easy to meet people thanks to the spatial transparency	Social interactions	Meaningfulness

glass partitions" was related to "exposure to visual stimuli and lack of control". This step was followed by a deductive coding process in step 3, in which the office environment features were related to the components of sense of coherence: comprehensibility [C], manageability [M], and meaningfulness [ME]. In the example given, the "exposure to visual stimuli" was related to manageability due to the lack of control over the stimuli.

The authors coded the transcription of one interview separately to discuss and develop a consistent coding strategy. The few differences were discussed until full agreement was reached to enable a consistent level of coding. The authors also regularly discussed the analysis, wave comparisons, and reporting strategy to ensure a consistent approach.

Data from the observations were analysed to support and complement the findings from the interviews. This involved reviewing and summarising observation field notes and occupancy data. Occupancy was calculated for office rooms, based on percentage of workstations occupied with respect to maximum number of workstations. Utilisation was calculated for back-up spaces, based on percentage of times the spaces were observed in use. The findings from the observations were compared with the interviewees' insights in the analysis.

The longitudinal analysis followed a convergent-parallel design (Figure 1.3), in which the two separate datasets from each wave were analysed independently and brought together during the interpretation (cf. Creswell, 2014). That is, the findings were contrasted with the perceptions extracted from both waves, to capture changes in the way various features were perceived over time and how they related to the sense of coherence framework.

Findings

In general, participants had a more positive perception of the office environment in Wave 1. The design features of new facilities (such as openness, brightness, and aesthetics) resulted in greater motivation, a stronger sense of belonging, more energy, and better social integration at a division level.

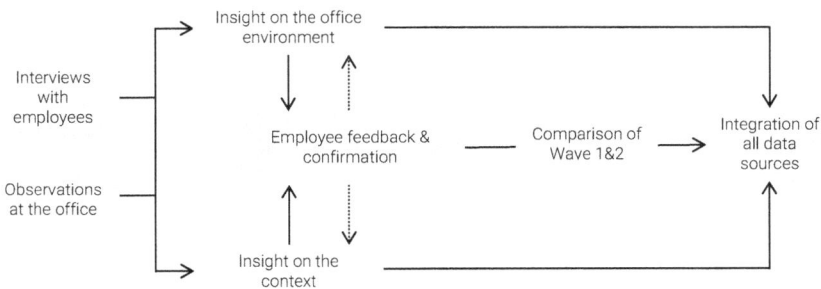

Figure 1.3 Research design.

In Wave 2, many of the positive influences of, say, social atmosphere and aesthetics deteriorated. Additionally, most of the negative perceptions such as exposure to environmental stimuli remained unresolved. The findings are presented in three sections: (1) long-lasting influences, (2) short-lived influences of the office environment, and (3) the contextual aspects the authors found relevant to better understand why office environment influenced interviewees' sense of coherence as it did.

Long-lasting influences on employees' sense of coherence

In general, several office environment features were found to have the same influence on employees' sense of coherence in both waves (Figure 1.4). Respondents indicated that meeting room availability, proximity to offices, diversity, furniture, and technical equipment supported them in managing their work. That said, the observation data showed low occupancy rates for meeting rooms for 4–6 people (30.3% in Wave 1), which remained almost at the same level (Table 1.3). Similarly, the breakout areas were perceived as diverse in size and type. In particular, the balconies were among the most popular spaces, as they offered a bright, relaxing environment with access to inspiring views *"It's a change of scenery there, you see the sky, you see people strolling by downstairs in the yard and you can sit down there and have a coffee, stretch your legs and talk"* (I13-W2). The interviewees appreciated the amount of daylight in Wave 1, thanks to the large windows, glass partitions, and use of light colours. Similarly, in Wave 2, the abundance of daylight created a positive mood for 11/17 interviewees, leading to a more meaningful environment: *"I think it affects everybody's mood in one way or another. [It is] very important and [I am] satisfied"* (I01-W2). However, the lack of control and (malfunctioning of) automated shades limited manageability for 6/17 interviewees: *"There is a good amount of daylight, but the sunshade usually blocks it and often we're forced to use artificial lighting"* (I15-W2).

Workspace personalisation had conflicting influences on employees. While the organisation had discouraged any personalisation pre-relocation, almost one-third of interviewees had a positive perception of the current arrangement: *"I have the possibility [to personalise my workspace], so even though they say we shouldn't, I did it anyway"* (I06-W1). Conversely, others perceived the space as impersonal which limited meaningful: *"Our office is quite empty ... it makes it less personal I think"* (I13-W2).

The building offered low levels of spatial seclusion for office rooms and back-up spaces, thanks to the large glass partitions and windows. Increased exposure to visual and acoustic stimuli limited manageability: *"what disturbs me the most is the big windows towards the corridors. It's completely open. It's not that I mind people passing by but, every time someone does, without being fully aware of it I turn my head and look up"* (I13-W2). In contrast, spatial openness increased the chances of social interactions

Design features	Reasons	Wave 1	Wave 2
Meeting rooms Positive→Positive	+ [M] [ME] Proximity to own workstation & territory + [ME] Sense of own territory + [M] Abundance & high availability + [M] Good ICT coverage + [M] [ME] Comfortable and high-quality furniture + [M] Good accessibility + [M] Variety of sizes		
Breakout areas Positive→Positive	+ [M] Abundance & high availability + [M] Access to coffee machines + [M] Spatial variety + [ME] Bright; Access to views + [ME] Signals luxury		
Daylight Positive →Divergent	+ [ME] Bright corridors & workspaces - [M] Daylight blocked due to the automated shade		
Workspace personalisation Divergent→Divergent	+ [MA] Freedom to add greenery & personal belongings - [ME] Limited opportunity for expression of identity in shared offices - [M] [ME] Discouragement by the organisation - [ME] Does not feel personal enough to personalise - [M] [C] Requires collective agreement		
Temperature Divergent→Divergent	+ [MA] Comfortable & not noticeable - [MA] Cool temperature, especially during summer		
Exposure to acoustic stimuli Divergent→Divergent	+ [ME] Good for exchanging information + [M] Easily modifiable (headphones, closing doors) + [M] Not sensitive to noise - [M] Background noise due to proximity to printers - [M] Proximity to high-traffic areas (breakout areas, printer rooms)		
Exposure to visual stimuli Divergent→Divergent	+ [ME] Easy to meet and interact with others - [M] [ME] Too open & transparent - [M] [ME] Lack of secluded back-up spaces - [M] Shared with eight people (too many people in one room)		

Aspects of sense of coherence in an architectural context. Comprehensibility [C], Manageability [M], Meaningfulness [ME]

The coloured bars illustrate the proportion of interviewees who reported positive, neutral or negative influence.

▦ Positive influence,　Neutral,　■ Negative influence.

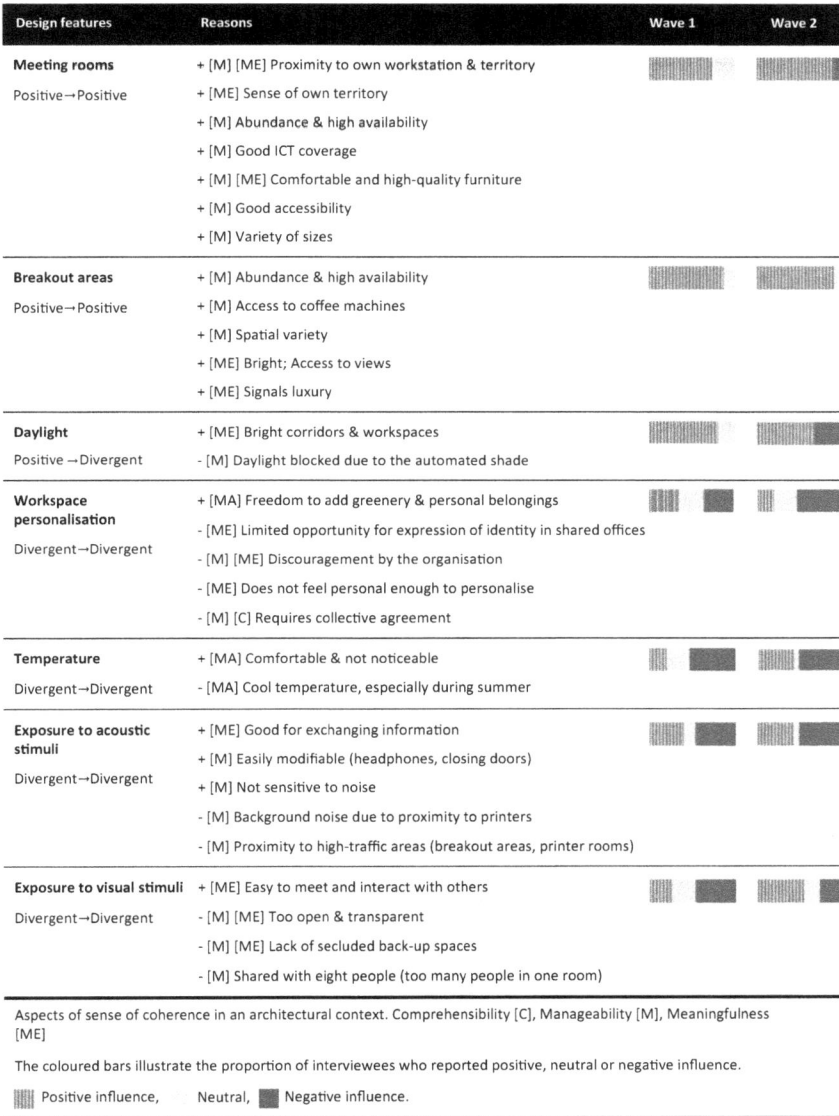

Figure 1.4 Long-lasting influences on employees' sense of coherence.

and was thought to be "*good for exchanging information*" (I05-W2), making the office environment more meaningful. The indoor temperature was perceived as cold by nearly half of interviewees, particularly in the summertime due to people wearing light clothing.

Table 1.3 Occupancy during a working week

Avg. occupancy*	Wave 1 (%)	Wave 2 (%)
Office rooms	31.4	32
Avg. utilisation**		
Meeting rooms 4–6p	30.3	25
Meeting rooms +6p	26.3	23.1
Quiet room with sofa	15.8	–
Quiet rooms with 2p	13.7	30.5
Quiet rooms with 6p	0	38.8
Flex room	44.7	66.6
Phone booths	6.6	13.1
Breakout areas	23.7	19.4
Lunchroom-fifth floor	94.4	88.8

Notes

* Percentage of workstations occupied with respect to maximum number of workstations.
** Percentage of times the spaces were observed in use of the total number of 19 and 18 observations in waves 1 and 2, respectively.

Short-lived influences in employees' sense of coherence

Several design features of the office environment had short-term influences on interviewees' sense of coherence and are presented as positive and negative changes (Figure 1.5).

Positive changes

While perceptions of personal storage were divided in Wave 1, many interviewees in Wave 2 indicated that the amount and location of personal storage helped them to manage their belongings in the office (13/17): *"There's more than enough space for me to store my stuff. It's accessible just by my workstation"* (I02-W2). That said, two interviewees remained dissatisfied with the amount of storage space. Another positive change was regarding the furniture that was found to signal luxury and status, and hence was associated with positive meaning: *"I also like the fancy meeting room … it feels luxurious"* (I16-W2). Furthermore, the functionality and quality of the furniture led to more comfort and manageability in Wave 2: *"I appreciate the fact those tables can go up and down, I can stand for a while … and the chair's comfortable"* (I19-W2).

Negative changes

Some of the positive features identified in Wave 1 were not appreciated in Wave 2. These included social interactions, aesthetics, spatial diversity, and (lack of a) sense of control and behavioural rules in the office.

Design features	Reasons	Wave 1	Wave 2
Personal storage Divergent→Positive	+ [M] Proximity to workstations + [M] Sufficient physical space		
Furniture Divergent→Positive	+ [M] Comfortable + [M] [ME] Of high quality + [ME] Signals luxury		
Social interactions Positive → Divergent	+ [ME] Easy to meet people thanks to spatial transparency - [ME] Lack of a division-specific space - [M] Limited capacity of breakout areas - [M] Floor layout and abundance of breakout spaces - [ME] Feeling of isolation		
Aesthetics Positive→Divergent	+[ME] Minimalistic design, neutral colours, modern, fancy - [ME] Lacks bright colours, textures and greenery; sterile - [ME] Lacks personal touch		
Spatial diversity Positive→Divergent	+ [M] Supports a variety of activities - [M] [ME] Lacks different level of spatial seclusion -[M] Lacks multi-functional spaces e.g., project work & creative work - [M] Lacks support facilities (sports, maternity facilities)		
Lack of behavioural rules Not reoccurring → Negative	+ [C] Relying on common sense - [C] Ambiguity concerning individual responsibilities - [C] [M] Cleanliness & visual clutter	-	
Control over environment Not reoccurring → Negative	+ [M] Secluded workstation/room + [M] Coping strategies - [M] Lack of control over climate system - [M] Lack of control over automated shades - [M] Lack of control over stimuli	-	

Aspects of sense of coherence in an architectural context. Comprehensibility [C], Manageability [M], Meaningfulness [ME]

The coloured bars illustrate the proportion of interviewees who reported positive, neutral or negative influence.

▦ Positive influence,   Neutral,   ▪ Negative influence.

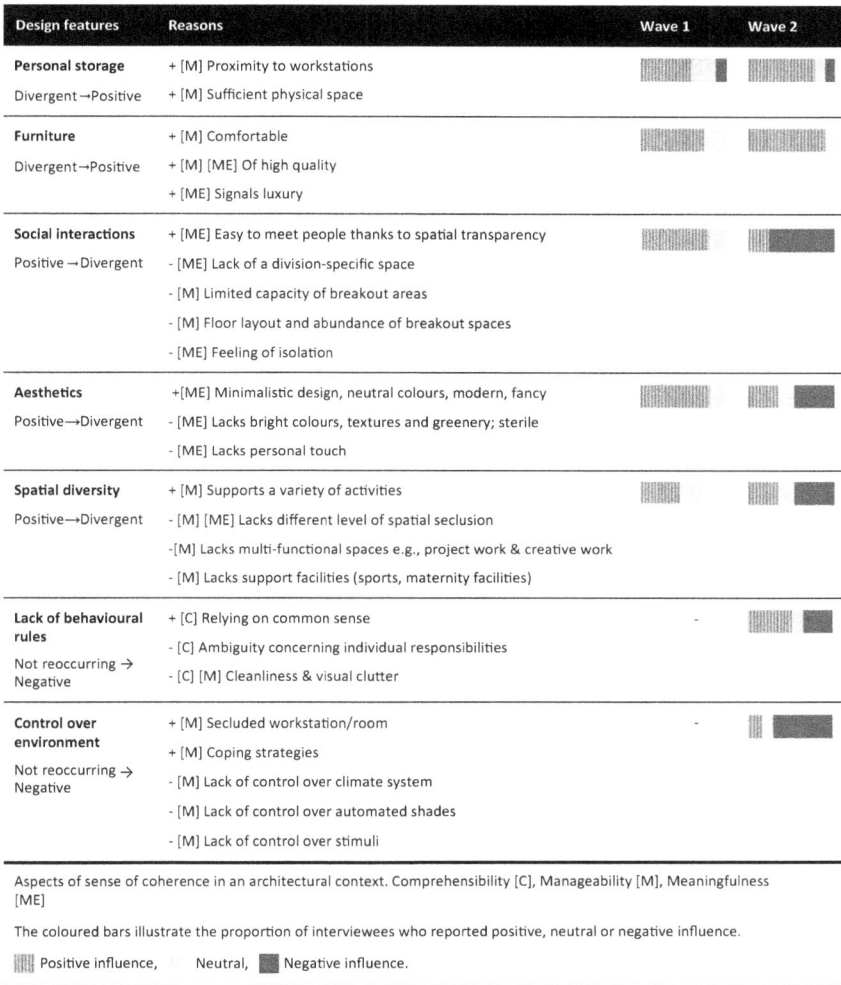

Figure 1.5 Short-lived influences on employees' sense of coherence.

The social atmosphere and increased opportunities for interaction were appreciated in Wave 1: "*social atmosphere is much, much, better than the previous one … because here, when you go to the coffee areas, you see more people and friends and start talking with them. I like it much more than the previous one*" (I03-W1). However, in Wave 2, most interviewees (10/17) expressed difficulty in meeting colleagues for coffee breaks due to the abundance of space which spread people around, plus the limited capacity of most breakout areas: "*We are more spread out in the division, and I think that's the most obvious drawback of the social atmosphere than before*"

(I13-W2). The negative perceptions also related to the lack of a division-specific space as a centralised meeting point: "*It was nice when someone could say 'brought birthday cake' and you had it all day or when people sent postcards and you put them up. You had your own space. I thought that was nice. Now, there's a lot of subgroups and we don't have just the one place to go*" (I06-W2). The perceived lack of opportunities for social interactions created a feeling of isolation, and thus leading to a less meaningful office environment: "*You're left there [in the office] and somehow forgotten … it's just a general feeling of isolation. That maybe in the long term can't be so good*" (I19-W2).

The aesthetics of the office was experienced as pleasurable and meaningful in Wave 1, making interviewees feel appreciated: "*It looks more modern, feels like you're treated as important if you work in a nice place*" (I05-W1). In Wave 2, perceptions varied with some appreciating the minimal look while others found it "sterile", "boring", and "homogenous" and thus less meaningful: "*There are only very boring colours in here [the office]. Some plants with flowers would be nice. We need more colours!*" (I18-W2). The observation data showed that the space became cluttered over time, with papers and books lying around on storage cupboards in the middle of corridors.

The diversity of workspaces was perceived as flexible and functional in Wave 1, which created a more manageable office environment: "*We have space for different types of meetings. We have a fancier one to have clients and some with video projectors … so I think we have flexibility. I haven't found a space that didn't match my work situation*" (I01-W1). However, in Wave 2, nearly half the interviewees found the office less supportive of individual or project work: "*I would like access to a room where I can spread things out and work more visually*" (I06-W2). Furthermore, the homogeneity of visual and acoustic seclusion in back-up spaces limited control over distractions, and consequently reduced office manageability.

The perceived limited opportunities to control the stimuli, temperature, and automated shades affected the manageability of the office. The high levels of spatial transparency thanks to the large glass partitions and windows limited control over visual and acoustic stimuli. That said, opinions varied among employees depending on personal preferences, workstation position, and room locations. Four interviewees who were dissatisfied with the lack of privacy and exposure to stimuli in Wave 1 had changed workstation position or offices to a more protected location. Hence, the various levels of work-station seclusion and coping strategies (such as noise-cancelling headphones or desk dividers) supported concentration for some: "*When I put my head-phones on and the wall [divider] up, that [concentration] is absolutely no problem*" (I02-W2). Whereas others were dissatisfied: "*To me, my environment includes a glass wall and window which I obviously can't control. I can't control visual distractions, nor can I control noise*" (I16-W2). The lack of control over the automated shades was also perceived as limiting and uncomfortable, as they restricted access to daylight.

Some interviewees were satisfied with not having any behavioural rules and preferred relying on common sense: "*With time, you sort of develop informal rules anyway, dependent on the group or room*" (I13-W2). However, the uncertainty and confusion over individual responsibilities made the office environment less comprehensible for others and subsequently led to feelings of frustration towards colleagues: "*The kitchen is dirty and there are so few people who feel responsible for its cleanliness. This makes me feel 'urgh'*" (I17-W2). Although signs were put up, these were not complied with, leading to visual clutter and mess, as apparent in the observations. An "in-house guidebook" had been shared with employees during the 2017 relocation, with practical information on space use and etiquette in the work environment. However, the book had not been updated since and was never mentioned by the interviewees.

Contextual aspects

The underlying explanation for the changed perceptions was, to some extent, associated with the contextual aspects of the office, including organisational working culture, facility management strategies, activity patterns, and individual preferences influencing different components of sense of coherence (Figure 1.6).

Organisational aspects

The organisation had a trust-based working model in which employees were free to choose when and where to work. Many interviewees (13/17) greatly valued their high level of autonomy, regarding it as beneficial to their work-life balance. For example, to improve concentration, some employees chose to work remotely or avoid peak hours in the office by coming in early. Regarding the facility management strategies, interviewees did not feel involved in the

Contextual aspects	Reasons
Organisation-related	+ [M] High level of autonomy
	- [C][M] Low level of user involvement
	- [C] Lack of responsiveness to faulty reports
Individual-related	± [M] [C] Personal preferences
	± [M] Previous experiences
Task-related	± [M] Task variety
	± [M] Level of interaction

Aspects of sense of coherence in an architectural context. Comprehensibility [C], Manageability [M], Meaningfulness [ME]

Figure 1.6 Influence of contextual factors on employees' sense of coherence.

change process, either before or after the relocation. Interviewees perceived that their opinions were disregarded and their ability to influence changes were limited. Subsequently, this had a negative influence on the manageability and meaningfulness of the office environment. Furthermore, the post-relocation interventions, such as installing curtains for some offices to cover glass partitions were implemented with neither communication nor involvement of the employees. Also, over one-third of the interviewees perceived the maintenance team unresponsive to reports of faults with the automated shades. This led to ambiguity and confusion about follow-up processes and hence reduced comprehensibility.

Task-related aspects

The choice of work setting and resources were partly influenced by the activity patterns of the interviewees. Nearly half of interviewees in Wave 2 indicated a rather low task variety mainly conducted at their workstations. Also, a few employees' tasks required more interaction with others, which would occasionally disturb colleagues in the same office. The task-related differences among the participants led to divergent perceptions of office manageability.

Individual aspects

Preferences varied among interviewees. Some interviewees indicated that they were more adaptable and/or less sensitive to stimuli and some had experienced better or worse conditions in their former workplaces, which influenced their expectations of the current office. Also, over two-thirds of interviewees preferred their workstations for most of their activities over the back-up spaces due to the provision of dual computer screens, proximity to personal storage and personal belongings, privacy, and the implied sense of ownership. Therefore, most interviewees preferred to modify their workstations by adopting coping strategies to concentrate better. This may explain the low occupancy of the back-up spaces (Table 1.3). Hence, the adaptation strategies indicate that the interviewees understood the potentials and shortcomings of the office environment (comprehensibility) and identified ways to craft a better working environment (manageability).

Discussion and conclusions

Office environment in relation to sense of coherence

The findings show that employees found the office equally manageable in both waves. This may be due to the high level of autonomy that allowed employees to cope with the lacking sense of control over the environment. Previous studies have associated autonomy with a positive impact on well-being, job satisfaction, and work motivation (Deci & Ryan, 2008; Gagné et al., 1997; Ilardi et al., 1993). That said, the increased demand on employees caused by lack of control may have influenced the positive perceptions of the office environment in Wave 1. Improving control options (e.g., curtains and screens for privacy and extra heaters for better temperature) may have resolved some of the issues. Concerning automated shades, future studies may investigate whether smart (automated) technologies would lead to energy gains or compromise user experience and a resulting performance gap.

The employees found the office environment less meaningful in the follow-up study due to difficulties in social interactions. The results of studies on the impact of spatial openness and transparency on communication and collaboration are mixed (Colenberg et al., 2021; De Croon et al., 2005; Engelen et al., 2019). Among longitudinal studies, the findings are also inconsistent. While Gerdenitsch et al. (2018) show that improvements in communication remained stable between the first and second measurement, our study confirms the findings from Haapakangas et al. (2019) that report a decrease in satisfaction with communication and the sense of belonging, three and 12 months post-relocation. A possible reason for this finding could be that the results on social relations in Wave 1 were positively influenced by a novelty effect of relocating from cellular offices to shared rooms, and/or the increase in spaces for breaks (Gerdenitsch et al., 2018). Over time, the accumulated negative influence of noise and visual distractions may have outweighed the initial positive experience. Future studies may investigate whether these changes mainly relate to novelty effects or if it would be different, for example, between organisations with different needs for collaboration and task interdependency. Another explanation could be that employees experienced a drift away from their group of colleagues because of the relocation and organisational merger. Organisations should be prepared to solve possible difficulties in socialisation and group cohesion in open and flexible offices, for example, with the help of scheduled coffee breaks and an allocated space. Furthermore, future research can benefit from exploring opportunities to strengthen challenges for social interactions in the office environment through spatial solutions.

The lack of opportunities for the personalisation of workspaces found in this study reduced the sense of ownership, and eventually meaningfulness of the office environment. This finding is in line with studies highlighting the importance of personalisation of space as a means of making sense of the environment and giving meaning to the workspace (Brunia & Hartjes-Gosselink, 2009). Our findings showed that some employees experienced their office environment as impersonal and sterile. Golembiewski (2010) indicates that drab and monotonous environments are linked to depression and confusion; on the other hand, personalised environments that are rich in details are associated with positive emotions, the expression of personal identities, and a sense of meaning (Ashkanasy et al., 2014; Brunia & Hartjes-Gosselink, 2009; Wells, 2000). Furthermore, the perceptions of aesthetic design can be attributed to the initial novelty that faded due to the increased clutter and mess. Opportunities to personalise breakout areas and workspace on a group level may create a sense of ownership over the space and help to maintain order and cleanliness.

The employees found the office environment less comprehensible. The lack of behavioural rules, an ambiguous facility management strategies/processes, and the maintenance system reduced comprehensibility of the office environment. The importance of having clear behavioural rules for successful implementations (Appel-Meulenbroek et al., 2011; Rolfö et al., 2018) as well as employee involvement in the change process (Hongisto et al., 2016; Lahtinen et al., 2015; Rolfö, 2018; Vischer, 2008) have been emphasised in previous research. Furthermore, the frustration caused by the maintenance system is consistent with other studies showing that a sense of resignation occurs when management does not address issues that disrupt employees' work (Babapour Chafi, 2019) and the role of management has been found to be crucial in creating comprehensibility, manageability, and meaningfulness in the office (Lahtinen et al., 2015). Hence, better comprehensibility may be achieved through constant open discussions between management and employees concerning the reasons, goals, and implications of change.

Limitations

The contextual nature of architectural design and health led the researchers to choose a qualitative case-study approach, which allowed the study of individuals and groups within their specific office context. While this approach has many strengths, it means that the results cannot be generalised to other cases, nor are they intended to. Instead, our findings are transferable (cf. criteria for ensuring the quality of qualitative studies by Miles & Huberman, 1994) in that perceptions of office environment evolve over time and the sense of coherence components can be experienced differently by different employees within an organisation, and this will likely occur in other cases. The qualitative approach was found to be a valuable approach to study employees' experience in relation to their perceived health over time in the same office (cf. Creswell, 2014). A key strength in applying the sense of coherence framework was its holistic perspective. This allowed the investigation of a range of aspects, from those causing illness to coping strategies, adaptations, and positive effects. Our findings can inform future research for developing survey instruments to assess sense of coherence in the office environment. This will allow for comparisons between different cases for achieving generalisable insights.

Several strategies contribute to the dependability/reliability of this qualitative case study: transparent and thorough description of the case context; triangulation and comprehensive use of multiple data sources. The measures taken to replicate the study design in Wave 2 and ensure credibility were the following: the discussions between the researchers to ensure a consistent analysis strategy; and dialogue with the interviewees for confirming the results.

The main advantage of this study is its longitudinal perspective on employees' experience of relocating from cellular offices to a combi office and its positive approach to health (not only focusing on the negative influences) using sense of coherence as a theoretical framework. Using the same mixed-method case study approach in both waves, six months and two years post-relocation, enabled the comparison of employee perceptions and gain a deep understanding of the influences of the physical environment on employees' sense of coherence. These time points are in line with other longitudinal studies of office environments in which one of the data collection procedures is often conducted within the first year post-relocation (Bergström et al., 2015; Haapakangas et al., 2019; Meijer et al., 2009). Therefore, studies investigating what makes an office design healthy or the interrelations between office environments and employees' health may benefit from adopting longitudinal approaches like the one presented in this chapter.

Practical implications

As a practical implication, the research provides a framework for architects, facility managers, corporate real estate owners, and occupational health professionals that illustrates an overview of the interrelations between office environment features and sense of coherence.

Designers can use the framework to explore how their designs can support comprehensibility, manageability, and meaningfulness for employees. Regarding comprehensibility aspects, incorporating design cues and information into the office space can support spatial readability and comprehensibility. To improve office manageability, designers should pay close attention to enabling control over visual and acoustic stimuli through, for example, curtains and screens that allow employees to craft preferred levels of visual and acoustic privacy. Meaningfulness can be supported by creating spatial solutions for efficient communication and interactions.

Facility managers should engage in recurring communication and dialogue with employees. Hence, management's role is crucial not only in the relocation but also in the operation phase to support health development within the office. Resources should be allocated for evaluation of office environment on a regular basis to identify emerging problems and avoid lingering problems over time. Our study showed that facility management plays an important role in creating a comprehensible work environment. Facilitating development of explicit behavioural rules, as well as regular maintenance of spaces seems to support how employees read and understand workspaces. Furthermore, the office environment can become less meaningful when employees have trouble with social interaction and hence an allocated space with opportunities for personalisation can support collective identity expression, a sense of community and group cohesion.

The COVID-19 pandemic and the subsequent increased interest for hybrid work have put new expectations on organisations to introduce new adaptations to offices. Providing office environments that promote health and wellbeing is therefore crucial to attract employees to the office and encourage them to stay in organisations. Providing such environments will need regular input from employees, such as the days employees work at the office, to allow activities to be scheduled and spatial solutions planned for varying occupancy rates.

Combining the conventional pathogenic perspective that focuses on identifying the risk factors, e.g., noise, with a salutogenic approach helps identifying characteristics that promote or hinder comprehensibility, manageability, and meaningfulness. These factors may include, for example, opportunities to craft an environment that matches one's needs and preferences (e.g., from the provision of noise-cancelling headphones to noise absorbing artefacts and quiet rooms). Instead of aiming for an idealistic environment and a state of "complete" wellbeing (World Health Organisation, 1948), office design should aim at a design that empowers individuals to adapt and self-manage actively and positively (Huber et al., 2011).

Concluding remarks

The research found that most of the positive perceptions of the office environment deteriorated over time. Employees found the office less meaningful in Wave 2, due to the reduced opportunities for social interactions and personalisation. The office was also experienced as being less comprehensible due to the lack of behavioural rules, ambiguous facility management strategies/processes, and a maintenance system that was perceived as unresponsive to the reporting of faults. Perceptions of the office manageability remained stable in both waves due to the flexible organisational work culture. Contextual aspects, such as tasks, flexible working culture, and the change processes, were identified that further elucidate how the changes in perceptions evolved over time.

This chapter has demonstrated that negative influences caused by poor design choices do not resolve themselves over time, without support from the facility management. When there is limited support for one component of sense of coherence, the initial observed benefits wear off and negative influences may spill over into other components. Therefore, office design should be approached with balanced attention to comprehensibility, manageability, and meaningfulness. Any move towards healthy office design should include mitigation of deficiencies and promotion of salutogenic resources to create and maintain health. The concept of a healthy office is therefore contextual, dynamic and evolves over time through active participation of employees, facilities managers, and organisations.

References

Antonovsky, A. (1979). *Health, stress, and coping: New perspective on mental and physical well-being*. Jossey-Bass Publishers.

Antonovsky, A. (1987). *Unraveling the mystery of health*. Jossey-Bass Publishers.

Antonovsky, A. (1993). The structure and properties of sense of coherence scale. *Social Science & Medicine, 36*(6), 725–733.

Appel-Meulenbroek, R., Clippard, M., & Pfnur, A. (2018). The effectiveness of physical office environments for employee outcomes: An interdisciplinary perspective of research efforts. *Journal of Corporate Real Estate, 20*(1), 56–80.

Appel-Meulenbroek, R., Groenen, P., & Janssen, I. (2011). An end-users perspective on activity-based office concepts. *Journal of Corporate Real Estate, 13*(2), 122–135.

Ashkanasy, N. M., Ayoko, O. B., & Jehn, K. A. (2014). Understanding the physical environment of work and employee behavior: An affective events perspective. *Journal of Organizational Behavior, 35*(8), 1169–1184.

Babapour Chafi, M. (2019). From fading novelty effects to emergent appreciation of activity-based flexible offices: Comparing the individual, organisational and spatial adaptations in two case organisations. *Applied Ergonomics, 81*, Article 102877.

Bauer, G. F., & Jenny, G. J. (2016). The application of salutogenesis to organisations. In M. B. Mittelmark, S. Sagy, M. Eriksson, G. F. Bauer, J. M. Pelikan, B. Lindström, & G. A. Espnes (Eds.), *The handbook of salutogenesis*. Springer.

Bergström, J., Miller, M., & Horneij, E. (2015). Work environment perceptions following relocation to open-plan offices: A twelve-month longitudinal study. *Work, 50*, 221–228.

Berlin, C., & Babapour Chafi, M. (2020). *Physical work environment for health, well-being and performance – A systematic review*. Swedish Agency for Work Environment Expertise. www.sawee.se

Blok, M., De Korte, E. M., Groenesteijn, L., Formanoy, M., & Vink, P. (2009). The effect of a task facilitating working environment on office space use, communication, concentration, collaboration, privacy and distraction. *Proceedings of the 17th World Congress on Ergonomics (IEA 2009)*, 9–14.

Braun-Lewensohn, O., Idan, O., Lindström, B., & Margalit, M. (2016). Salutogenesis: Sense of coherence in adolescence. In *The handbook of salutogenesis* (pp. 123–136). Springer Cham.

Brennan, A., Chugh, J. S., & Kline, T. (2002). Traditional versus open office design: A longitudinal field study. *Environment and Behavior, 34*(3), 279–299.

Brunia, S., & Hartjes-Gosselink, A. (2009). Personalization in non-territorial offices: A study of a human need. *Journal of Corporate Real Estate, 11*(3), 169–182.

Candido, C., Thomas, L., Haddad, S., Zhang, F., Mackey, M., & Ye, W. (2019). Designing activity-based workspaces: Satisfaction, productivity and physical activity. *Building Research & Information, 47*(3), 275–289.

Clements-Croome, D. (2018). Effects of the built environment on health and well-being. In D. Clements-Croome (Ed.), *Creating productive workplace* (3rd ed., pp. 3–40). Routledge.

Colenberg, S., Jylhä, T., & Arkesteijn, M. (2021). The relationship between interior office space and employee health and well-being – A literature review. *Building Research & Information, 49*(3), 352–366.

Creswell, J. (2014). *Research design: Qualitative, quantitative and mixed methods approaches* (4th ed.). Sage.

Danko, S., Eshelman, P., & Hedge, A. (1990). A taxonomy of health, safety, and welfare implications of interior design decisions. *Journal of Interior Design Education and Research, 16*(2), 19–30.

Davis, M. C., Leach, D. J., & Clegg, C. W. (2011). The physical environment of the office: contemporary and emerging issues. In G. P. Hodgkinson & J. K. Ford (Eds.), *International review of industrial and organizational psychology, 2012* (pp. 193–235). John Wiley & Sons.

De Croon, E., Sluiter, J., Kuijer, P. P., & Frings-Dresen, M. (2005). The effect of office concepts on worker health and performance: A systematic review of the literature. *Ergonomics, 48*(2), 119–134.

Deci, E. L., & Ryan, R. M. (2008). Self-determination theory: A macrotheory of human motivation, development, and health. *Canadian Psychology, 49*(3), 182–185.

Engelen, L., Chau, J., Young, S., Mackey, M., Jeyapalan, D., & Bauman, A. (2019). Is activity-based working impacting health, work performance and perceptions? A systematic review. *Building Research & Information, 47*(4), 468–479.

Eriksson, M., & Lindström, B. (2006). Antonovsky's sense of coherence scale and the relation with health: A systematic review. *Journal of Epidemiology & Community Health, 60*(5), 376–381.

Eriksson, M., & Lindström, B. (2007). Antonovsky's sense of coherence scale and its relation with quality of life: A systematic review. *Journal of Epidemiology and Community Health, 61*(11), 938–944.

Gagné, M., Senécal, C. B., & Koestner, R. (1997). Proximal job characteristics, feelings of empowerment, and intrinsic motivation: A multidimensional model. *Journal of Applied Social Psychology, 27*(14), 1222–1240.

Gerdenitsch, C., Korunka, C., & Hertel, G. (2018). Need–supply fit in an activity-based flexible office: A longitudinal study during relocation. *Environment and Behavior, 50*(3), 273–297.

Golembiewski, J. A. (2010). Start making sense: Applying a salutogenic model to architectural design for psychiatric care. *Facilities, 28*(3/4), 100–117.

Golembiewski, J. A. (2016). Salutogenic architecture in healthcare settings. In *The handbook of salutogenesis* (pp. 267–276). Springer Cham.

Groen, B. H., Jylhä, T., & van Sprang, H. (2018). Healthy offices: An evidence- based trend in facility management? *Transdiciplinary Workspace Research Conference Tampere 2018.*

Haapakangas, A., Hallman, D. M., Mathiassen, S. E., & Jahncke, H. (2019). The effects of moving into an activity-based office on communication, social relations and work demands – A controlled intervention with repeated follow-up. *Journal of Environmental Psychology, 66*(August), 101341.

Heerwagen, J. H., Heubach, J. G., Montgomery, J., & Weimer, W. C. (1995). Environmental design, work, and well being. *AAOHN Journal, 43*(9), 458–468.

Hongisto, V., Haapakangas, A., Varjo, J., Helenius, R., & Koskela, H. (2016). Refurbishment of an open-plan office – Environmental and job satisfaction. *Journal of Environmental Psychology, 45*, 176–191.

Huber, M., André Knottnerus, J., Green, L., Van Der Horst, H., Jadad, A. R., Kromhout, D., Leonard, B., Lorig, K., Loureiro, M. I., Van Der Meer, J. W. M., Schnabel, P., Smith, R., Van Weel, C., & Smid, H. (2011). How should we define health? *BMJ (Online), 343*(7817).

Idan, O., Braun-Lewensohn, O., Lindström, B., & Margalit, M. (2017). Salutogenesis: Sense of coherence in childhood and in families. In M. B. Mittelmark, S. Sagy, M. Eriksson, G. F. Bauer, J. M. Pelikan, B. Lindström, & G. A. Espnes (Eds.), *The Handbook of Salutogenesis*. Springer.

Ilardi, B. C., Leone, D., Kasser, T., & Ryan, R. M. (1993). Employee and supervisor ratings of motivation: Main effects and discrepancies associated with job satisfaction and adjustment in a factory setting. *Journal of Applied Social Psychology*, *23*(21), 1789–1805.

Inalhan, G., & Finch, E. (2004). Place attachment and sense of belonging. *Facilities*, *22*(5), 120–128.

Jambroes, M., Nederland, T., Kaljouw, M., Van Vliet, K., Essink-Bot, M. L., & Ruwaard, D. (2016). Implications of health as "the ability to adapt and self-manage" for public health policy: A qualitative study. *European Journal of Public Health*, *26*(3), 412–416.

Jensen, P. A., & van der Voordt, T. (2019). Healthy workplaces: What we know and what else we need to know. *Journal of Corporate Real Estate*, *22*(2), 95–112.

Kämpf-Dern, A., & Konkol, J. (2017). Performance-oriented office environments – Framework for effective workspace design and the accompanying change processes. *Journal of Corporate Real Estate*, *19*(4), 208–238.

Koelen, M., Eriksson, M., & Cattan, M. (2016). Older people, sense of coherence and community. In *The handbook of salutogenesis* (pp. 137–149). Springer.

Kupritz, V. W. (1998). Environmental psychology privacy in the work place: The impact of building design. *Journal of Environmental Psychology*, *18*(4), 341–356.

Lahtinen, M., Ruohomäki, V., Haapakangas, A., & Reijula, K. (2015). Developmental needs of workplace design practices. *Intelligent Buildings International*, *7*(4), 198–214.

Lamb, S., & Kwok, K. C. S. (2016). A longitudinal investigation of work environment stressors on the performance and wellbeing of office workers. *Applied Ergonomics*, *52*(2016), 104–111.

Meijer, E. M., Frings-Dresen, M. H. W., & Sluiter, J. K. (2009). Effects of office innovation on office workers' health and performance. *Ergonomics*, *52*(9), 1027–1038.

Miles, M. B., & Huberman, A. M. (1994). *Qualitative data analysis: An expanded sourcebook*. SAGE Publications, Inc.

Oseland, N. (2009). The impact of psychological needs on office design. *Journal of Corporate Real Estate*, *11*(4), 244–254.

Rolfö, L. (2018). Relocation to an activity-based flexible office – Design processes and outcomes. *Applied Ergonomics*, *73*(May), 141–150.

Rolfö, L., Eklund, J., & Jahncke, H. (2018). Perceptions of performance and satisfaction after relocation to an activity-based office. *Ergonomics*, *61*(5), 644–657.

Roskams, M., & Haynes, B. (2019). Salutogenic workplace design: A conceptual framework for supporting sense of coherence through environmental resources. *Journal of Corporate Real Estate*, *22*(2), 139–153.

Ruohomäki, V., Lahtinen, M., & Reijula, K. (2015). Salutogenic and user-centred approach for workplace design. *Intelligent Buildings International*, *7*(4), 184–197.

Sander, E. (Libby) J., Caza, A., & Jordan, P. J. (2019). Psychological perceptions matter: Developing the reactions to the physical work environment scale. *Building and Environment*, *148*(2018), 338–347.

Timmermans, S., & Tavory, I. (2012). Theory construction in qualitative research: From grounded theory to abductive analysis. *Sociological Theory*, *30*(3), 167–186.

van der Voordt, T. J. M., Vrielink, D., & van Wegen, H. B. R. (1997). Comparative floorplan-analysis in programming and architectural design. *Design Studies*, *18*(1), 67–88.

Vischer, J. C. (2008). Towards an environmental psychology of workspace: How people are affected by environments for work. *Architectural Science Review*, *51*(2), 97–108.

Vogt, K., Hakanen, J. J., Jenny, G. J., & Bauer, G. F. (2016). Sense of coherence and the motivational process of the job-demands-resources model. *Journal of Occupational Health Psychology*, *21*(2), 194–207.

Wells, M. M. (2000). Office clutter or meaningful personal displays: The role of office personalization in employee and organizational well-being. *Journal of Environmental Psychology*, *20*(3), 239–255.

Wijk, K., Bergsten, E. L., & Hallman, D. M. (2020). Sense of coherence, health, well-being, and work satisfaction before and after implementing activity-based workplaces. *International Journal of Environmental Research and Public Health*, *17*(14), 1–15.

Wilson, E. O. (1984). *Biophilia*. Harvard University Press.

Wohlers, C., & Hertel, G. (2018). Longitudinal effects of activity-based flexible office design on teamwork. *Frontiers in Psychology*, *9*(OCT), 1–16.

World Health Organisation. (1948). *Constitution of the World Health Organisation*. The World Health Organisation.

2 The productivity of office occupants in relation to the indoor thermal environment

Jaime Soto Muñoz, Maureen Trebilcock Kelly, Vicente Flores-Alés, and Raúl Ramírez-Vielma

Introduction

The assessment of productivity in built spaces is particularly complex. Studies indicate that occupant perceptions can reflect thermal conditions and are therefore an important factor to consider. In office buildings, the architectural design creates spaces and arrangements that influence how people may feel and act. These spaces form an environment composed of different building elements, for example, office type, its furnishings, the environmental conditioning systems, and the occupants' own adaptive comfort elements. Studies have attempted to examine the link between occupant thermal satisfaction and self-rated productivity in office buildings. However, there is still a need to push for new work to enrich knowledge of the phenomenon. It is necessary to improve physical and perceptual metrics, and how these can incorporate more variables to improve understanding of what happens to individuals in their workspaces.

The concept of productivity is often used interchangeably with performance, although they are not the same (Zhang et al., 2019). Workplace outcomes generally focus on individual performance or output, which is different from organisational productivity (Campbell & Wiernik, 2015; Groen et al., 2019). For Parsons (2000), productivity is an organisation's systematic achievement in activities that generate useful results. This definition integrates production and adds other social, organisational, and personal dimensions. For organisations, occupants and their requirements regarding built space are an important issue because occupants who are comfortable in their workspaces tend to contribute more to the corporation's objectives (Agha-Hossein et al., 2013; Altomonte et al., 2020; Clements-Croome, 2015), i.e., they tend to be more productive. Nonetheless, expectations and reality do not always go hand in hand. There are many buildings that do not function as expected, thereby affecting occupant satisfaction, and with it individual and organisational performance.

Office buildings are complex flexible entities focused on an organisation's needs. Layout varies between cellular and open plan offices, with varying degrees of flexibility, aimed at promoting an effective and productive

DOI: 10.1201/9781003344711-3

work culture. There is community and organisational access to information and associated resources. Within this framework, offices have meeting places that are usually available to the entire organisation. However, spontaneous meetings or the use of shared devices among workers can occur. In this environment, the concept of workspace or workplace emerges, which is distinct from that of workstation. The workspace depends on the interior design, organisational policies, social relationships, and occupant functions. According to Ayoko and Ashkanasy (2020), work design, interpersonal and team processes, and other factors predict a change in workspaces that will have to adapt to flexible and agile spatial arrangements. Although the open floor plan is the most common, implicit boundaries may emerge where occupants usually work with more technologies and in a more interactive way. Today's designs attempt to resolve these and other current issues through open plan offices, and to a lesser extent with fewer individual and shared offices, depending primarily on the information workers handle and the degree of confidentiality it requires.

An office occupant is a person who usually works Monday to Friday. In the United Kingdom or Spain, the average workweek is around 40 hours and 45 hours in Chile. Nevertheless, depending on national legislation and organisational availability criteria, workweeks can be much longer as is the case in Japan, where individuals may work up to 12 hours a day. Contracts may impose different cognitive and emotional demands on workers, which affect them in various ways, for example, in the use or availability of resources, dress codes, or prohibited behaviours. Workload also varies between and within organisations, with levels of creativity and individual autonomy differing with function and employer.

In relation to space and the environmental conditions, occupants interact based on what the spatial arrangement allows, as noted in Chapter 1. However, understanding people and their behaviour is challenging. Studies in this regard have improved understanding of occupant behaviour (Li & Liu, 2020; Šujanová et al., 2019; Yan et al., 2017). For example, for Yan and Hong (2018), this is a complex phenomenon with many variables, which requires an interdisciplinary approach to be fully understood. It is relevant to keep in mind that everyone's behaviour may affect other office occupants. On the one hand, each occupant is influenced by external factors such as culture, economy, and climate, as well as by internal factors such as environmental comfort preferences, and personal physiology and psychology (Altomonte et al., 2020; Gunay et al., 2013). On the other hand, the interactions of individual occupants with building systems strongly influence building operations and thus building energy use and indoor comfort. This can give rise to a non-virtuous cycle of difficulties for organisational productivity if not carefully attended to.

Alternatively, the mechanisms of thermoregulation and thermal behaviour of human beings can generate discomfort and lead to disease if the environmental conditions are not satisfactory (Havenith, 2005; Schlader et al., 2009).

As a homeotherm, human beings have a complex system to maintain their average internal temperatures, which is made up of three components. The afferent thermoreceptor pathways collect thermal information and direct it to the integration centres. Then, the integration centres are responsible for the coordinated processing of the afferent information. They generate a response in body temperature by changing or maintaining it as needed. There are also the thermoeffective efferent pathways, which provide feedback and raise or lower body temperature according to the response of the regulatory centres (Arens & Zhang, 2009; Flouris, 2011). This thermoregulatory system is based on the interrelation and cooperation of several seemingly independent systems that actually interact together: nervous, immune, cardiovascular, musculoskeletal, endocrine and adipose tissue, and skin, among others (Morrison & Nakamura, 2019). All are linked to the brain, which controls these physicochemical actions according to an individual's psychological condition. For example, it is interesting to analyse the thermal inequality that occurs in offices according to sex. Parkinson et al. (2021) suggest that overcooling is a common problem in offices, and the associated impacts of these circumstances pervasively affect wellbeing and performance predominantly for women.

It is important, therefore, to consider office thermal conditions because they affect occupant perception of the workspace, and undesirable variations, however small, can translate into dissatisfaction, distraction or the need for adaptation that may impact work. In this chapter, the self-assessed productivity of office occupants in relation to the thermal environment is examined in a Chilean context. Environmental parameters and the arrangement of office spaces are analysed in contrast to occupants' perceptions based on cross-sectional and retrospective questionnaires.

The indoor office environment

Office design aims to provide workspaces that are conducive to keeping occupant body temperature relatively constant and moderate. However, in modern office environments, it is difficult for traditional HVAC system design to meet the increasing demands of individual worker preferences in their microclimates (Chao & Wan, 2004). This takes into consideration daily and seasonal variations that cause the temperature outside of a building to fluctuate. This phenomenon and its impact have been studied internationally (Frontczak et al., 2012; Huizenga et al., 2003; Ornetzeder et al., 2016; Schulte et al., 2015) in different locations and building types. According to Rupp et al. (2015), different thermal comfort models have been developed that give meaning to the physical conditions of building occupants. They analyse an individual's thermal state using intuitive perception categories, such as cold, neutral, or warm, which is equivalent to being comfortable or uncomfortable in the thermal environment. Other stationary and transient models exist that do not focus on the overall thermal state of the human body, but rather on certain parts, such as the limbs or the back (Enescu, 2019; Wang et al., 2007).

Spatial arrangement

Today's dynamic work environments demand flexible, multifunctional spatial designs. In this sense, office design is constantly evolving, seeking to adapt to employee requirements. However, to analyse the thermal environment and its relation to productivity it is possible to subdivide offices into three categories: individual, shared private, and open plan. In the first type, the occupant acts freely with respect to the spatial arrangement and use of the environmental conditioning systems. In the case of open plan offices, it is very difficult for workers to agree on conditions for the whole group and the freedom to do so can lead to complications in the work environment. Therefore, the design of this kind of office means that workers do not manage the climate control systems. Between these two types, is the shared private office with a maximum of eight occupants, where workers may be able to reach an understanding of the spatial layout, the use of the thermostat, or the opening of windows.

Associated factors

When designing office buildings, a simple premise is generally followed regarding thermal comfort: buildings should be designed to operate at between 20.0 and 25.0 °C (Al Horr et al., 2017; Šujanová et al., 2019). Nonetheless, according to ISO 15251 (2008), the situation is a bit more complex. It states that the indoor environment affects the health, productivity, and wellbeing of occupants. Alternately, Mishra et al. (2016) and Yan et al. (2017) mention that the heterogeneous and dynamic nature of the daily work reality of the occupants of a given building and their resulting adaptive actions have been recognised in literature showing that the workplace environment is complex. Additionally, the effect of other indoor environmental variables such as noise, glare, or poor air quality must be taken into account, since when they are unacceptable to workers they influence occupants' thermal perception (Mulville et al., 2016; Pellerin & Candas, 2003; Thomas, 2017). That is, the perspective presented in ISO 10551 (2019) is very relevant here: thermal sensation can have more than one meaning. It encompasses psychological factors such as a motivation to express satisfaction with the situation or occupant's mood, so that preference and acceptability collaborate to specify the context of thermal conditions. It is also worth noting that according to a review by Bueno et al. (2021), there are few studies both with sufficient participants and that relate multiple workspace variables, for example, that examine demographic realities in different countries, as well as the personal characteristics of occupants, and how they perceive their environment and report their degree of satisfaction.

In Chile, a highly seismic country, structures are usually robust and most of the time designed using reinforced concrete construction. Also, the glazing ratio of envelopes differs in each individual design. In general terms, occupants recognise that building characteristics are favourable, but affect their

Table 2.1 General characterisation of the occupants

	Winter	Summer
Predominant age 26–45 years (% of occupants)	66.1	65.8
Votes male/female	930/922	840/859
Average metabolic activity (MET)	1.25	1.24
Average clothing (clo)	0.89	0.66
Time in workspace (% of day)	90.7	88.6

perception of the thermal environment. That is to say, Chilean workers, like those in other countries, show a high degree of satisfaction with their workspaces, which is in line with other studies of office buildings (Rijal et al., 2017). Soto-Muñoz et al. (2022a, 2022b) studied 18 office buildings in the cities of Santiago and Concepción, Chile. The general characterisation of the participants showed that they remained in their workspaces approximately 90% of the workday. Therefore, it can be said that the occupants are aware of the reality of their offices. This differs greatly from Akimoto et al. (2010) who suggest that office workers spend 40% of the day in their workspaces. The predominant metabolic activity was found to be "active sitting" accompanied by brief movements. The average metabolic rate was 1.25 MET, which is to be expected according to the ASHRAE 55 (2017) and ISO 8996 (2005) standards, since most of the time office workers perform sedentary administrative tasks and their duties mainly require upper limb dexterity. There was no explicit dress code for the majority of the workers in the organisations studied. However, casual dress was observed with a mean clo of 0.89, which corresponds to light work clothes. Metabolic activity and other characterisation data for winter and summer are shown in Table 2.1.

The clothing of office occupants was similar in both cities, with a difference between winter and summer of 0.26 clo for Concepción and 0.21 clo for Santiago. The seasonal variation observed in both cities is related to a decrease in insulation to improve individual thermal comfort. The standard work chair employed was of the conventional desk or executive type with an estimated insulation of 0.15 clo in the seat and backrest.

Perception of the thermal environment

To examine occupant perception, three quantitative data collection instruments were used. First, the participating offices and workers were characterised. Next, a questionnaire with different scales was used to ascertain the occupants' perceptions. Workers were surveyed using this cross-sectional instrument in their workspace during one day in winter and another in summer, thereby resulting in 3,551 completed questionnaires. Since the time of responses was recorded, it was possible to relate this data to the environmental monitoring data from the offices, which was obtained simultaneously during the workday. In addition, the workers responded to a general retrospective questionnaire about their individual subjective experience over the past winter and summer season. Data were collected with this instrument once in spring and 535 valid responses were obtained. This made it possible to prioritise environmental factors, as occupants retrospectively rated the influence of environmental parameters on productivity.

Regarding the analysis of operative temperatures in the buildings, in winter the minimum in Concepción was 20.2 °C and the maximum 22.8 °C, and in Santiago the corresponding temperatures were 21.0 °C and 24.0 °C. Whereas in summer, the minimum in Concepción was 21.5 °C and the maximum 24.5 °C and in Santiago the minimum was 23.0 °C and the maximum 24.4 °C. The average operating temperature in Concepción was 21.4 °C in winter and 22.9 °C in summer, versus Santiago where the average was 22.4 °C in winter and 23.7 °C in summer. Considering all the buildings studied, the neutral temperature range was found to be 19.5–24.6 °C and the preferred temperature range was 19.9–24.6 °C (Trebilcock et al., 2020). The thermal conditions observed in the offices were in alignment with ASHRAE 55 (2017) and ISO 15251 (2008) for human occupancy in winter. However, in some cases in Concepción in summer, temperatures were found to be slightly below the recommended standards for 0.5 clo. The temperature variation between the two cities can be explained by their different climates and the preferred temperature range by the effect of the occupants' long-term climate history (Wu et al., 2020). Buildings in Santiago have mostly mechanical conditioning systems, unlike those in Concepción that are mainly free-running. Workers reported a nearly neutral thermal sensation for operating temperatures above and below the lower limit of the range recommended by the standards (Wagner et al., 2007). This sense of wellbeing or hedonic pleasure by occupants is linked to frequent comfort experiences, which seems reasonable in these cases and implies adequate productivity conditions (Anderson & French, 2010).

As Figure 2.1 shows, occupants perceive a slightly higher level of comfort in winter than in summer. This may suggest that there are opportunities to improve the design and management of environmental conditioning strategies. However, specific situations vary by organisation. It should be noted that differences may exist in summer compared to winter, due to, for example, seasonal conditions such as the impact of vacations or workload fluctuations, among others.

In the 18 office buildings studied, environmental conditions were very similar, with organisational criteria focused on avoiding discomfort, technical criteria favouring mechanical systems, and decreasing human involvement in the control of environmental conditions. There were many cases of conflict between occupants involving the control of air conditioning systems, windows, fans, heaters, remote control of equipment, thermostats, curtains and the like. Each of the buildings had different policies for the operation of thermal conditioning elements, which affected the workspaces. Nonetheless, care must be taken since it was observed that rigid

How would you describe the typical conditions in your work area in winter/summer?

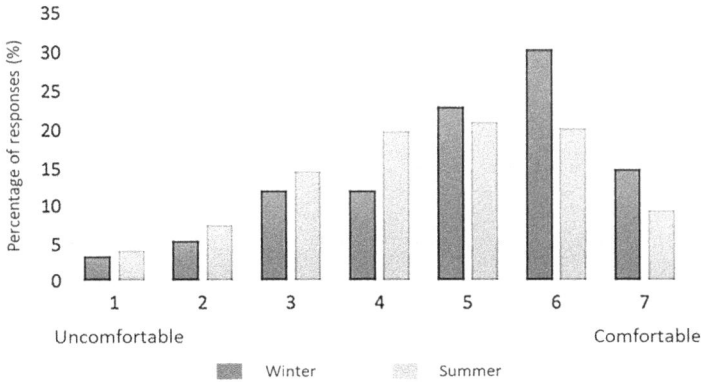

Figure 2.1 Retrospective perceived comfort in the workspace.

organisational policies related to energy savings had undesired effects. In this regard, de Dear et al. (2013) mention that this situation can generate a rebound effect based on the use of personal thermal conditioning elements that workers introduce in the office environment. Thermal dissatisfaction that causes an individual to take an adaptive action could be understood as a distraction from their work tasks. Therefore, matching the design and management of the work environment to the needs of employees may be essential to obtain the greatest contribution from workers towards orga-nisational goals (Heydarian et al., 2020).

In contrast, from the perspective of eudaimonic wellbeing, greater personal control of the workspace enables occupants to achieve comfort through adaptation, and at the same time self-actualisation, as workers feel that thermal conditions are adequate and allow them to function fully (Anderson & French, 2010). In this case, the individual autonomy that a workspace can provide has a positive effect on occupant productivity. This autonomy can occur according to the degree of control present, or the possibility that occupants have to use the thermal control elements in the environment (Table 2.2). It could also be observed that elements such as lamps, fans, and individual heaters are absent in more than 60.0% of the cases, which is due to restrictive institutional policies. However, as shown in Table 2.3, occupants give different importance to having specific conditioning elements in their workspaces, which coincides with Brager et al. (2004) who emphasise the importance of occupant control.

As shown in Tables 2.2 and 2.3, the degree of occupant control over the elements and their relative importance are evident, which is consistent with André et al. (2020). In cases where the different elements are present, greater

Table 2.2 Degree of control over environmental conditioning elements in the work-space

What degree of personal control do you have over the following elements in your workspace?

Environmental conditioning elements	No control 1	Percentage of responses (%)					Total control 7
		2	3	4	5	6	
Window	21.2	1.9	3.3	6.0	3.7	5.2	15.4
Blinds or curtains	12.8	6.1	5.2	6.7	6.9	6.7	28.0
Door	17.5	3.7	4.9	4.3	4.3	4.1	12.0
Personal lamp	12.7	0.8	0.6	1.2	0.4	0.6	5.1
General lighting	32.7	6.2	6.8	8.9	5.2	3.3	9.5
Personal fan	10.8	1.4	0.6	1.0	0.6	1.0	10.8
Shared fan	13.4	3.5	3.5	5.1	3.3	1.8	4.3
Personal heater	9.4	1.6	0.6	0.8	0.4	0.4	6.1
Shared heater	16.6	3.9	3.3	6.1	3.5	2.9	5.5
Thermostat	24.7	5.1	7.3	10.5	6.1	3.0	7.9

Table 2.3 Importance of control over environmental conditioning features in the work environment

How important is it for you to have control over the following elements in your work environment?

Environmental conditioning elements	Not important 1	Percentage of responses (%)					Very important 7
		2	3	4	5	6	
Window	16.6	3.1	7.5	7.5	8.7	8.7	26.2
Blinds or curtains	13.1	5.4	5.2	10.2	12.5	9.1	29.5
Door	19.7	5.7	6.6	7.6	6.3	5.7	16.0
Personal lamp	15.6	3.9	3.7	4.1	3.4	3.2	9.9
General lighting	20.4	7.9	10.1	11.5	10.5	8.7	16.2
Personal fan	12.4	3.4	3.0	4.8	3.8	3.6	16.4
Shared fan	12.6	4.4	6.0	6.8	7.2	6.8	8.8
Personal heater	13.0	3.8	2.2	5.6	3.2	4.0	10.8
Shared heater	14.0	4.0	5.6	7.4	9.2	6.4	10.8
Thermostat	14.3	5.8	6.2	13.3	13.3	10.1	15.7

importance is given to control over windows and blinds or curtains, while less importance is given to control over general lighting and doors. In this sense, the level of occupant satisfaction with the degree of control can be seen in Table 2.4. In this regard, in contrast to what was reported in the cross-sectional survey shown in the previous tables, in the retrospective evaluation it was observed that only 7.4% of the occupants stated they were very satisfied with the degree of control they have over the thermal environment of their

Table 2.4 Occupant satisfaction with degree of control

In general, how satisfied are you with the degree of control you have over the environment in your office?

Very dissatisfied	Percentage of response (%)					Very satisfied
1	2	3	4	5	6	7
8.9	8.9	14.5	26.2	18.3	15.9	7.4

workspace. These results demonstrate that occupants desire more opportunities for adaptation.

However, it was also observed that the number of occupants in an office affects perceived control, which is consistent with the findings of (Schweiker & Wagner, 2016). In this research, behavioural changes were identified in records of occupants' reported adaptive actions in their workspaces. In retrospective and cross-sectional evaluations, workers recognise the effect of the thermal environment on productivity, either by access to, or control or relative use of the thermal conditioning elements, including windows, blinds, fans, lights, and heating and cooling systems. This is in line with Haldi and Robinson (2010) and Nicol and Roaf (2005) who mention that through the operation of these elements the desired indoor conditions can be obtained. When well thought out, these office design features also contribute to improved worker performance (Vischer, 2017).

Office temperature is a characteristic of the indoor environment. An appropriate range can lead to greater worker satisfaction in the workspace and therefore to more productive behaviour. However, a greater understanding of its effects on productivity and drivers goes beyond temperature. Other office factors that affect worker perceptions are key and translate into adjusting the workplace depending on the available resources in order to achieve a better balance in the thermal environment.

The concept of thermal comfort has been defined by various standards as the state of mind that expresses satisfaction with the thermal environment (ASHRAE 55, 2017; ISO 7730, 2005). These regulations indicate that six environmental and personal factors should be considered when evaluating human responses to thermal conditions: air temperature, average radiant temperature, air velocity, humidity, and the clothing and activity of building occupants. Studies have shown that their combined effects and the workspace environment can have considerable consequences on the acceptability of conditions for occupants and their work performance (Huang et al., 2012; Rupp et al., 2015).

In Chile, there are few building standards related to indoor thermal comfort management, only the *Sistema de Certificación de Edificación Sustentable* (CES) or Sustainable Building Certification System (Instituto de la Construcción, 2014), which is based on ASHRAE 55, and the *Términos de*

Referencia sobre Confort Ambiental y Eficiencia Energética (TDRe) or Terms of Reference on Environmental Comfort and Energy Efficiency (CITEC, 2012). Thermal comfort control depends on the building and its environmental conditioning strategy or system (Seppänen et al., 2006). A number of models exist to predict and measure the thermal comfort of occupants. Among them is that developed by Fanger (1973), which assumes stationary conditions and considers the six previously mentioned variables that influence the thermal exchanges between a person and his or her environment, thereby affecting their feeling of comfort. Nevertheless, assuming that office thermal conditions are constant overlooks the interactions between the building, the possibility of natural ventilation, the climate, the occupancy, and the environmental conditioning system. Consequently, this model is normally only used for the design of buildings without natural ventilation.

In the office environment, indoor thermal variations should be considered, since occupants perceive them and hence interpret work processes in relation to space and time (Lan et al., 2012). Over the workday or different seasons of the year it is unreasonable to think that expected productivity patterns and actual productivity will coincide. When thermal conditions are unsuitable, workers become distracted (Wyon & Wargocki, 2006). Consequently, their immediate goals change, and they take actions that produce thermal changes and affect them and their coworkers.

For organisations, expected productivity may not be well defined or there may even be a difference in the impact of the components of the thermal environment on the occupant, which originates from design and operational considerations. Different studies such as Lan et al. (2007), Tanabe et al. (2007), and Wargorcki and Seppänen (2006) present the idea that many times when office temperature is within the comfort range, occupants may feel comfortable, but prefer to change the thermal conditions to avoid lethargy or sleepiness. Also, occupants frequently prefer greater air movement, as dissatisfaction is quite common (Brager et al., 2015; Zhang et al., 2007). In this regard, research on individuals in real time in their workspace provides data suggesting that thermal preferences have intrinsic, as well as geographical and cultural components (Antoniadou & Papadopoulos, 2017; Chappells & Shove, 2005; Kenawy & Elkadi, 2013).

A potential for productivity gains may lie in adjusting design and operational strategies by recognising occupants' environmental preferences and delving into ways of measuring productivity in relation to expectations and the reality of indoor built space. A review of the results of previous studies on thermal sensation and preference reveals discrepancies: the preferred sensation of respondents systematically changes depending on the situation (Haldi & Robinson, 2010; Humphreys & Nicol, 2007; Mishra et al., 2016). In this sense, for Kosonen and Tan (2004), Romero Herrera et al. (2020), and Thomas (2017), occupant responses differ at similar temperatures depending on the building, whether it is naturally ventilated or air-conditioned. Also, the influence of other indoor environmental variables should be taken into account when they are unacceptable and alter occupants' thermal perception, such as noise, glare, or stuffy air (Frontczak et al., 2012; Geng et al., 2017; Jung & Jazizadeh, 2019; Mulville et al., 2016).

Variations in occupant preference can be caused by sociocultural and economic differences, in addition to physiological, anthropometric (Antoniadou & Papadopoulos, 2017), and functional factors (Vischer & Wifi, 2017). However, to manage occupant satisfaction in conventional buildings, facility managers generally believe that operative temperature and air humidity are the appropriate metrics to use. Nonetheless, some studies have demonstrated that physical measurements are only moderately related to thermal comfort (Reeve, 2018). From a holistically integrated perspective, a human being interacts emotionally and rationally with a given thermal environment in their workspace. Thermal comfort is a personal experience and should primarily be assessed through subjective evaluation. In this context, productivity interacts with the thermal comfort in different ways. In most cases, the components that comprise it cannot be separated without consequences. To better understand this phenomenon, it must be recognised that objective and subjective evaluation of the indoor built environment have different roles that are fundamentally complementary (Geng et al., 2019).

Before continuing, it is necessary to define the terms "thermal sensation", "thermal acceptability", and "thermal preference", which are part of thermal comfort. Thermal sensation is a subjective response that assesses an individual's satisfaction in a specific thermal environment. It involves a person's conscious interpretation of sensory data resulting from exposure to the environment. In contrast, thermal acceptability refers to a state of mind that expresses the ability to tolerate the thermal conditions of the environment up to a certain limit. Thermal acceptability is an occupant response to the relationship between body heat and the maximum amount of it that can be lost or accepted under the prevailing conditions. It is influenced by organisational context and personal motivation. Lastly, thermal preference is the desired condition based on thermal sensation. As mentioned by de Dear and Brager (1998), this concept goes beyond human physiology and is based on the idea of an occupant as an active receiver of thermal conditions.

Methods for measuring work productivity

Measuring productivity as affected by the thermal environment can enable an organisation to recognise the importance of the proper management of environmental conditioning systems. Understanding which factors may be responsible for variation in productivity can lead to operational and personnel changes that improve the company or institution's performance results. However, it is reasonable to begin a study with the most stable conditions, thereby improving classification of the permanent variables related to the phenomenon being examined. One situation to consider when studying productivity throughout the year is what happens in spring and fall. In summer the human body makes changes in its physiology to resist the heat, such as sweating more easily, and in winter, the body sends a bit more blood to exposed areas such as the face and hands to keep the skin warm. However, in these transitional seasons, the body takes time to adapt, and this affects the perception of how cool or warm the person feels, resulting in discomfort in the workspace (Sawka et al., 2002). The change of season highlights the problems of air conditioning systems. In temperate climates, it is common during the spring or fall, for one side of a building to require heating while another requires cooling, or more complex still, two similar adjacent offices may require different degrees of heating or cooling because one office is densely occupied while the other is not. Ideally, each indoor space in a building would need its own HVAC system (Rock, 2018). Notwithstanding, such an approach is often cost prohibitive, so trade-offs must be made in organisations. This change can cause underlying problems with thermal conditioning systems that went unnoticed during the previous season to suddenly become evident and uncomfortable for office workers.

Several studies (de Dear et al., 2013; McArthur & Powell, 2020; Rupp et al., 2015) examined elements of this management and thermal comfort. Their differing results showed various response actions by occupants. Hence, when an organisation imposes a narrow temperature range, workers often use their own personal thermal conditioning devices. Likewise, when control of air conditioning systems is ceded to occupants, it can affect the working climate or create serious energy savings problems. For example, in open plan offices where some workstations face towards the sun and others are always in the shade, individual preferences will not always be the same and please everyone. If a single worker controls the temperature, others may feel undervalued, thereby leading to disagreements in the organisation. What is certain is that the temperature of the air surrounding the occupant is an important consideration (Table 2.5). Although other environmental factors also play a role, from the studies conducted it is evident that temperature is the main variable affecting long-term productivity.

Table 2.5 Influence of environmental parameters on winter/ summer productivity

What parameters do you think most affect your productivity in your workspace in winter/summer?

Parameters	Winter	Summer
Temperature (T)	45.9%	51.1%
Noise (N)	25.8%	25.0%
Indoor air quality (IAQ)	15.2%	14.5%
Glare (G)	3.6%	5.4%
Lighting (L)	9.5%	4.0%

It should be kept in mind that authors such as Geng et al. (2017), Pellerin and Candas (2003), and Tiller et al. (2010) mention that noise can distort the effect of thermal satisfaction for occupants. Nevertheless, the situation is usually brief or temporary. This is because noise is so distracting that the occupant immediately takes effective actions to correct the situation and continue working.

In contrast, the permanent daily load of work stressors and strain experienced by office occupants leads to burnout (Sonnentag, 2018). Another factor that results in day-to-day variability and should be taken into account when surveying office occupants is the effect of positive allesthesia produced by transient thermal conditions from occasional stimuli (André et al., 2020; de Dear, 2011). These temporary conditions can cause brief changes in occupant perceptions, thus biasing cross-sectional worker responses. In contrast, retrospective responses may be more rational and reflective regarding conditions, and can indicate plausible causes, occurrences, and aspects of behaviour through hindsight (Mangal & Mangal, 2013). Therefore, to assess and understand perceived productivity in relation to the thermal environment, it is important to recognise that the method used, or temporal perspective of a questionnaire, may yield different perspectives.

In addition, there is the difference of how to measure the phenomenon, either objectively or subjectively. Different studies (Feige et al., 2013; Roelofsen, 2002) mention that in order to measure the productivity of workers in relation to the thermal environment, objective data on the physical-environmental conditions of their workspaces should be used. This involves collecting data such as air temperature, radiant temperature, relative humidity, and air speed. Readily available data collection instruments such as the Delta OHM data logger are frequently used by researchers. In recent years, they have become increasingly accurate and practical for successful fieldwork.

It is possible to examine productivity objectively by measuring the achievement of objectives. This requires key information for data analysis and should be part of a detailed assessment of individual worker by their corresponding human resources department. Alternately, when relating productivity to the thermal environment, it is appropriate to incorporate subjective assessment. From this point of view, the thermal environment represents the characteristics of the space and surroundings that affect a person's heat loss or gain in their workspace, as well as their preference to change that condition when deemed unfavourable. It should be remembered that according to (ASHRAE 55, 2017), thermal sensation is defined as the mental condition that expresses satisfaction with the thermal environment. It is explored through subjective evaluation and implicitly considers the person's climatic history for the response. Thus, in a variety of office situations each occupant seems to be the best source of feedback on their own thermal perception in the workspace and how it affects their productivity.

According to the above, thermal perception is a mental condition that in offices makes it possible to analyse occupant acceptance of the workspace.

Similarly, self-assessment of work productivity can be used in relation to information on the thermal environment. Perhaps the underlying rationale is based on Humphreys and Nicol (2007), who indicate that office work involves a variety of complex tasks and therefore that the occupants of a building are the best judges of their own efficiency in the thermal environment. In this regard, Haapakangas et al. (2018a) indicate that an objective measurement of worker performance is often not feasible in office work and that researchers must rely on self-assessments as a useful and holistic mechanism to understand occupants and their productivity. Nevertheless, it is difficult to distinguish which variables are most meaningful and interrelated with the built environment and truly matter.

Self-perceived productivity

The relationship between work performance and the thermal environment

In fields such as organisational psychology, the relationship between the design of workspace conditions and normal worker productivity is still an area with unresolved questions (de Dear et al., 2013; Ramírez-Vielma & Nazar, 2019). In line with different authors (Akimoto et al., 2010; Al Horr et al., 2016; Lin et al., 2015), it was found that the perceived work productivity of individual office occupants is affected by temperature and the building systems that regulate it.

Organisations seem to be aware of this phenomenon. Nevertheless, they often experience difficulties in judgement when developing methods to determine productivity according to office environmental conditions. In this sense, the criterion problem is a phenomenon that accounts for difficulties related to the development and measurement of outcome constructs for organisations due to their multidimensional nature, as is the case with performance, production, and productivity. It is explained by factors such as measurement limitations or the intervention of situational factors (Bedford & Speklé, 2018). The criterion problem must be considered when interpreting the results of self-perceived productivity (Austin & Villanova, 1992; Viswesvaran & Ones, 2000). In the offices studied, occupant responses reveal a lack of diagnosis of workspace functionality. This is mainly due to the diversity of tasks carried out in the same workspace.

The relationship between self-perceived productivity and adaptation in the workspace

In office buildings, such as those studied, environmental conditions are often similar. It is common to find organisational criteria focused on avoiding discomfort, technical criteria favouring mechanical systems, and decreasing human involvement in the control of environmental conditions. There were many disagreements between occupants involving control of air conditioning systems, windows, fans, heaters, equipment remote controls, thermostats, curtains, and the like. Each of the buildings had different policies for the operation of thermal conditioning elements, which affects the workspaces. However, care must be taken, since rigid organisational energy-saving policies can result in a rebound effect caused by the use of personal thermal conditioning devices that workers introduce into the office environment. Every behaviour or adaptive action performed by an individual can be understood to be a distraction from work tasks. Therefore, matching the design and management of the work environment to the needs of employees is essential to obtain the greatest contribution from workers towards the organisation's goals (Heydarian et al., 2020). In contrast, from the perspective of eudaimonic wellbeing, greater personal control of the workspace allows occupants to achieve comfort through adaptation, and at the same time self-actualisation, as workers feel that thermal conditions are adequate and enable them to function fully (Anderson & French, 2010). In this case, the autonomy provided by a given workspace has a positive effect on productivity. The degree of control or the opportunity occupants have to operate the thermal control devices in their environment was unsatisfactory in the buildings studied. However, the results indicate that the occupants attach the greatest importance to having this type of thermal conditioning elements in their workspaces, which coincides with Brager et al. (2004), who emphasise the importance of occupant control. They also observed that the number of occupants in an office affected perceived control. In the research conducted in Chile, behavioural changes were identified in the records of adaptive actions reported by occupants in their workspaces. Thus, retrospective and cross-sectional evaluations recognised the effect of the thermal environment on productivity based on access, control, or relative use of thermal conditioning features, including windows, blinds, fans, lights, and heating and cooling systems. In this way, through the operation of these devices, the desired indoor conditions can be obtained. When foreseen, they contribute to improve the performance of the workers.

The effect of "work normality" on occupants

Normality in offices should not be considered an absolute and/or universal concept. This is even less true after the COVID-19 pandemic that affected the reality of workplaces worldwide. However, it is possible to understand that normality is a condition that encompasses all that occurs frequently on a day-to-day basis in the workplace. That is to say, normal work situations conform to a regulated framework and are within the common-sense expectations of workers. In this context, there are no extraordinary circumstances that positively or negatively affect productivity. Alternately, offices tend to have moderate environmental conditions, resulting only in temporary discomfort. However, temporary disturbances can occur that workers manage with a kind of mental buffering capacity. According to Zhang et al. (2019), occupants appear to possess a certain cognitive reserve or sense of normalcy that involves adaptive actions caused by discomfort from the thermal environment.

In this regard, occupants were asked to evaluate their self-perceived productivity cross-sectionally in relation to the thermal environmental conditions of their workspaces. They intuitively compared their responses with other workdays and considered their habitual activities and frequent daily stressors. The results show that "normal" corresponds to that usual condition occupants naturally took on while performing their duties. No significant variations were observed between the responses given in Santiago and Concepción, either in winter or in summer. Taking into consideration all the data and that the state of "normal" represented neutrality (0) on an ordinal scale from −3 to +3, the mean productivity was +0.03, with a standard deviation of 0.53 (Table 2.6). These results are similar to those reported by Humphreys and Nicol (2007). Moreover, the results also appear to align with Vischer and Wifi's (2017) concept of functional comfort, in which occupants' perceptions of comfort and its effects are grounded in the use of the thermal conditioning elements in workspaces, along with their knowledge of them and the conditions essential for worker tasks.

As illustrated in Table 2.7, the results indicate that noise (N) is the main influence on productivity since it is a distractor. Likewise, Haapakangas et al. (2018b) mention that distractions in the office are essentially environmental

Table 2.6 Distribution of occupant's cross-sectional right-now perceived productivity votes

Based on your self-evaluation and according to the environmental conditions, what do you think of your current productivity in your workspace?	Percentage of responses (%)
Much less than normal (−2)	0.8
A little less than normal (−1)	8.4
Normal (0)	81.0
A little more than normal (+1)	8.5
Much more than normal (+2)	1.8

Table 2.7 Degree of influence of parameters on retrospective perceived productivity

How much influence do the following parameters have on your productivity?

Parameters	Percentage of responses (%)					
	No influence	Very little	Little	Moderate	High	Very high
Temperature (T)	3.8	6.5	11.9	27.3	30.2	20.3
Noise (N)	6.4	4.7	14.8	23.4	27.9	22.8
Indoor air quality (IAQ)	3.7	7.0	13.0	30.6	28.7	17.1
Glare (G)	11.2	11.0	21.8	31.5	16.0	8.5
Lighting (L)	7.6	7.4	15.0	32.7	27.3	9.8

Table 2.8 Retrospective perceived productivity versus cross-sectional perceived productivity (n = 240)

(Number of responses)			*Cross-sectional productivity*					
			-2 Much less than normal	-1 A little less than normal	0 Normal	1 A little more than normal	2 Much more than normal	*Total*
Retrospective productivity	-4	40% or more decrease	0	0	3	0	0	3
	-3	30% decrease	0	1	10	0	1	12
	-2	20% decrease	0	5	29	0	0	34
	-1	10% decrease	0	5	30	0	0	35
	0	Not affected (0%)	0	1	37	1	1	40
	1	10% increase	0	2	27	1	0	30
	2	20% increase	0	0	43	1	1	45
	3	30% increase	0	1	23	3	0	27
	4	40% or more increase	0	0	14	0	0	14
		Total	0	15	215	6	3	240

demands that can produce other negative effects. In addition, environmental dissatisfaction can influence worker attitudes towards changes in conditions, which in turn affects perception of the thermal environment and influences the self-evaluated productivity of office occupants. Workers completed a retrospective assessment that asked them to estimate the degree to which their productivity increases or decreases due to thermal environmental conditions. As shown in Table 2.8, 42.5% of the participants believe that their productivity increases between 10.0% and 40.0%, and 38.6% state that their productivity decreases between 10.0% and 40.0% due to thermal environmental conditions.

Concerning the retrospective assessment of the overall productivity perceived by workers during the twelve months prior to data collection, it was found that respondents do in fact recognise that the thermal environmental conditions of their workspaces have a positive effect on their productivity. This is in line with most studies on the subject (Al Horr et al., 2016; Leaman & Bordass, 2001; Lipczynska et al., 2018).

Nevertheless, to assess how related the cross-sectional and retrospective productivity responses are, the retrospective questionnaire responses of 240 participants were analysed, as these were the occupants who consistently remained in their workspaces. The results are shown below.

Table 2.8 shows that most of the participants who reported their productivity as "normal" in the cross-sectional survey declared higher productivity in the retrospective evaluation. This would seem to indicate that occupants tend to evaluate their daily productivity within a context of normality. However, this translates into a positive perception of productivity in a retrospective evaluation.

This difference in participant opinions may be due to a better understanding of an initial perception, which comes with time. Before assigning an absolute value, perceptions must be processed by the mind for completeness. A cross-sectional evaluation may not be the best way to determine the perceived productivity of occupants if it is not complemented by a retrospective assessment.

Since thermal comfort is a mental assessment, considering the thermal conditions and workspace adaptation described above, the cross-sectional responses given in the context of perceived work normality can be associated with a certain mental resilience or cognitive reserve that enables psychological acceptance of variation in moderate environmental conditions. This concept used by Zhang et al. (2019) recognises that building occupants possess a buffering capacity, with little or no detrimental effect on their work, but with limits that depend on each individual's situation. In Chile, thermal conditions do not significantly interfere with office workers' cross-sectional perceived productivity responses and workers are slightly uncomfortable, which is in line with Akimoto et al. (2010) and Oliveira et al. (2015). Nonetheless, if this cognitive reserve includes opportunities for adjustment and control, it implies that occupants of office buildings may not express minor thermal discomfort, as they may be subject to work responsibilities or obligations. In other words, cognitive reserve can be considered part of work normality. Regarding the influence of the thermal environment on perceived productivity, 71.2% of the occupants stated in the retrospective evaluation that the temperature in their workspace affects the thermal environment, 22.0% indicated that it is detrimental to their mood, 19.1% that it causes illness, and 13.4% that it increases the amount of time wasted on actions to improve thermal comfort. At the same time, 8.7% reported that temperature increases the frequency of ailments, 5.1% indicated that it negatively affects their commitment to work, and 2.9% stated that it increases their absenteeism.

To better understand the observed variables from the cross-sectional and retrospective evaluations, categorical principal component analysis can be conducted, and structural equation models can be generated using software such as IBM SPSS AMOS version 22.0. Operating temperature and cross-sectional thermal sensation were found to be related to seasonal thermal perception and this in turn to perceived productivity. Parameters for the evaluation of occupant perception were identified and estimated. In this way, exogenous variables were progressively removed to focus on the relationship of the main variables and to compare both self-reporting techniques. Responses were contrasted in two seasons of the year and under the perception of different mental perspectives: one cross-sectional and one retrospective. Structural equation modelling will be discussed in more detail in the next section.

The relationship between cross-sectional perceived productivity and retrospective perceived productivity

The relationship between cross-sectional perceived productivity and retrospective perceived productivity structural equation modelling has increasingly been used to examine people and aspects of the built environment in order to evaluate the relationships of multiple variables with each other. The analysis contrasted the occupants' perceptions over time in the cross-sectional and retrospective evaluations using a structural equation model of self-reported productivity and the effect of the thermal environment.

Considering that both the cross-sectional perceived productivity and retrospective perceived productivity measurements are ordinal, Spearman's correlation coefficient was calculated. The rho value obtained was 0.192, with a p-value of 0.14, which confirms that there is a positive (although weak) and statistically significant relationship. This may imply that such a relationship does not exist between cross-sectional perceived productivity and retrospective perceived productivity responses. However, the reduced number of responses used and the diversity of organisations from which they were obtained may lead to a weak relationship between the perceived productivity responses. Nonetheless, it should not necessarily be assumed that there is a weak or non-existent relationship between the variables because the correlation is small (Bland & Altman, 2011) and thus these results should be taken with caution.

Given the previous, a categorical principal components analysis was employed using scatter diagrams with 95.0% confidence ellipses for winter and summer to examine the dependence of the cross-sectional perceived productivity responses; operative temperature in the morning, at midday, and in the afternoon; and the retrospective perceived productivity responses. To this end, data on operative temperature were pooled every 0.5 °C to obtain ordinal data sets. The 95.0% confidence ellipse plots that show the findings are presented in Figures 2.2 and 2.3. The location of the variables is represented geometrically by identifying each variable with a vector, and the non-association of two variables is shown by the orthogonality between the corresponding vectors. In winter, both perceived productivity assessments are close to each other and their relative right-angle position differs, thereby indicating a relationship between these variables; this does not occur in summer. Alternately, in all the cases analysed the operative temperature lies outside this relationship.

This can be interpreted as the absence of perceived productivity dependence on temperature. However, it is not easy to measure the effect of the thermal environment on human performance, especially when there are differences in and complexities specific to the work done at each organisation. This research is consistent with Zhang et al. (2019), since although there are similar work patterns, thermal conditions, metabolism, and clothing in the

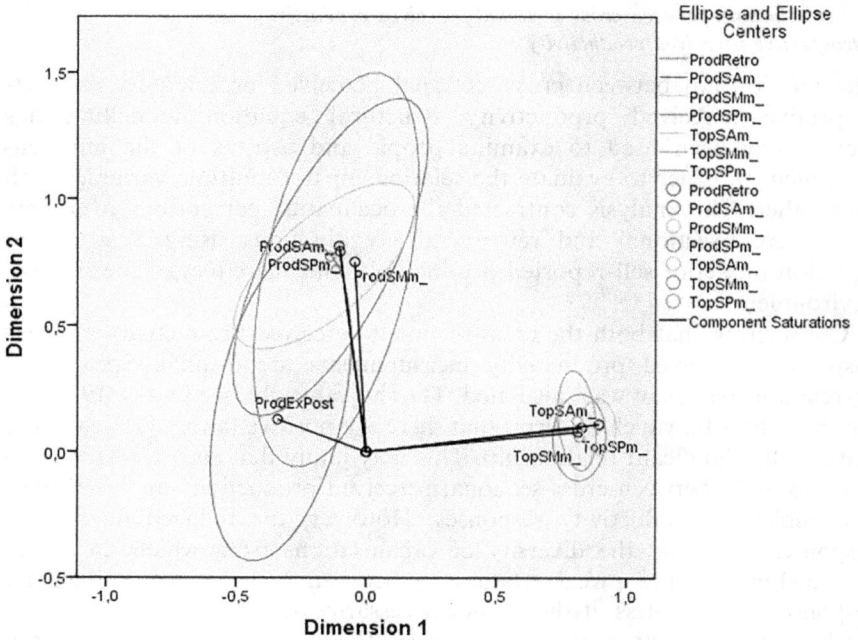

Figure 2.2 Principal component analysis with 95.0% confidence ellipses in winter.

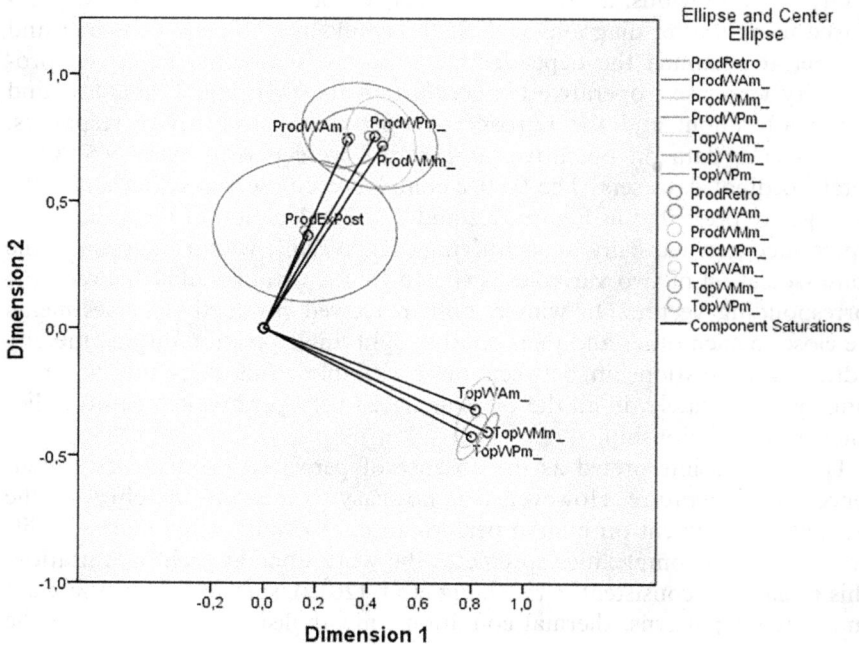

Figure 2.3 Principal component analysis with 95.0% confidence ellipses in summer.

buildings studied, there are also other variables related to specific tasks in particular contexts that cannot be adequately explained at present, and the adoption of reductionist approaches may lead to incorrect conclusions.

The analysis shows that the variables are effectively correlated according to Spearman's rho, as shown in Tables 2.9 and 2.10. That is to say, in winter it is evident that there is indeed a link between the perceived productivity assessments, while in summer this is not so, except at midday. However, it is not possible to affirm that non-significant findings imply there is no effect. This could be caused by measurement difficulties in summer due to omitted-variable bias. As such, this is an opportunity for future research, which can improve sample selection and consider additional variables such as workload.

Table 2.9 Winter correlations of cross-sectional and retrospective perceived productivity

Winter correlations			Retrospective productivity
Spearman's rho Cross-sectional productivity	Winter – morning	Correlation coefficient	0.260[**]
		Sig. (bilateral)	0.000
		N	240
	Winter – midday	Correlation coefficient	0.166[*]
		Sig. (bilateral)	0.010
		N	240
	Winter – afternoon	Correlation coefficient	0.298[**]
		Sig. (bilateral)	0.000
		N	240

Notes
[**] The significance level is <0.01 (two-tailed).
[*] The significance level is < 0.05 (two-tailed).

Table 2.10 Summer correlations of cross-sectional and retrospective perceived productivity

Summer correlations			Retrospective productivity
Spearman's rho Cross-sectional productivity	Summer – morning	Correlation coefficient	0.120
		Sig. (bilateral)	0.630
		N	240
	Summer – midday	Correlation coefficient	0.166[**]
		Sig. (bilateral)	0.009
		N	240
	Summer – afternoon	Correlation coefficient	0.057
		Sig. (bilateral)	0.381
		N	240

Note
[**] The significance level is <0.01 (two-tailed).

Taking all of the previous analyses into account, structural equation models were used to simultaneously estimate each of the pathways between the cross-sectional and retrospective assessments in winter and summer, while taking into consideration correlations between multiple variables (Figure 2.4). As can be seen in Table 2.11, the results of the goodness-of-fit indices show that the model is a good representation of the proposed relationships.

As in Peng et al. (2019), the structural equation method uses path analysis to examine the direct and indirect effects of various factors on subjective comfort. The greatest dependencies were found in the following relationships. Cross-sectional thermal perception in summer has a negative influence on cross-sectional perceived productivity in summer (r = −0.329). In addition, retrospective thermal perception in winter directly influences retrospective perceived productivity (r = 0.165). Also, cross-sectional perceived productivity in winter directly influences the retrospective assessment of perceived productivity (r = 0.259). In the model, two important relationships emerge:

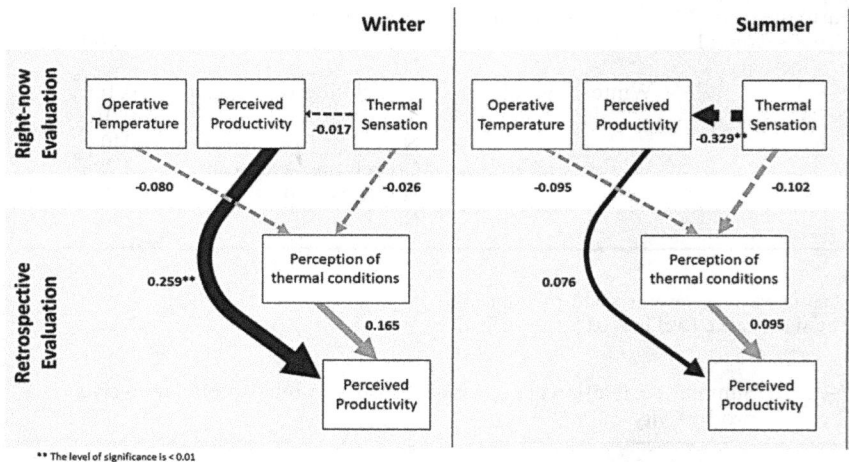

Figure 2.4 Model of structural equations of perceived productivity affected by the thermal environment.

Table 2.11 Goodness of fit of the model

index	Reference values	Model
X^2/df	2–5	1.434
CFI	≥0.950	0.952
TLI	≥0.900	0.939
SRMR	≥0.090	0.065
RMSEA	≤0.080	0.043

first, the influence of cross-sectional thermal perception on cross-sectional perceived productivity in both seasons had a minimal effect on retrospective perceived productivity. Secondly, the following phenomenon occurs: in summer, cross-sectional thermal perception significantly negatively affects cross-sectional perceived productivity, while in winter this does not occur and retrospective perceived productivity is directly influenced by both retrospective thermal perception and cross-sectional perceived productivity. Structural equation modelling can analyse a large amount of non-experimental data to validate complex constructs that emerge between the built interior space and building occupants.

Conclusions

This study suggests that impressions and the senses predominately emerge from the cross-sectional evaluation, whereas the results of the retrospective assessment reflect the effects of greater rationality and judgement. Indeed, retrospective self-evaluation would appear to be the best method for measuring perceived productivity, since for different tasks, occupant functions, and organisations, using a single field metric seems to be quite problematic.

The use of structural equations is a stronger method to evaluate multiple causes and effects, make comparisons by group, study the structure of covariances, and verify factorial structures. Unlike other techniques such as simple linear regression, factor analysis or correlation, the structural equation technique has many more relevant implications for the explanation of the phenomenon of perceived productivity. The use of multiple correspondence analyses has the advantage of explaining the statistical relationship between perceived productivity levels and describing those patterns in order to suppose the existing relationships, which can then be tested using Spearman's rho coefficient.

A better understanding of office thermal environment variables can identify their effects on occupant productivity. Certain factors act as drivers, which are key to workers' perceptions. Recognising these drivers can help to inform the redesign of workspaces and the allocation of available resources to achieve a better balance in the thermal environment. The results show that in office buildings constructed in Chile, individuals reported being comfortable in their workplaces with moderate temperatures and recognised that temperature is a very relevant parameter in the workplace, and in the search for adequate productivity conditions. While specific to Chile, the findings and the approach taken provide a benchmark for future research.

Acknowledgements

This work was supported by the Chilean National Fund for Scientific and Technological Development, FONDECYT, under research grants 1171497 and 1201456. The authors would also like to thank the Research Group in

Integrated Building Design and Management and Internal Research Project DIUBB 2120538 IF/R at the Universidad del Bío-Bío.

References

Agha-Hossein, M. M., El-Jouzi, S., Elmualim, A. A., Ellis, J., & Williams, M. (2013). Post-occupancy studies of an office environment: Energy performance and occupants' satisfaction. *Building and Environment, 69*, 121–130.

Akimoto, T., Tanabe, S. ichi, Yanai, T., & Sasaki, M. (2010). Thermal comfort and productivity - Evaluation of workplace environment in a task conditioned office. *Building and Environment, 45*(1), 45–50.

Al Horr, Y., Arif, M., Kaushik, A., Mazroei, A., Elsarrag, E., & Mishra, S. (2017). Occupant productivity and indoor environment quality: A case of GSAS. *International Journal of Sustainable Built Environment, 6*(2), 476–490.

Al Horr, Y., Arif, M., Kaushik, A., Mazroei, A., Katafygiotou, M., & Elsarrag, E. (2016). Occupant productivity and office indoor environment quality: A review of the literature. In *Building and Environment* (Vol. 105, pp. 369–389). Elsevier Ltd.

Altomonte, S., Allen, J., Bluyssen, P. M., Brager, G., Heschong, L., Loder, A., Schiavon, S., Veitch, J. A., Wang, L., & Wargocki, P. (2020). Ten questions concerning well-being in the built environment. *Building and Environment, 180*, 106949.

Anderson, J., & French, M. (2010). Sustainability as promoting well-being: Psychological dimensions of thermal comfort. In *Personal communication, Institute of Well-Being*.

André, M., De Vecchi, R., & Lamberts, R. (2020). User-centered environmental control: a review of current findings on personal conditioning systems and personal comfort models. In *Energy and Buildings* (Vol. 222, p. 110011). Elsevier Ltd.

Antoniadou, P., & Papadopoulos, A. M. (2017). Occupants' thermal comfort: State of the art and the prospects of personalized assessment in office buildings. In *Energy and Buildings* (Vol. 153, pp. 136–149). Elsevier Ltd.

Arens, E. A., & Zhang, H. (2009). *The skin's role in human thermoregulation and comfort.*

ASHRAE 55. (2017). *Standard 55 – Thermal environmental conditions for human occupancy.* https://www.ashrae.org/technical-resources/bookstore/standard-55-thermal-environmental-conditions-for-human-occupancy

Austin, J. T., & Villanova, P. (1992). The criterion problem: 1917–1992. *Journal of Applied Psychology, 77*(6), 836–874.

Ayoko, O. B., & Ashkanasy, N. M. (2020). The physical environment of office work: Future open plan offices. *Australian Journal of Management, 45*(3), 488–506.

Bedford, D. S., & Speklé, R. F. (2018). Construct validity in survey-based management accounting and control research. *Journal of Management Accounting Research, 30*(2), 23–58.

Bland, J. M., & Altman, D. G. (2011). Correlation in restricted ranges of data. *BMJ, 342.*

Brager, G., Paliaga, G., & De Dear, R. (2004). Operable windows, personal control and occupant comfort. *ASHRAE Transactions, 110*, 17–35. www.ashrae.org

Brager, G., Zhang, H., & Arens, E. (2015). Evolving opportunities for providing thermal comfort. *Building Research & Information, 43*(3), 274–287.

Bueno, A. M., de Paula Xavier, A. A., & Broday, E. E. (2021). Evaluating the connection between thermal comfort and productivity in buildings: A systematic literature review. *Buildings, 11*(6).

Campbell, J. P., & Wiernik, B. M. (2015). The modeling and assessment of work performance. *Annual Review of Organizational Psychology and Organizational Behavior*, *2*(1), 47–74.

Chappells, H., & Shove, E. (2005). Debating the future of comfort: Environmental sustainability, energy consumption and the indoor environment. *Building Research & Information*, *33*(1), 32–40.

Chao, C. Y. H., & Wan, M. P. (2004). Airflow and air temperature distribution in the occupied region of an underfloor ventilation system. *Building and Environment*, *39*(7), 749–762.

CITEC. (2012). *TDRe: Términos de Referencia Estandarizados con Parámetros de Eficiencia Energética y Confort Ambiental, para Licitaciones de Diseño y Obra de la Dirección de Arquitetura, Según Zonas Geográficas del País y Según Tipología de Edificios, Términos de Refere.*

Clements-Croome, D. (2015). Creative and productive workplaces: A review. *Intelligent Buildings International*, *7*(4), 164–183.

de Dear, R. (2011). Revisiting an old hypothesis of human thermal perception: Alliesthesia. *Building Research & Information*, *39*(2), 108–117.

de Dear, R., & Brager, G. (1998). Developing an adaptive model of thermal comfort and preference. *ASHRAE Transactions*, *104*(Part 1), 1–18.

de Dear, R., Akimoto, T., Arens, E., Brager, G., Candido, C., Cheong, K., Li, B., Nishihara, N., Sekhar, S., Tanabe, S., Toftum, J., Zhang, H., & Zhu, Y. (2013). Progress in thermal comfort research over the last twenty years. *Indoor Air*, *23*(6), 442–461.

Enescu, D. (2019). Models and indicators to assess thermal sensation under steady-state and transient conditions. *Energies*, *12*(5), 841.

Fanger, P. (1973). Assessment of man's thermal comfort in practice. *British Journal of Industrial Medicine*, *30*(4), 313–324.

Feige, A., Wallbaum, H., Janser, M., & Windlinger, L. (2013). Impact of sustainable office buildings on occupant's comfort and productivity. *Journal of Corporate Real Estate*, *15*(1), 7–34.

Flouris, A. D. (2011). Functional architecture of behavioural thermoregulation. In *European Journal of Applied Physiology* (Vol. 111, Issue 1, pp. 1–8). Springer.

Frontczak, M., Schiavon, S., Goins, J., Arens, E., Zhang, H., & Wargocki, P. (2012). Quantitative relationships between occupant satisfaction and satisfaction aspects of indoor environmental quality and building design. *Indoor Air*, *22*(2), 119–131.

Geng, Y., Ji, W., Lin, B., & Zhu, Y. (2017). The impact of thermal environment on occupant IEQ perception and productivity. *Building and Environment*, *121*, 158–167.

Geng, Y., Ji, W., Wang, Z., Lin, B., & Zhu, Y. (2019). A review of operating performance in green buildings: Energy use, indoor environmental quality and occupant satisfaction. In *Energy and Buildings* (Vol. 183, pp. 500–514). Elsevier Ltd.

Groen, B., van der Voordt, T., Hoekstra, B., & van Sprang, H. (2019). Impact of employee satisfaction with facilities on self-assessed productivity support. *Journal of Facilities Management*, *17*(5), 442–462.

Gunay, H. B., O'Brien, W., & Beausoleil-Morrison, I. (2013). A critical review of observation studies, modeling, and simulation of adaptive occupant behaviors in offices. *Building and Environment*, *70*, 31–47.

Haapakangas, A., Hallman, D. M., Mathiassen, S. E., & Jahncke, H. (2018a). Self-rated productivity and employee well-being in activity-based offices: The role of environmental perceptions and workspace use. *Building and Environment*, *145*, 115–124.

Haapakangas, A., Hongisto, V., Varjo, J., & Lahtinen, M. (2018b). Benefits of quiet workspaces in open-plan offices – Evidence from two office relocations. *Journal of Environmental Psychology, 56*, 63–75.

Haldi, F., & Robinson, D. (2010). On the unification of thermal perception and adaptive actions. *Building and Environment, 45*(11), 2440–2457.

Havenith, G. (2005). Temperature regulation, heat balance and climatic stress. *Extreme Weather Events and Public Health Responses*, 69–80.

Heydarian, A., McIlvennie, C., Arpan, L., Yousefi, S., Syndicus, M., Schweiker, M., Jazizadeh, F., Rissetto, R., Pisello, A. L., Piselli, C., Berger, C., Yan, Z., & Mahdavi, A. (2020). What drives our behaviors in buildings? A review on occupant interactions with building systems from the lens of behavioral theories. *Building and Environment, 179*, 106928.

Huang, L., Zhu, Y., Ouyang, Q., & Cao, B. (2012). A study on the effects of thermal, luminous, and acoustic environments on indoor environmental comfort in offices. *Building and Environment, 49*(1), 304–309.

Huizenga, C., Zagreus, L., Arens, E., & Lehrer, D. (2003). *Measuring indoor environmental quality: A web-based occupant satisfaction survey*. Indoor Environmental Quality. http://www.cbe.berkeley.edu/research/pdf_files/Huizenga2003_USGBC.pdf

Humphreys, M., & Nicol, J. F. (2007). Self-assessed productivity and the office environment: Monthly surveys in five European countries. *ASHRAE Transactions, 113*, 606–616.

Instituto de la Construcción. (2014). *Manual de Evaluación y Calificación CES*.

ISO 10551. (2019). *ISO 10551:2019 - Ergonomics of the physical environment — Subjective judgement scales for assessing physical environments*, 28.

ISO 15251. (2008). *ISO 15251 Indoor environmental input parameters for design and assessment of energy performance of buildings addressing indoor air quality, thermal environment, lighting and acoustics*.

ISO 7730. (2005). *ISO 7730 – Ergonomics of the thermal environment – Analytical determination and interpretation of thermal comfort using calculation of the PMV and PPD indices and local thermal comfort criteria*, 52.

ISO 8996. (2005). *ISO 8996 ergonomics of the thermal environment – Determination of metabolic rate*.

Jung, W., & Jazizadeh, F. (2019). Human-in-the-loop HVAC operations: A quantitative review on occupancy, comfort, and energy-efficiency dimensions. *Applied Energy, 239*, 1471–1508.

Kenawy, I., & Elkadi, H. (2013). The impact of cultural and climatic background on thermal sensation votes. *PLEA 2013: Proceedings of the 29th Sustainable Architecture for a Renewable Future Conference*, 1–6.

Kosonen, R., & Tan, F. (2004). Assessment of productivity loss in air-conditioned buildings using PMV index. *Energy and Buildings, 36*(10 SPEC. ISS.), 987–993.

Lan, L., Lian, Z., Pan, L., Samuel, D. G. L., Nagendra, S. M. S., Maiya, M. P., Tanabe, S., Nishihara, N., Haneda, M., Wong, L. T., & Mui, K. W. (2007). Indoor temperature, productivity, and fatigue in office tasks. *HVAC&R Research, 13*(4), 623–633.

Lan, L., Wargocki, P., & Lian, Z. (2012). Optimal thermal environment improves performance of office work. *Indoor Environment, January*, 12–17.

Leaman, A., & Bordass, B. (2001). Assessing building performance in use 4: The Probe occupant surveys and their implications. *Building Research & Information, 29*(2), 129–143.

Li, J., & Liu, N. (2020). The perception, optimization strategies and prospects of outdoor thermal comfort in China: A review. *Building and Environment, 170*, 106614.

Lin, Y., Yang, L., Zheng, W., & Ren, Y. (2015). ScienceDirect study on human physiological adaptation of thermal comfort under building environment. *Procedia Engineering, 121*, 1780–1787.

Lipczynska, A., Schiavon, S., & Graham, L. T. (2018). Thermal comfort and self-reported productivity in an office with ceiling fans in the tropics. *Building and Environment, 135*, 202–212.

Mangal, S. K., & Mangal, S. (2013). *Research methodology in behavioural sciences.* PHI Learning Pvt. Ltd.

McArthur, J. J., & Powell, C. (2020). Health and wellness in commercial buildings: Systematic review of sustainable building rating systems and alignment with contemporary research. *Building and Environment, 171*, 106635.

Mishra, A. K., Loomans, M. G. L. C., & Hensen, J. L. M. (2016). Thermal comfort of heterogeneous and dynamic indoor conditions—An overview. *Building and Environment, 109*, 82–100.

Morrison, S. F., & Nakamura, K. (2019). Central mechanisms for thermoregulation. *Annual Review of Physiology, 81*(1), 285–308.

Mulville, M., Callaghan, N., & Isaac, D. (2016). The impact of the ambient environment and building configuration on occupant productivity in open-plan commercial offices. *Journal of Corporate Real Estate, 18*(3), 180–193.

Nicol, F., & Roaf, S. (2005). Post-occupancy evaluation and field studies of thermal comfort. *Building Research & Information, 33*(4), 338–346.

Oliveira, E. A. S. d., Xavier, A. A. d. P., Michaloski, A. O., Torres, F., & Pizyblskia, E. M. (2015). Subjective productivity in different states of thermal comfort. *Revista ESPACIOS, 36*(07), *Año 2015*.

Ornetzeder, M., Wicher, M., & Suschek-Berger, J. (2016). User satisfaction and well-being in energy efficient office buildings: Evidence from cutting-edge projects in Austria. *Energy and Buildings, 118*, 18–26.

Parkinson, T., Schiavon, S., de Dear, R., & Brager, G. (2021). Overcooling of offices reveals gender inequity in thermal comfort. *Scientific Reports 2021 11:1, 11*(1), 1–7.

Parsons, K. C. (2000). Environmental ergonomics: A review of principles, methods and models. *Applied Ergonomics, 31*(6), 581–594.

Pellerin, N., & Candas, V. (2003). Combined effects of temperature and noise on human discomfort. *Physiology and Behavior, 78*(1), 99–106.

Peng, Y., Feng, T., & Timmermans, H. (2019). A path analysis of outdoor comfort in urban public spaces. *Building and Environment, 148*, 459–467.

Ramírez-Vielma, R., & Nazar, G. (2019). Factores motivacionales de diseño del trabajo y su relación con desempeño laboral. *Revista Psicologia Organizações e Trabalho, 15*(4), 791–799.

Reeve, J. (2018). *Understanding motivation and emotion* (7th ed.). Wiley.

Rijal, H. B., Humphreys, M. A., & Nicol, J. F. (2017). Towards an adaptive model for thermal comfort in Japanese offices. *Building Research & Information, 45*(7), 717–729.

Rock, B. A. (2018). Thermal zoning For HVAC design. *ASHRAE Journal.* www.ashrae.org.

Roelofsen, P. (2002). The impact of office environments on employee performance: The design of the workplace as a strategy for productivity enhancement. *Journal of Facilities Management, 1*(3), 247–264.

Romero Herrera, N., Doolaard, J., Guerra-Santin, O., Jaskiewicz, T., & Keyson, D. (2020). Office occupants as active actors in assessing and informing comfort: A context-embedded comfort assessment in indoor environmental quality investigations. *Advances in Building Energy Research*, *14*(1), 41–65.

Rupp, R. F., Vasquez, N. G., & Lamberts, R. (2015). A review of human thermal comfort in the built environment. *Energy and Buildings*, *105*, 178–205.

Sawka, M. N., Castellani, J. W., Pandolf, K. B., & Young, A. J. (2002). *Human adaptations to heat and cold stress*. Defense Technical Information Center.

Schlader, Z. J., Prange, H. D., Mickleborough, T. D., & Stager, J. M. (2009). Characteristics of the control of human thermoregulatory behavior. *Physiology and Behavior*, *98*(5), 557–562.

Schulte, P., Guerin, R., Schill, A., Bhattacharya, A., Cunningham, T., Pandalai, S., Eggerth, D., & Stephenson, C. (2015). Considerations for incorporating "well-being" in public policy for workers and workplaces. *American Journal of Public Health*, *105*(8), 31–44.

Schweiker, M., & Wagner, A. (2016). The effect of occupancy on perceived control, neutral temperature, and behavioral patterns. *Energy and Buildings*, *117*, 246–259.

Seppänen, O., Fisk, W., & Lei, Q. (2006). Effect of temperature on task performance in office environment. *Lawrence Berkeley National Laboratory*, 11.

Sonnentag, S. (2018). The recovery paradox: Portraying the complex interplay between job stressors, lack of recovery, and poor well-being. In *Research in Organizational Behavior* (Vol. 38, pp. 169–185). JAI Press.

Soto-Muñoz, J., Trebilcock-Kelly, M., Flores-Alés, V., & Caamaño-Carrillo, C. (2022a). Recognizing the effect of the thermal environment on self-perceived productivity in offices: A structural equation modeling perspective. *Building and Environment*, *210*(108696).

Soto Muñoz, J., Trebilcock Kelly, M., Flores-Alés, V., & Ramírez-Vielma, R. (2022b). Understanding the perceived productivity of office occupants in relation to workspace thermal environment. *Building Research & Information*, *50*(1–2), 152–170.

Šujanová, P., Rychtáriková, M., Sotto Mayor, T., & Hyder, A. (2019). A healthy, energy-efficient and comfortable indoor environment: A review. *Energies*, *12*(8), 1414.

Tanabe, S. I., Nishihara, N., & Haneda, M. (2007). Indoor temperature, productivity, and fatigue in office tasks. *HVAC and R Research*, *13*(4), 623–633.

Thomas, L. E. (2017). Combating overheating: mixed-mode conditioning for workplace comfort. *Building Research & Information*, *45*(1–2), 176–194.

Tiller, D., Wang, L., Musser, A., & Radik, M. (2010). AB-10-017: Combined effects of noise and temperature on human comfort and performance (1128-RP). *Architectural Engineering –Faculty Publications*. https://digitalcommons.unl.edu/archengfacpub/40

Trebilcock, M., Soto-Muñoz, J., & Piggot-Navarrete, J. (2020). Evaluation of thermal comfort standards in office buildings of Chile: Thermal sensation and preference assessment. *Building and Environment*, *183*, 107158.

Vischer, J. C. (2017). Building-in-use assessment: Foundation of workspace psychology. In *Building Performance Evaluation: From Delivery Process to Life Cycle Phases* (pp. 129–139). Springer International Publishing.

Vischer, J. C., & Wifi, M. (2017). The effect of workplace design on quality of life at work. In *Handbook of environmental psychology and quality of life research*. Cham: Springer.

Viswesvaran, C., & Ones, D. S. (2000). Perspectives on models of job performance. In *International Journal of Selection and Assessment, 8*(4), 216–226.

Wagner, A., Gossauer, E., Moosmann, C., Gropp, T., & Leonhart, R. (2007). Thermal comfort and workplace occupant satisfaction: Results of field studies in German low energy office buildings. *Energy and Buildings, 39*(7), 758–769.

Wang, D., Zhang, H., Arens, E., & Huizenga, C. (2007). Observations of upper-extremity skin temperature and corresponding overall-body thermal sensations and comfort. *Building and Environment, 42*(12), 3933–3943.

Wargorcki, P., & Seppänen, O. (2006). *REVHA Guidebook N°6. Indoor environment and productivity in office environment. How to integrate productivity in life-cycle cost analysis of building services.*

Wu, Y., Liu, H., Chen, B., Li, B., Kosonen, R., Jokisalo, J., & Chen, T. (2020). Effect of long-term thermal history on physiological acclimatization and prediction of thermal sensation in typical winter conditions. *Building and Environment, 179,* 106936.

Wyon, D. P., & Wargocki, P. (2006). Room temperature effects on office work. In *Creating the productive workplace* (Taylor & Francis, pp. 181–192).

Yan, D., & Hong, T. (2018). *Definition and simulation of occupant behavior in buildings annex 66 final report operating agents of annex 66.* www.iea-ebc.org

Yan, D., Hong, T., Dong, B., Mahdavi, A., D'Oca, S., Gaetani, I., & Feng, X. (2017). IEA EBC annex 66: Definition and simulation of occupant behavior in buildings. *Energy and Buildings, 156,* 258–270.

Zhang, F., de Dear, R., & Hancock, P. (2019). Effects of moderate thermal environments on cognitive performance: A multidisciplinary review. *Applied Energy, 236,* 760–777.

Zhang, H., Arens, E., Fard, S. A., Huizenga, C., Paliaga, G., Brager, G., & Zagreus, L. (2007). Air movement preferences observed in office buildings. *International Journal of Biometeorology, 51*(5), 349–360.

3   Use of portable air purifiers, occupant behaviour, and indoor air quality in homes in three European cities

Elizabeth Cooper, Yan Wang, Samuel Stamp, and Dejan Mumovic

Introduction

Levels of outdoor air pollution, cultural and behavioural patterns, and perhaps even perceptions of wellbeing vary widely across Europe. However, home, for most people, is a place of comfort and safety, and people spend up to 65% of their time there (Klepeis, 2001). Therefore, it is important to understand place-specific differences in the quality of the air in homes, people's responses to it and how best to mitigate it when it is poor.

Substantial research has been published on the effectiveness of air purifiers in reducing indoor $PM_{2.5}$, in laboratory settings and through computer modelling, as well as limited short-term monitoring in homes (Allen, 2011; Barn et al., 2018; Zhan et al., 2018). However, little evidence is available that explains the actual use of the equipment by occupants, or what the motivations are for HAP use. This work aimed to explore the impact of commercially available home air purifiers (HAPs) used in bedrooms on indoor $PM_{2.5}$ concentration and perceived indoor air quality (IAQ). As well as, to better understand how and why portable air purifiers are used by occupants in three European cities (Eindhoven, NL; Helsinki, FL; and London, UK).

Building standards have changed to meet requirements for energy efficiency and carbon reduction which has lowered infiltration rates, making intentional ventilation paramount to the dilution of indoor generated pollutants to provide acceptable IAQ (Shrubsole, 2014). According to a review article by Dimitroulopoulou (2012), ventilation rates in Europe often fall below 0.5 h^{-1} (a common regulatory standard) which can lead to an accumulation of indoor generated air pollutants, and consequently increased pollutant exposure risks. Although there are several ways to achieve the required air change rate, including continuous mechanical extract, or supply and extract with heat recovery, residences in many places have relied primarily, or entirely, upon natural ventilation (i.e., windows and doors) and uncontrolled ventilation has been common.

In the UK, background ventilators (e.g., trickle-ventilators) remain a common approach but, as with other types of natural ventilation, they do not

DOI: 10.1201/9781003344711-4

have filtration capacity, and leave the IAQ heavily dependent upon the quality of the outdoor air. In addition to the reliance upon good outdoor air quality, for events of high indoor pollutant generation (e.g., cooking), ventilation through natural ventilation alone may be inadequate. The results of a Building Research Establishment (BRE) study found that 68% of homes had a whole house ventilation rate below the minimum design value of 0.5 h^{-1} in the winter, and in summer 30% of homes failed to reach this standard (Dimitroulopoulou et al., 2005). As more than two-thirds of the homes in the work presented here (and all of those located in London and Helsinki) were apartments, it is notable that, in the same BRE study (ibid), flats performed even more poorly than other types of homes monitored.

In cold climates, such as Finland, airtightness of buildings is critical in maintaining thermal comfort efficiently, and as a consequence mechanical ventilation is essential in providing acceptable IAQ in the heating season. However, occupant behaviour, such as opening windows and doors, cooking, burning candles, etc., will influence the ultimate indoor to outdoor ratio. Flats monitored in this study were equipped with mechanical ventilation with heat recovery (MVHR), and although their performance was not measured in the work presented here, previous studies in Finnish homes found that the recommended ventilation rate (>0.5 h^{-1}) was achieved by only 57% of newly constructed dwellings with MVHR (Kurnitski et al., 2007).

By decree the required ventilation rate in Dutch homes is 300 m^3/h, and studies have reported that this is often achieved (van der Wal, 1991). However, low-energy homes, monitored in another study, which primarily used mechanical ventilation had lower ventilation rates than those required by the Dutch Building Code (Balvers et al., 2012).

This research focusses on PM$_{2.5}$ indoors for two main reasons. First, it is widely recognised in the literature as having a negative impact on health outcomes. Secondly, air purifiers such as the type used in this study are designed to filter particles in this size range and have a limited impact on gaseous pollutants. Therefore, other indoor air pollutants, such as nitrogen dioxide (NO$_2$) and volatile organic compounds (VOCs), are not included in the scope of this work.

IAQ and health

Particulate matter of less than 2.5 μm in diameter (PM$_{2.5}$) is known to have negative health effects (Pope et al., 2020), and more than 4 million deaths globally are estimated to be associated with indoor exposure (WHO, 2019). Exposure to PM$_{2.5}$ may be especially high at home because (1) it is where people spend most of their time, (2) there are many indoor sources (e.g., cooking, smoking, cleaning) in addition to the contribution from outdoors, and (3) people have not been found to perceive PM$_{2.5}$ and therefore may not act to mitigate unhealthy levels. Additionally, home is different from most other indoor settings as it is where people sleep. Sleep being a time of special vulnerability because people cannot take action to remedy poor air quality. It is therefore important to understand ways to improve the IAQ in homes, and the occupant behaviours that impact IAQ.

Air pollution concentrations, including particulate matter, can, in many locations, exceed health-based guidelines developed by the World Health Organisation (WHO) for both chronic and acute exposure (Logue et al., 2012; WHO, 2006). Prior studies have demonstrated the contribution of indoor air pollution to total exposure (Samet, 1993; Weisel et al., 2005), as well as the negative health impacts associated with exposure. Atmospheric particulate matter less than 2.5 μm in aerodynamic diameter has been explicitly implicated in multiple health outcomes including cardiovascular diseases (Ostro, 1989), asthma (Schwartz, 1993), bronchitis (Anderson et al., 2012), premature mortality (Crouse et al., 2012; Laden et al., 2006; Pope & Dockery, 2006) and lung cancer (Pope, 2002).

Perception of air quality

There is little evidence to indicate that people readily perceive poor air quality due to $PM_{2.5}$. The perception of air quality has been shown to be most strongly influenced by the thermal conditions and relative humidity (RH) of a space (Fang, 2004). A study by Rotko et al. (2002) found that, although people expressed annoyance with air pollution, there was poor association between annoyance and measured $PM_{2.5}$ concentrations. A study in France assessed the perception of air quality in homes and found that there was little correlation between occupants' perceived air quality and the measured parameters (including particulate matter) (Langer et al., 2017). In the Langer et al. study, occupants generally described their home more favourably than visitors, who did a better job of assessing air quality, as compared to measured pollutants such as VOCs. However, neither occupants' nor visitors' perceptions were strongly associated with $PM_{2.5}$.

Thermal stimuli affect the way that occupants experience comfort and control of their environment indoors. A review by Day et al. (2020) provides a good description of the way in which occupants interact with different components of the built environment and the drivers behind those behaviours. Thermal comfort is explored as an occupant motivation for window operations and thermostat use in the Day et al. review, and is further explored in work by Calì et al. (2016) and by Jeong et al. (2016), among others. Very little work was found that included occupant interactions with building environmental controls other than windows and thermostats. One study by Rijal et al. (2008) developing adaptive algorithms that included the operation of fans to predict thermal comfort, and noted that increased mean globe temperatures were associated with more fan use.

HAPs

Previous studies have considered the health benefits of different methods of particulate filtration (Batterman et al., 2012; Fisk, 2018; Fisk & Chan, 2017b), and the adoption of technologies to mitigate indoor air pollution is increasingly common ("Global Residential Air Purifiers Market: Growth, Trends, COVID-19 Impact and Forecasts", 2021). HAPs which utilise high-efficiency particulate air (HEPA) filtration as the primary mechanism of air cleaning are one of the most common devices currently available for in-home use. Simple installation without the requirement of a central air handling system, flexibility in location and the lack of harmful by-products give these devices advantages over other air cleaning methods.

Substantial reductions in $PM_{2.5}$ in spaces using these devices, from as much as 82.7% (Zhan et al., 2018) to as little as 29% (Barn et al., 2018), were reported in previous studies, with most studies finding reductions of around 50% (McNamara et al., 2017; Shao et al., 2017). A crossover study in Denmark reported a median reduction in $PM_{2.5}$ of 54.5% in locations using HEPA filtration (Spilak et al., 2014), and a 43% reduction in $PM_{2.5}$ was shown in an intervention study in the United States (Park et al., 2017). In a modelling study by Fisk and Chan (2017a), a number of scenarios were simulated, including using portable air purifiers in homes without forced air systems, which closely resembles many of the dwellings monitored in the work presented here. The results of models of homes with continuously operating portable air purifiers showed a reduction of 45% in $PM_{2.5}$ concentrations (Fisk & Chan, 2017a).

However, past research was, for the most part, not inclusive of typical ambient air quality conditions and healthy adults. Rather, outdoor pollution events, such as wildfires, and occupants with specific health conditions, such as lung disease, and children were the focus of the studies (Brugge et al., 2017; Maestas et al., 2019; Park et al., 2017; Spilak et al., 2014; Vyas et al., 2016; Weichenthal et al., 2013).

Use of HAPs

As with IAQ perception, there is a paucity of research available on occupant use of HAPs. Factors affecting both IAQ and the performance of HAPs, such as, building ventilation systems, building infiltration rates, personal behaviour (e.g., window/door opening, smoking, etc.) and location of the air purifier in the residence (Novoselac & Siegel, 2009; Shaughnessy & Sextro, 2006; Whitby, 1983), have been documented. However, there exists little work in the literature that describes how or why people use HAPs, or how that might affect performance.

A study in China by Pei et al. (2019) found that of 43 households provided with portable air purifiers more than 80% did not use the device at all, and the rest used them only intermittently. These patterns of use, they concluded, would be insufficient to adequately reduce indoor $PM_{2.5}$ levels. A study from the California Air Resources Board (Piazza, 2006) found very different use patterns to those in China. Although the devices in this study were not monitored, in surveys conducted by the researchers, 57% of owners of air purifiers claimed to use them continuously every day. Little evidence is available to explain the significant difference between these two studies, but the authors speculated that the motivation of participants in California for frequent air purifier use was due to the perceived health benefits of their use. It seems unlikely, however, that owners of HAPs in China would be unaware of similar potential health benefits of cleaner air. Any differences in air purifier use across countries, cultures, and climates have the potential to be important factors in the effectiveness of HAPs.

Kaviany et al. (2022) reported on the use of HAPs in an intervention study in homes of asthmatic children in the USA. This study monitored not only the utilisation of HAPs (i.e., power ON or OFF), but also the fan speed, to determine adherence to the intervention's protocol. The authors reported that participants used the purifiers 80% of the time, with adherence to the fan settings 60% of the time. However, this study used financial incentives (US $50) and weekly reminder calls to participants to encourage adherence to the prescribed air purifier regime. Higher rates of HAP use are therefore not unexpected. Interestingly, in their multivariable analysis model, winter season was found to be the main driver of HAP use. There was a 21% decrease in adherence to the high and turbo fans speeds in winter which the authors attribute to the cold draught produced by the devices (Kaviany et al., 2022).

Schweiker et al. (2020) reviewed multidomain approaches to investigate indoor environment behaviour and found that studies remain limited despite recognition by many that the stimuli that influence occupants' behaviour and perception are multifactorial and varied (e.g., thermal, visual, and IAQ). In the work presented here, physical (i.e., IAQ measurements, temperature, and RH), contextual (i.e., country and season), and personal (i.e., thermal sensation, IAQ preferences, perception of control over environment) variables were included in the analysis of HAP operating behaviour. This method yielded new insights into occupants' perceptions of their homes and behaviours that may impact air quality.

Methods

Context

The study utilised a convenience sample for both the cities and monitored households with a target of 20 households in each of three cities, Eindhoven, The Netherlands, Helsinki, Finland, and London, UK. Participants had to be adults, and no specific health status (e.g., healthy, asthma, etc.) was required. Children or pets in the home were both allowed, as was smoking or wood-burning stoves. Demographic information for all participants can be found in Table 3.1. After some exclusions and drop-out of participants there were 18 households in London, 19 households in Eindhoven, and 20 households

Table 3.1 Demographics of participating households in each city

	Helsinki				London				Eindhoven				Overall			
Demographic	Value	Frequency	%		Value	Frequency	%		Value	Frequency	%		Value	Frequency	%	
Gender (of lead participant)	Male	6	30.0		Male	10	55.6		Male	13	68.4		Male	29	50.9	
	Female	14	70.0		Female	8	44.4		Female	6	31.6		Female	28	49.1	
Age (of lead participant)	Under 30	3	15.0		Under 30	3	16.7		Under 30	0	0.0		Under 30	6	10.5	
	Over 30	17	85.0		Over 30	15	83.3		Over 30	19	100.0		Over 30	51	89.5	
Years at residence	<1 years	18	90.0		<1 years	0	0.0		<1 years	0	0.0		<1 years	18	31.6	
	>1 years	2	10.0		>1 years	18	100.0		>1 years	19	100.0		>1 years	39	68.4	
Household size	1	3	15.0		1	4	22.2		1	3	15.8		1	10	17.5	
	2 to 4	15	75.0		2 to 4	8	44.4		2 to 4	16	84.2		2 to 4	39	68.4	
	>4	2	10.0		>4	6	33.3		>4	0	0.0		>4	8	14.0	
<18 y.o. in household	0	8	40.0		0	10	55.6		0	15	78.9		0	33	57.9	
	1 to 2	10	50.0		1 to 2	3	16.7		1 to 2	4	21.1		1 to 2	17	29.8	
	>2	2	10.0		>2	5	27.8		>2	0	0.0		>2	7	12.3	
Smoking status	Yes	2	10.0		Yes	6	33.3		Yes	5	26.3		Yes	13	22.8	
	No	18	90.0		No	12	66.7		No	14	73.7		No	44	77.2	
Cooking (per week)	1	0	0.0		1	0	0.0		1	2	10.5		1	2	3.5	

(*Continued*)

Table 3.1 (Continued)

Helsinki				London				Eindhoven				Overall			
Demographic	Value	Frequency	%	Demographic	Value	Frequency	%	Demographic	Value	Frequency	%	Demographic	Value	Frequency	%
	2 to 5	1	5.0		2 to 5	6	33.3		2 to 5	2	10.5		2 to 5	9	15.8
	>5	19	95.0		>5	12	66.7		>5	15	78.9		>5	46	80.7
Cleaning (per week)	not reported			Cleaning (per week)	1	4	22.2	Cleaning (per week)	1	6	31.6	Cleaning (per week)	1	10	17.5
					2 to 5	9	50.0		2 to 5	11	57.9		2 to 5	20	35.1
					>5	5	27.8		>5	2	10.5		>5	7	12.3
Air freshener use (per week)	never	16	80.0	Air freshener use (per week)	never	2	11.1	Air freshener use (per week)	never	13	68.4	Air freshener use (per week)	never	31	54.4
	1	3	15.0		1	6	33.3		1	1	5.3		1	10	17.5
	2 to 5	0	0.0		2 to 5	1	5.6		2 to 5	3	15.8		2 to 5	4	7.0
	>5	1	5.0		>5	9	50.0		>5	2	10.5		>5	12	21.1
Candle use (per week)	never	9	45.0	Candle use (per week)	never	4	22.2	Candle use (per week)	never	8	42.1	Candle use (per week)	never	21	36.8
	1	10	50.0		1	11	61.1		1	6	31.6		1	27	47.4
	2 to 5	1	5.0		2 to 5	1	5.6		2 to 5	3	15.8		2 to 5	5	8.8
	>5	0	0.0		>5	2	11.1		>5	2	10.5		>5	4	7.0
Pets in home	Yes	9	45.0	Pets in home	Yes	0	0	Pets in home	Yes	11	57.9	Pets in home	Yes	20	35.1
	No	11	55.0		No	18	100		No	8	42.1		No	37	64.9
Wood/pellet stove	Yes	0	0	Wood/pellet stove	Yes	0	0	Wood/pellet stove	Yes	6	31.6	Wood/pellet stove	Yes	6	10.5
	No	20	100		No	18	100		No	13	68.4		No	51	89.5

in Helsinki (a total of 57 dwellings). Both Eindhoven and London are located in the Cfb Köppen Climate Classification subtypes (marine west coast climate) with winter temperatures between 2 °C and 6 °C, and summer temperatures between 17 °C and 20 °C. Helsinki is located in the Dfb subtype (warm-summer, humid continental climate) with a coldest month average temperature of −3 °C, and the warmest month average of approximately 17 °C. Heating Degree Days (HDD) at 15.5 °C are 1,973, 1,724, and 3,504 for Eindhoven, Helsinki, and London, respectively.

Eindhoven dwellings included in the work were the most varied in size, type, location, and construction. Participants were selected from throughout the city, and housing types included ten townhouse/terraced houses, three apartments/flats, three semi-detached, and two detached houses. The smallest home was a flat of approximately 90 m^2 and the largest were detached houses of about 270 m^2. Seven were classified as being located in a "town with or without a small garden", four were described as "city centre, densely packed housing", and the other were reported as "suburban with larger garden". Nine of the homes utilised mechanical ventilation while the other ten relied upon natural ventilation alone. Bedrooms ranged in volume from approximately 23–60 m^3. None of the homes provided social or subsidised housing.

In Helsinki, the monitored site was in Jätkäsaari, a new urban district next to the city centre by the sea. All 20 residences were flats located in a recently constructed high-rise apartment building in the southeast part of the city, described as "city centre, densely packed housing". Light vehicular traffic, building construction, and harbour traffic were noted in the immediate area. Flats used MVHR, as well as window openings, for ventilation, and bedrooms were typically 30–40 m^3 in volume. As in Eindhoven, none of the housing was subsidised.

In the UK, the 18 residences were located within three high-rise apartment buildings at two sites (Sites A and B) in east London. Site A in London included 11 units, all of which had some level of social housing subsidy. Both buildings were constructed within the last 15 years and relied primarily upon natural ventilation in the non-heating season. At Site B, trickle-ventilators provided ventilation in the heating months. Site A used MVHR during the heating season with a by-pass mode for use in non-heating times. However, most residents reported that the MVHR was turned off during the warmer months. The MVHR units were decentralised, one unit per flat, with fan efficiencies between 75% and 77%, and heat exchanger performance compliance of 92–93%. Filtration provided in the MVHR was minimal (ISO Coarse 45%), and filter changing and maintenance was intermittent, at best. None of the flats had any air conditioning systems. Previous work at Site A included a pressure test which found an air permeability of 2–3 m^3/(h.m^2) at 50 Pa. Given the age and characteristics of the other building, the infiltration rate is estimated to also be less than 5 m^3/(h.m^2) at 50 Pa. Bedrooms in which the HAPs were located, ranged in size from approximately 28–34 m^3, and typically had one operable window approximately 1.6 m^2.

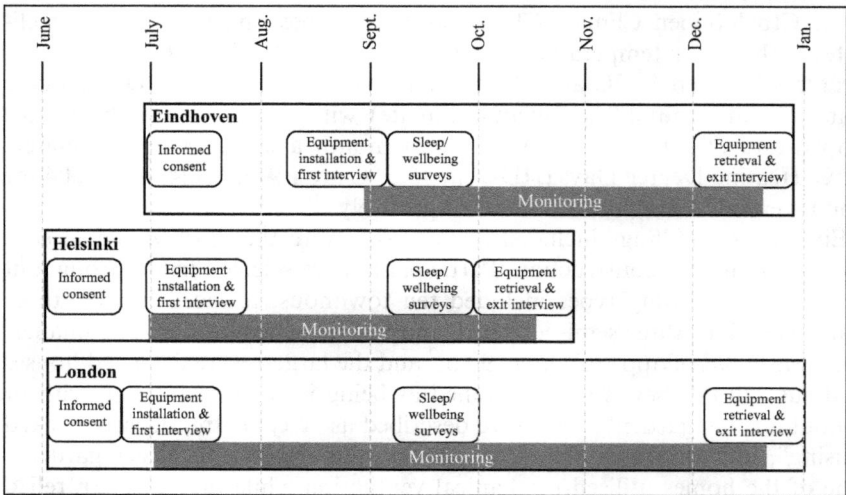

Figure 3.1 Diagram of study dates and timeline at each city.

The HAPs used in this study had a pre-filter, an activated carbon filter, and a HEPA filter with a clean air delivery rate (CADR) of 500 m^3/hour with a 0.3-μm particle removal efficiency of 99.97%, for room sizes up to 130 m^2. Each HAP had a built-in sensor for measuring $PM_{2.5}$ (μg/m^3) and sent information via the cloud to the manufacturer regarding ON/OFF status, operation mode (e.g., fan speed), and $PM_{2.5}$ levels. Surveys were conducted of the households to gather information about occupancy, physical character-istics of the dwelling (e.g., area, carpeted, etc.), and occupancy patterns and behaviours.

Flats in Eindhoven and London were monitored for six months, from July until the end of December, to measure conditions across three seasons, and Helsinki was monitored from July through October. Informed consent was obtained from all individual participants included in the study. A diagram of the study timeline is shown in Figure 3.1.

Air quality monitoring

Air quality data in Eindhoven was collected using bespoke sensors developed by IMEC. The sensor box consisted of commercially available environmental (temperature, RH) and air quality ($PM_{2.5}$, PM_{10}, and NO_2) sensors on custom developed sensor boards and the OCTA prototype platform. The particulate matter sensor (Alphasense OPC-N3) was an optical particle counter (OPC) with a fan-based sampling flow rate of 1.2 L/min, it optically (658-nm laser scattering) quantified particles within the 0.38–17 μm particle size range, defined in 16 different size bins (Mie scattering theory). From these particle counts, particle mass concentrations of PM_1, $PM_{2.5}$, and PM_{10} were calculated from the particle size spectra and concentration data, assuming a particle density of 1.65 g/ml and refractive index (RI) of 1.5. An electrochemical sensor for NO_2 (Alphasense NO2-A43F) was included as well. The Alphasense NO_2 sensors were capable of detecting NO_2 concentrations at ppb (outdoor) level. A Farnell SHT31 environmental sensor measured ambient temperature (°C) and RH (%). According to the technical specifications, this sensor exhibits a typical accuracy tolerance of 2% for RH and 0.2 °C for air temperature. The raw sensor data were collected at a 1/7 Hz temporal resolution and BLE-transmitted to an ethernet connected gateway (raspberry pi) at a 1/30 Hz resolution and subsequently averaged to five-minute readings. Sensor measurements were corrected for temperature (°C) and RH (%) and subsequently calibrated online against the regulatory reference monitoring stations of the Dutch National Institute for Public Health and the Environment (RIVM).

In Helsinki, the air quality sensors were the AQBurk, a self-contained, compact setup monitoring box. These monitors collected data on temperature, RH, PM_{10}, and $PM_{2.5}$. Boxes incorporated two sensor units, one unit for particles (Nova Fitness SDS011) and one for temperature (°C) and RH (%) (Bosch BME280). The AQBurk were installed inside and outside one bedroom of each monitored flat. The AQBurk connected to existing WiFi networks and sent data via MQTT to a server in one-second intervals. Data were held in an Influx database and five minutes averages were delivered to an Azure installation. The apparatus had previously been deployed in several unpublished air quality studies. Compensation parameters for the sensors were computed on the basis of data collected during a calibration session at Helsinki Region Environmental Services Authority measurement site at Mäkelänkatu in Helsinki.

Indoor and outdoor air quality sensors in London were Eltek TU1082 – AQ110/112. This device is equipped with Alphasense PM (OPC-N2) and gas (NO2-A43F) sensors (similar to the units used in Eindhoven). Overall, 18 living rooms, 17 bedrooms, and 60 opening areas (18 doors and 42 windows) were monitored by sensors which worked in a clustered sensor network. After testing the onsite transmission signal strength, all 18 flats were allocated to 11 Eltek Squirrel SRV250 data loggers. This architecture enabled real-time data collection from each flat to be sent and stored to an online server every five minutes using available 3G networks. Due to the availability of a constantly updated database, a core part of data quality assurance work was automated to check for power-off, signal loss, or other issues. Problems were quickly identified, and the appropriate action was taken to minimise data loss to the greatest extent. The Eltek IAQ transmitters, AQ110/112, were placed at a height of 1.5–1.7 m above the finished floor in the living room of each flat to avoid disruptions in occupants' use of their homes. Eltek GD47B sensors were located at the same height in the bedroom where the HAP was used to measure air temperature, RH, and CO_2. An AQ110/112 sensor was deployed outside of each building to measure the real-time outdoor environmental pollutant level. The buildings were all located in relatively dense urban mixed-use areas adjacent to high traffic roads. Full specifications for all the sensors used in the study are available in previous work (Cooper et al., 2021).

Crossover study design

The cross-over structure of the study was developed to answer research questions regarding the performance of the HAP with respect to $PM_{2.5}$ indoors, its relationship to outdoor concentrations, and to people's perceptions of air quality in their homes. The World Health Organisation Air Quality Guidelines (2008) were used as a reference for both outdoor and indoor air in this study. This recommendation is for a short-term exposure limit of 25 $\mu g/m^3$ 24-hour mean, and long-term limit of 10 $\mu g/m^3$ annual mean (WHO, 2006). The HAP turned on to fan speeds 1, 2, 3, or turbo (HAP ON) was compared with respect to using no purification device (HAP OFF) as well as using the HAP always ON but on the lowest fan speed setting (HAP BACKGROUND).

Pollutant levels, and operational status of the HAP, were collected and recorded every five minutes. In addition to the data on use collected from the devices themselves, use was evaluated through interviews when installing (baseline) and when collecting the HAPs at the end of the study (final). The cohorts in each city were divided into four roughly equal tracks, three with alternating configurations of HAP use: always off, always on at the lowest fan speed, or freely operated. Each phase of the crossover period lasted a minimum of three weeks. For one week of each phase, participants were sent short surveys each day that asked them about the quality of their sleep and wellbeing during the previous day.

Semi-structured interviews

Semi-structured interviews were conducted at the first site visit to establish a baseline of the occupants' overall satisfaction with the dwelling, their general health and wellbeing, and sleep quality. A part of the Building Users' Survey (BUS) Methodology (Arup, 2020) was used to determine the occupants' opinions on various aspects of their home, including air quality, thermal comfort, and control of the environment (Cohen et al., 2001). The Short Form health survey (SF-12) was employed to assess the self-reported mental and physical health of the participants (Jenkinson et al., 1997). Additionally, participants were asked about their sleep quality using the Pittsburgh Sleep Quality Index (PSQI) (Buysse et al., 1989). At the first interview, the monitoring equipment was installed and participants were introduced to the use of the air purifier. After the nine-week crossover period, another semi-structured interview was performed in an effort to determine if there were any changes to participants' sleep and wellbeing, as well as to understand how the air purifiers were perceived and utilised. Some of the households in London and Eindhoven agreed to continue with monitoring after the cross-over study period to the end of the calendar year. This extension allowed the capture of data during the heating season. Due to agreements with study participants in Helsinki, data were collected only until mid-October.

Statistical analysis

Summary statistics (means, medians, ranges) were generated for $PM_{2.5}$, indoor and outdoor temperature and RH using the open source statistical software R (R Core Team, 2018). The tests of statistical significance and correlations that were used in the analysis are specified in the results. BUS survey results were analysed through the Usable Buildings Trust, information about which can be found at the BUS Methodology website (Arup, 2020).

A logistic regression model was used to explore correlations between environmental parameters and HAP use. This type of model has been used to describe occupant behaviour related to window operations, and is one approach to discerning operational behaviour of binary actions (ON/OFF) in relation to another variable (Andersen et al., 2013). In this model, outdoor temperature was used as an explanatory variable to simulate whether the HAP was ON or not. The coefficients for this model are represented by the following expressions, and are significant to the level of 0.05:

Eindhoven: Logit (probability of HAP ON) = $\log(p/(1-p)) = -4.93 + 0.14 *$ Outdoor Temperature

Helsinki: Logit (probability of HAP ON) = $\log(p/(1-p)) = -0.21 + 0.063 *$ Outdoor Temperature

London: Logit (probability of HAP ON) = $\log(p/(1-p)) = -2.83 + 0.082 *$ Outdoor Temperature

Results

IAQ

Homes monitored during the study period had good air quality when compared against WHO guidelines. Indeed, there were few times or days during the study period where indoor or outdoor air exceeded the limits (10 and 25 $\mu g/m^3$). It is worth noting, however, no safe exposure limits have been established for $PM_{2.5}$ (WHO, 2013), and as almost two-thirds of our time is spent at home, even small reductions in concentrations are expected to be impactful.

The typical daily patterns of $PM_{2.5}$ concentrations indoors and outdoors illustrate the daily dynamics between indoor and outdoor sources, as well as when the internal generation of pollutants may occur. Figure 3.2 shows average hourly values across a day, aggregated for all days and all homes for

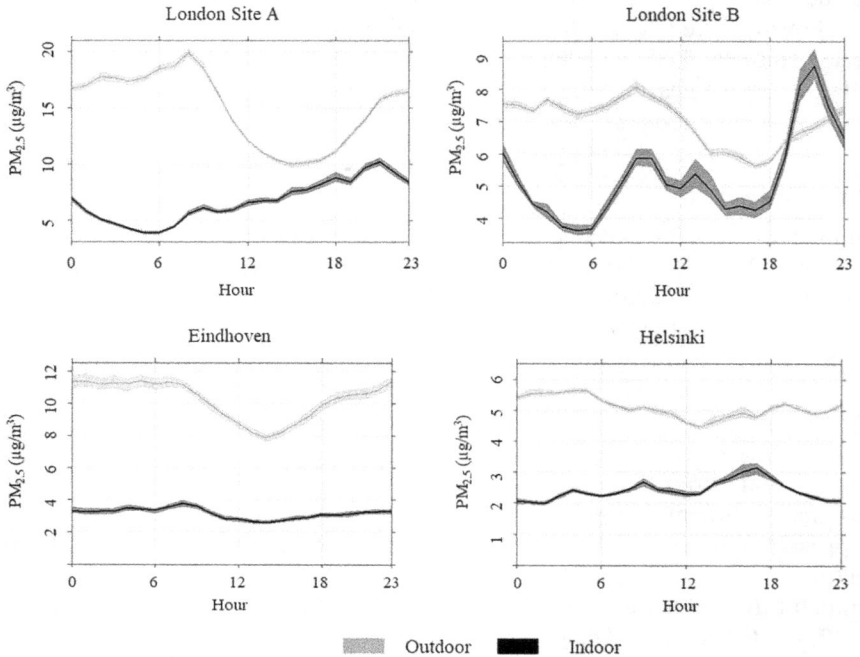

Figure 3.2 Typical daily patterns of outdoor and indoor PM$_{2.5}$ at all sites in three cities.

the three cities (four sites). In London, particulate matter levels outside at both sites show a peak around 8 am, most likely associated with road traffic, before dropping in the afternoon. Indoor levels at London site B show a morning peak correlated with outdoor levels, and a large evening peak attributable to cooking activities. London Site A concentrations are relatively flat throughout the day with a small increase in the evening. PM$_{2.5}$ concentrations outdoors in Eindhoven have relatively equivalent levels in the morning and evenings, with a drop midday, once again most likely reflecting traffic conditions. Indoor levels in Eindhoven remain very constant throughout the day. In Helsinki, outdoor levels are relatively flat across the day, illustrating that the building is located in a low-traffic area. Indoor levels in Helsinki show a small rise in the evenings, most likely coinciding with the preparation of evening meals. Although the average IAQ is consistently better than what is experienced outside, short-lived peak events occasionally far exceed outdoor concentrations.

When measurements from participants' bedrooms are combined, clear decay curves can be seen from the onset of HAP use to 100 minutes run time (Figure 3.3). The decay curves represent the aggregated performance of the HAP; however, it is important to note that not all run cycles resulted in the

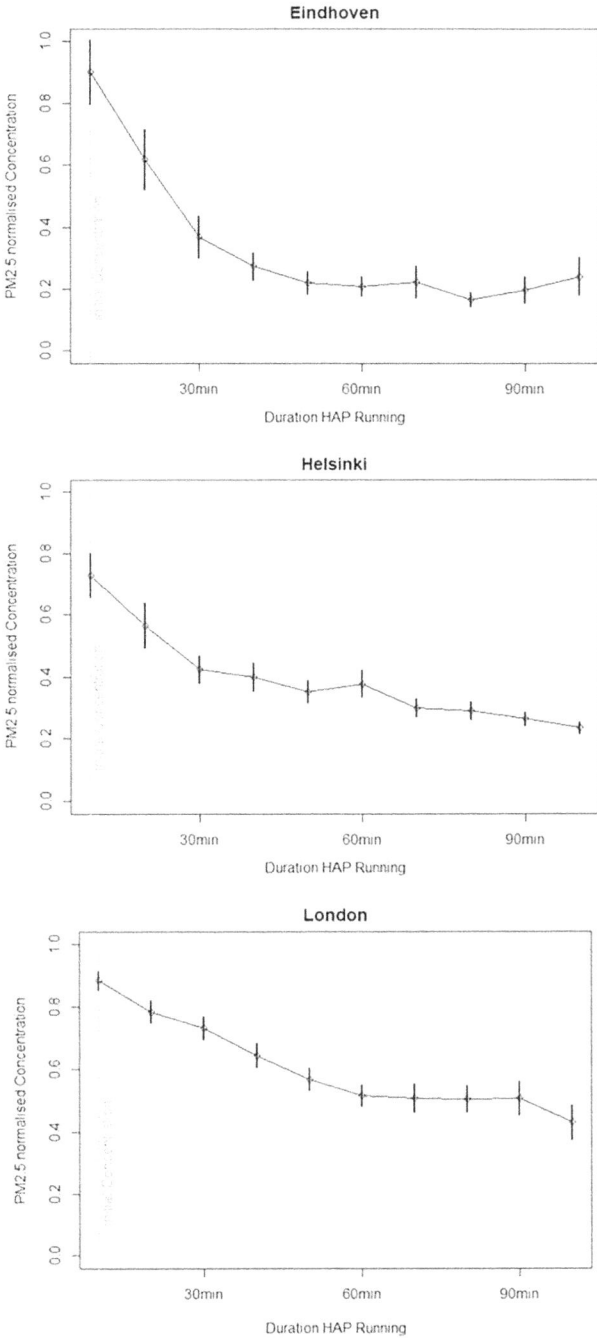

Figure 3.3 Change in the mean concentration of $PM_{2.5}$ in bedrooms using home air purifiers. Start measurements at time 0, with minutes of run time shown. Top: Eindhoven. Middle: Helsinki. Bottom: London.

Table 3.2 Air purifier flow rate and clean air delivery rate (CADR) by mode

Mode	Flow (m³/hour)	CADR (m³/hour)
Sleep	117.6	115
Mode 1	210.8	207
Mode 2	308.7	303
Mode 3	416.8	408
Turbo	509.8	500

same reduction pattern, particularly in the presence of continued internal sources, re-suspension, etc. In Eindhoven after 90 minutes of operation, $PM_{2.5}$ concentrations were reduced by a mean of 69%. In Helsinki after 90 minutes of operation, $PM_{2.5}$ concentrations were reduced by a mean of 68%. In London after 90 minutes of operation, $PM_{2.5}$ concentrations were reduced by a mean of 45%. Differences between sites may be attributable to differing use in regard to fan speed, different window operations and ventilation, and differing indoor source generation.

Normalised concentrations were used for the decay curves because data from the internal HAP sensors were used in this analysis. This was to avoid conflicts or differences between the different types of external sensors deployed in each city. The HAP sensors could not be fully calibrated however, calibrated sensors collocated with the HAPs were in strong agreement with the levels measured by the air purifiers ($R^2 = 0.9$, RMSE = 4.5 µg/m³, MBE = −0.16 µg/m³). Technical specifications that include CADR by fan speed are shown in Table 3.2. Hourly patterns indicated that the concentration of particulate matter is correlated with fan speed. That is, the higher the fan speeds the lower the concentration of $PM_{2.5}$.

Indoor concentrations of $PM_{2.5}$ were typically below WHO guidelines in all cities (measured by outdoor and indoor instruments), with the homes in Helsinki exhibiting the lowest outdoor and indoor (mean: 2.3 µg/m³) $PM_{2.5}$ levels, London and Eindhoven had very similar median $PM_{2.5}$ concentrations; however, the range in Eindhoven was greater. This difference could be explained as Eindhoven included 19 different locations, and London had only two sites. The mean in London was higher (6.6 µg/m³) compared with 5.1 µg/m³ in Eindhoven (Figure 3.4).

Indoor temperatures in all three cities ranged from a high near 30 °C (in London) to a low of nearly 17 °C (Figure 3.5). RH in all locations remained within an acceptable range for occupant comfort (40–60%), and results from the BUS survey indicate that there was general satisfaction with the humidity of the homes in winter. There were no reports of problems with condensation, and no visible moisture or mould in any of the residences at the baseline or exit interviews. Correlations between temperature, or RH, and $PM_{2.5}$ were generally very weak, with Pearson's correlation factors all below +/−0.5.

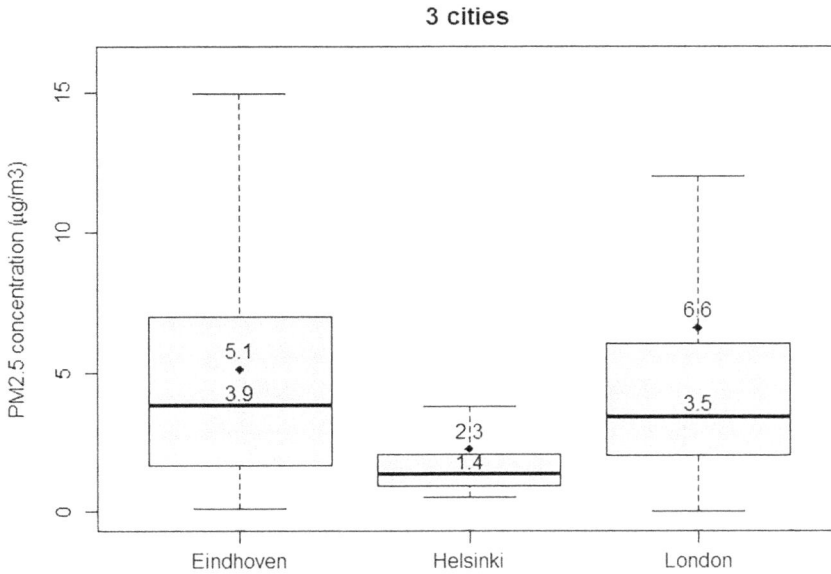

Figure 3.4 Measured indoor $PM_{2.5}$ concentration range in each of the partner cities, mean (diamonds), median (horizontal lines), and range for all three sites.

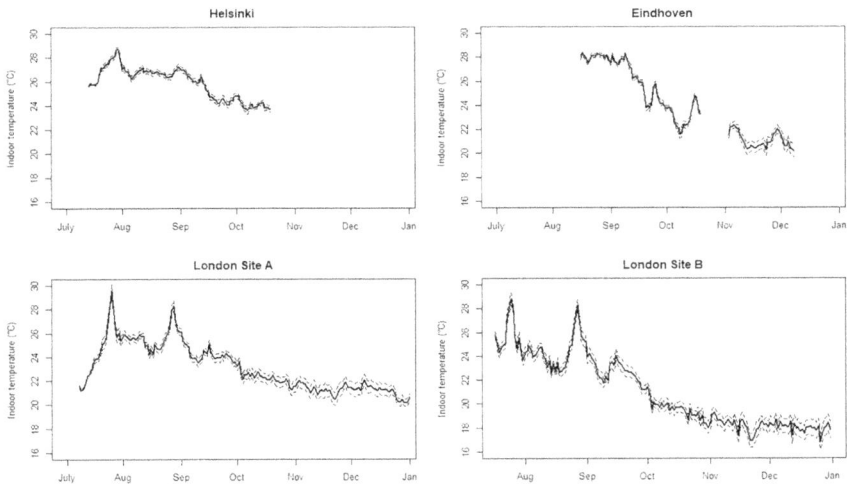

Figure 3.5 Indoor daily mean temperature is shown by the solid lines for each site. Dashed lines are 95% confidence intervals. (Missing temperature data in Eindhoven due to a server failure.)

Perceived IAQ

Sections of the BUS (Arup, 2020) were used to assess the satisfaction of occupants on a number of indoor environmental factors. Of the 22 factors that were scored, five were considered satisfactory in all cities: stillness of the air in winter, overall condition of the air in winter, control over lighting and noise, and the stability of the temperature in winter. Ten factors were marginal including odour of the air in summer and winter, overall condition of the air in summer, dryness of the air in winter, freshness of the air in winter, overall comfort, control over heating, stability of the temperature in summer, overall winter temperature, and the coldness of the winter temperature. Notably, seven factors were unsatisfactory including humidity of the air in summer, stuffiness of the air in summer, stillness of the air in summer, control over cooling and ventilation, temperature in summer (too hot), and the overall comfort of temperature. A list of parameters and aggregate scores is shown in Table 3.3.

Table 3.3 A summary of parameters and scores (upper and lower limits) from the Building Users' Survey (BUS)

Parameter (long name)	Eindhoven study mean score	Helsinki study mean score	London study mean score	Benchmark score (limits)
Air in summer: dry/humid	3.6	3.7	4.4	3.5 (3.3–3.7)
Air in summer: fresh/stuffy	4.5	4.1	4.9	3.5 (3.2–3.7)
Air in summer: odourless/ smelly	2.5	2.9	3.4	2.6 (2.9–3.4)
Air in summer: overall	4.2	4	3.9	5.4 (5.1–5.6)
Air in summer: still/draughty	2.3	2.7	2.4	2.8 (2.5–3.1)
Air in winter: overall	6.1	4.6	5.6	5.5 (5.3–5.7)
Air in winter: dry/humid	3.3	2.4	3.3	3.3 (3.1–3.5)
Air in winter: fresh/stuffy	2.4	4.5	3.8	3.3 (3.1–3.6)
Air in winter: odourless/smelly	2.1	3.1	2.5	2.8 (2.5–3.0)
Air in winter: still/draughty	3.3	3.3	2.9	3.1 (2.7–3.4)
Comfort: overall	5.6	4.7	4.9	5.9 (5.7–6.0)
Control: over cooling	4.2	3	3.2	4.4 (4.0–4.7)
Control: over heating	6.1	3.2	6.5	5.2 (4.9–5.6)
Control: over lighting	6.7	5.4	6.2	5.7 (5.4–6.0)
Control: over noise	4.2	4.8	3.2	3.9 (3.6–4.2)
Control: over ventilation	4.9	2.9	4.5	5.1 (4.8–5.4)

(Continued)

Table 3.3 (Continued)

Parameter (long name)	Eindhoven study mean score	Helsinki study mean score	London study mean score	Benchmark score (limits)
Temp in summer: hot/cold	2.9	2.5	2.4	3.3 (3.2–3.5)
Temp in summer: overall	4.2	4	3.1	4.9 (4.6–5.1)
Temp in summer: stable/ variable	2.9	4	3.8	4.2 (3.9–4.4)
Temp in winter: hot/cold	4.6	3.9	4.6	4.3 (4.1–4.4)
Temp in winter: overall	5.1	5	5.7	5.5 (5.3–5.8)
Temp in winter: stable/ variable	2.6	2.7	3.4	3.8 (3.6–4.1)

Generally, occupants rated the IAQ poor in the summer with a very high rate of dissatisfaction with the temperature, stuffiness and stillness of the air, as well as control over the cooling and ventilation.

HAP operation behaviour

Given that residents across all sites expressed some dissatisfaction with the temperatures in their homes in summer, and that many felt that there was inadequate control over cooling and ventilation, and that the HAPs' internal fans generate a "cooling" effect, the pattern of use displayed in Figure 3.6 is perhaps not surprising. A clear correlation between increasing temperatures and increasing HAP use is shown in the logistic regression model. As there was no mechanical cooling available in the homes, the correlation between the outdoor and indoor temperatures was strong, suggesting that it is actually indoor temperature that influences HAP use.

It is clear that the probability that the HAP was operating was greater with increasing outdoor temperatures, although the degree of use differed across the sites irrespective of temperature. For example, the predicted probability that the HAP was ON in London was approximately 0.42 when it was 30 °C outside, while in Eindhoven at the same temperature the predicted probability was only about 0.35, but in Helsinki at 30 °C the probability that the HAP was ON was nearly 0.82. The model provides good statistical evidence for the anecdotal finding that participants' HAP use is driven by the perceived cooling effects of the devices. However, it does not provide insights into why the use, or temperature thresholds for use, differs between cities.

From interviews, people in all three cities generally expressed more satisfaction with the overall air quality and comfort in the cooler months which could contribute to a decline in the perceived utility of an air purifier, and decreased utilisation. For participants in the group that was allowed to use

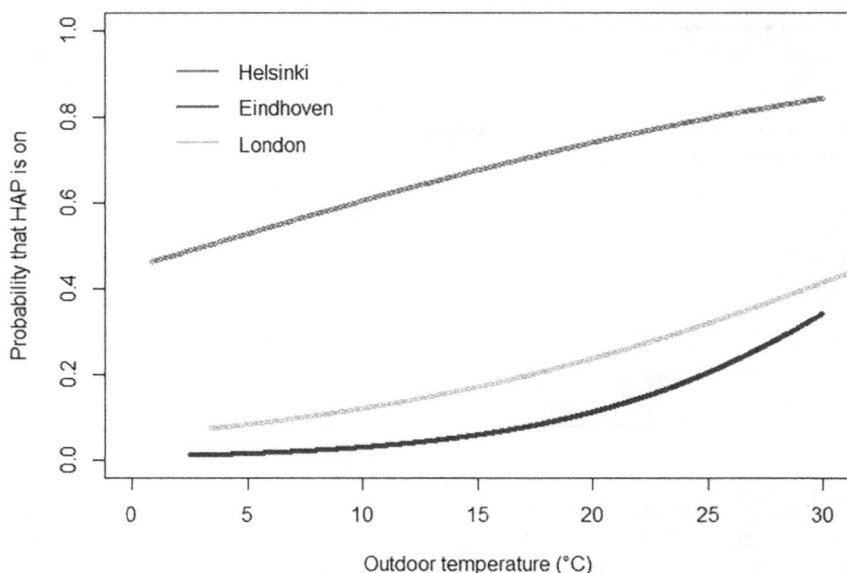

Figure 3.6 Probability of air purifier use in relation to mean outdoor temperature (p < 0.05).

the HAP in any manner they pleased during the entirety of the study period mean hours per day the HAP was ON (any speed) was 7.5, 14.1, and 10.4 for Eindhoven, Helsinki, and London, respectively. These usage means are also reflected in the logistic regression model shown in Figure 3.6.

Another possible motivation for HAP use could include the health status of occupants. Healthy adults were recruited, however having specific health conditions did not prevent people from participating. Of the participants, 33 (58%) reported having allergies, 10 (18%) reported having asthma, 12 (21%) reported frequent respiratory infections, and 3 (5%) had been diagnosed with COPD. Only 13 participants reported no symptoms of allergies, asthma, frequent respiratory infections, or COPD. However, no statistical associations between frequency of use, or duration of use, of the devices and any of the health conditions were found.

Discussion

Principal findings

The results of the work presented here demonstrate the effectiveness of HEPA air purifiers to reduce indoor $PM_{2.5}$ concentrations. Although reductions are reported for running times of 90 minutes, it is worth noting that the actual running time of air purifiers was typically much longer. This was the case especially in warmer weather, which could lead to larger reductions for longer periods of time. However, there were also many conditions and times, either due to thermal comfort or perceived air quality, in which residents did not use their HAPs at all.

The participants in this study generally reported dissatisfaction with several aspects of their indoor environment, in particular during the warmer months. The combination of the residents' opinions that the quality of the indoor environment of their homes was better in the cooler months and that the air purifiers had a cooling effect, may lead residents to use the air purifier less often, or inconsistently, in the heating months, irrespective of the actual air quality.

Many of the standards of practice for ventilation are based upon what is perceived as acceptable air quality by occupants; however, there is little evidence that people's perception correlates with actual air quality. The evidence presented here indicates it does not. Notably, although Helsinki had the lowest median daily $PM_{2.5}$ concentration (1.4 $\mu g/m^3$), they had the highest daily mean HAP use (14.1 hours), with London use at 10.4 and Eindhoven occupants using HAPs only 7.5 hours daily. The perception of IAQ is influenced by many factors including RH, noise, and most importantly, temperature. Those participants in the work presented here who reported their motivations for HAP use did not, in large measure, use the HAPs for their intended benefit of reduction in particulate matter.

In The Netherlands, the types of homes in this study varied widely; flats, semi-detached, and detached houses with mechanical and natural ventilation systems were included in the monitoring campaign. Perhaps as a consequence of this variety, the median $PM_{2.5}$ concentrations spanned a larger range, and the use of the air purifiers also varied more widely, than in the flats in Helsinki or London. Due to the heterogeneity of the Dutch cohort, as well as different monitoring setup in The Netherlands, interpreting the results of this study presents some challenges. However, given the recognised shortcomings of some ventilation strategies, the measured indoor $PM_{2.5}$ concentration and the effectiveness of the HAPs is noteworthy.

Relation to similar research

The reduction in $PM_{2.5}$ seen in the work presented here, with means of 45–69% after 90 minutes, is in line with reductions found in other studies. This study differed from many previous studies in the length of the studied period of approximately six months. Most other research on HAPs monitored for only days or weeks, no other similar work was found that monitored for more than 21 days.

There is very little published research on occupants' operation of air purifiers and the two studies that were found differed substantially in their findings. Personal health motivations were suggested by one study (Pei et al., 2019) as the reason for the substantial difference in the use patterns found in their study and those reported by Piazza et al. (2006). The findings from the work presented here do not support that supposition. No correlation between reported health conditions and HAP use was seen, despite many of the participants saying in the baseline interviews that they were concerned about the impact of air pollution on their personal health.

Limitations

Due to the agreements and coordination between the different sites and cities, the monitoring times and durations were not the same (Figure 3.1). As a result, unlike in London and Eindhoven, data in Helsinki were only collected from July until the middle of October. Therefore, information for occupant use of HAPs during the coldest time of the year is missing for Helsinki. Patterns still emerge, however, that are consistent across all three sites.

Another potential limitation of this study was the lack of a sham device. Participants were aware when the HAP was off and therefore may have believed that the air quality was poor when it was not. An additional limitation of the work presented here was that the devices used to measure the IAQ were not the same in all three cities. The difference between the sensors could lead to differences in absolute concentrations. Some of this limitation was overcome in the analysis of the $PM_{2.5}$ decay through the use of the sensors internal to the HAPs, which were all the same make and model. It should also be noted that this study used only one type of HAP from one manufacturer (Philips); however, similar results are expected from devices with equivalent specifications from other manufacturers.

A potential factor that should be considered in HAP utilisation, and may be a limitation in this study, was the cost of operating the device. Participants were provided with the HAPs for the duration of the study at no cost, but electricity to operate the device was paid for by the occupants. Although operational costs were relatively low, at approximately €2–4 per month, they were not negligible for some participants, and remain a limitation in our understanding of the motivations that could influence occupant behaviour. Additionally, the first-time cost of purchasing an air purifier may also be beyond the financial capacity of many people.

Implications and impact

CO_2 was monitored in this study in London (both living room and bedroom). The London data were presented in a previous publication (Cooper et al., 2021). Those findings showed typical patterns of CO_2 concentrations for the bedrooms of naturally ventilated buildings, that is, lower concentrations in the non-heating season and higher concentrations in the heating season, due to window operations. These findings support the conclusion that because occupants' use of HAPs is positively correlated with temperature, as is window opening, the benefits of reduced $PM_{2.5}$ from indoor sources using HAPs may be reduced, especially in the heating season. The winter period is typically associated with (1) higher outdoor air pollution levels, (2) lower natural ventilation rates (i.e., opening of windows), and (3) potential additional indoor emissions (e.g., wood stoves, candles). There is therefore a greater risk that low rates of HAP utilisation in the heating season could lead to unacceptable IAQ when ventilation rates from natural ventilation are typically very low. If users prioritise thermal comfort over IAQ, they may not respond appropriately to the actual risk of $PM_{2.5}$ exposure.

In the rooms in which they are located, commercially available HAPs utilising HEPA filtration, do a good job of reducing $PM_{2.5}$ levels in the indoor air. However, if occupants fail to use them because of a misperception of risk, or due to a misunderstanding of their utility, solutions that automate functionality are one reasonable approach to ensure the devices are working as intended and to their full capacity. Recommendations to provide internal sensors (a feature that is currently available), default ON (user must opt-out of HAP use), and integration with outdoor air quality data are also options that could allow the HAPs to function more effectively to reduce $PM_{2.5}$.

The present study collected evidence on indoor and outdoor $PM_{2.5}$ dynamics at different households in each of the partner cities. Generally, indoor $PM_{2.5}$ levels were much lower than outdoor levels. Nevertheless, indoor concentrations reflected outdoor concentrations and recurrent events of indoor $PM_{2.5}$ generation could often be observed that exceeded outdoor concentrations (e.g., cooking). The timing, size, and periodicity of these events were found to be household specific. Participants reported dissatisfaction with many of the conditions in their homes in summer, in particular high temperatures, stillness and stuffiness of air, and insufficient control over cooling. These conditions may be affected by the use of air purifiers due to the fan-driven air. However, poor air quality persists throughout the year, and may increase in the non-heating season in naturally ventilated homes due to reduced window opening. Therefore, it is important to consider other motivations of air purifier use, or other control solutions, if air purifiers are to be used for year-round removal of particulate matter.

If occupant behaviour towards the air purifiers could be better managed to reflect indoor air pollution levels rather than thermal conditions, better HAP performance (higher and more consistent $PM_{2.5}$ reductions) is achievable, ultimately aiding in the mitigation of the negative health effects of exposure while at home.

Conclusions

Unanswered questions and future work

This study included questions on sleep and wellbeing at both the baseline and exit interviews to try to better understand the impact the HAPs might have. Although there were trends that indicated reported improvement in sleep quality, they did not reach statistical significance in most cases. Questions regarding associations between sleep quality and wellbeing remain important areas of inquiry and future work should be undertaken in this area.

As with the questions of sleep and wellbeing, additional work should be done to understand any connections between HAP use and perceived improvements in health, as the evidence found in the literature remains weak. The level of reduction found in this work, and reported elsewhere, suggests that health outcomes of conditions such as asthma, lung cancer, stroke, ischemic heart disease, and chronic lung disease could be improved with consistent and long-term use of HAPs in homes. More work should be done to understand the impact of HAP use on population health and mortality.

COVID-19 has brought wider attention to issues of IAQ, and the use of HAPs has been an area of new interest for airborne infection control. Future research will likely include a greater focus on the design and operation of buildings that reduce the risk of infection, and HAPs could play a role in the mitigation of this risk. More research should be done across multiple settings (e.g., offices, schools) with different building ventilation system types. The work presented here could contribute to this work and provide insights into why or when people choose to operate HAPs. Indoor operating temperature should be considered when specifying any occupant-controlled device, especially when part of a critical infection control system.

This study had one of the longest study periods of any found in the literature; however, additional research would benefit from a longer study period (a full year), with a greater number of participants, and a range of measured pollutants (e.g., NO_2 and TVOCs). That being said, the results presented here remain important due to the demonstrated adverse health impacts of $PM_{2.5}$. This research considered homes with low outdoor and indoor $PM_{2.5}$ levels and it is not known that the reported findings on air quality perception and device use hold true for areas or homes where $PM_{2.5}$ levels are very high. Additional studies in locations with high ambient $PM_{2.5}$ concentrations, as well as different climatological conditions (e.g., in Southern Europe, North America, and South Asia), should be undertaken to better understand these relationships.

As was noted earlier in this chapter, although the HAPs in this study were lent to the participants at no cost, they were still responsible for the cost of electricity. Given that even this relatively small monthly financial outlay presented a nonnegligible burden for some, the cost of acquiring a new device along with maintenance and operation may be too much of a barrier to adoption for many people. This economic reality may be especially true for areas of the world that have the worst outdoor air conditions which impact indoor air. Therefore, although these devices may provide health benefits to those that have them, a reliance upon expensive devices to mitigate poor IAQ could exacerbate existing inequalities globally.

Acknowledgements

The authors would like to acknowledge the contributions of Forum Virium Helsinki, imec and Philips.

Support was provided by the European Institute of Technology Digital (EIT-Digital Award No. 19144).

All aspects of the work involving human participants were in accordance with, and approved by, the ethical standards of the institution (University College London) and with the 1964 Helsinki declaration and its later amendments or comparable ethical standards.*Declaration of interest statement*: The authors declare that they have no known competing financial interests or personal relationships that could have appeared to influence the work reported in this chapter.

References

Allen, R., Carlsten, C., Karlen, B., Leckie, S., van Eeden, S., Vedal, S., Wong, I., & Brauer, M. (2011). The impact of portable air pilters on indoor air pollution and cardiovascular health in awoodsmoke-impacted community in British Columbia, Canada. *Epidemiology, 22*.

Andersen, R., Fabi, V., Toftum, J., Corgnati, S. P., & Olesen, B. W. (2013). Window opening behaviour modelled from measurements in Danish dwellings. *Building and Environment, 69*, 101–113.

Anderson, J. O., Thundiyil, J. G., & Stolbach, A. (2012). Clearing the air: A review of the effects of particulate matter air pollution on human health. *Journal of Medical Toxicology, 8*(2), 166–175.

Arup. (2020). Occupant satisfaction evaluation. Retrieved from https://busmethodology.org.uk/

Balvers, J., Bogers, R., Jongeneel, R., van Kamp, I., Boerstra, A., & van Dijken, F. (2012). Mechanical ventilation in recently built Dutch homes: Technical shortcomings, possibilities for improvement, perceived indoor environment and health effects. *Architectural Science Review, 55*(1), 4–14.

Barn, P., Gombojav, E., Ochir, C., Laagan, B., Beejin, B., Naidan, G., & Allen, R. W. (2018). The effect of portable HEPA filter air cleaners on indoor PM2.5 concentrations and second hand tobacco smoke exposure among pregnant women in Ulaanbaatar, Mongolia: The UGAAR randomized controlled trial. *Science of the Total Environment, 615*, 1379–1389.

Batterman, S., Du, L., Mentz, G., Mukherjee, B., Parker, E., Godwin, C., & Lewis, T. (2012). Particulate matter concentrations in residences: An intervention study evaluating stand-alone filters and air conditioners. *Indoor Air, 22*(3), 235–252.

Brugge, D., Simon, M. C., Hudda, N., Zellmer, M., Corlin, L., Cleland, S., & Durant, J. L. (2017). Lessons from in-home air filtration intervention trials to reduce urban ultrafine particle number concentrations. *Building and Environment, 126*, 266–275.

Buysse, D., Reynolds, C., Monk, T., Berman, S., & Kupfer, D. (1989). The Pittsburgh Sleep Quality Index: A new instrument for psychiatric practice and research. *Psychiatry Research*, 193–213.

Calì, D., Andersen, R. K., Müller, D., & Olesen, B. W. (2016). Analysis of occupants' behavior related to the use of windows in German households. *Building and Environment, 103*, 54–69.

Cohen, R., Standeven, M., Bordass, B., & Leaman, A. (2001). Assessing building performance in use 1: The Probe process. *Building Research & Information, 29*(2), 85–102.

Cooper, E., Wang, Y., Stamp, S., Burman, E., & Mumovic, D. (2021). Use of portable air purifiers in homes: Operating behaviour, effect on indoor PM2.5 and perceived indoor air quality. *Building and Environment, 191*, 107621.

Crouse, D. L., Peters, P. A., van Donkelaar, A., Goldberg, M. S., Villeneuve, P. J., Brion, O., & Burnett, R. T. (2012). Risk of nonaccidental and cardiovascular mortality in relation to long-term exposure to low concentrations of fine particulate matter: A Canadian national-level cohort study. *Environmental Health Perspectives, 120*(5), 708–714.

Day, J. K., McIlvennie, C., Brackley, C., Tarantini, M., Piselli, C., Hahn, J., & Kjærgaard, M. B. (2020). A review of select human-building interfaces and their relationship to human behavior, energy use and occupant comfort. *Building and Environment, 178*, 106920.

Dimitroulopoulou, C. (2012). Ventilation in European dwellings: A review. *Building and Environment, 47*, 109–125.

Dimitroulopoulou, C., Crump, D., Coward, S., Brown, B., Squire, R., Mann, H., & Ross, D. (2005). Ventilation, air tightness and indoor air quality in new homes. *BR477, BRE Bookshop.*

Fang, L., Wyon, D., Clausen, G., & Fanger, P. (2004). Impact of indoor air temperature and humidity in an office on perceived air quality, SBS symptoms and performance. *Indoor Air, 14*, 74–81.

Fisk, W. J. (2018). How home ventilation rates affect health: A literature review. *Indoor Air, 28*(4), 473–487.

Fisk, W. J., & Chan, W. R. (2017a). Effectiveness and cost of reducing particle-related mortality with particle filtration. *Indoor Air, 27*(5), 909–920.

Fisk, W. J., & Chan, W. R. (2017b). Health benefits and costs of filtration interventions that reduce indoor exposure to PM2.5 during wildfires. *Indoor Air, 27*(1), 191–204.

Global Residential Air Purifiers Market: Growth, Trends, COVID-19 Impact and Forecasts (2021). *Business Wire*, 7 July.

Jenkinson, C., Layte, R., Jenkinson, D., Lawrence, K., Petersen, S., Paice, C., & Stradling, J. (1997). A shorter form health survey: Can the SF-12 replicate results from the SF-36 in longitudinal studies? *Journal of Public Health, 19*(2), 179–186.

Jeong, B., Jeong, J.-W., & Park, J. (2016). Occupant behavior regarding the manual control of windows in residential buildings. *Energy and Buildings, 127*, 206–216.

Kaviany, P., Brigham, E. P., Collaco, J. M., Rice, J. L., Woo, H., Wood, M., & Koehler, K. (2022). Patterns and predictors of air purifier adherence in children with asthma living in low-income, urban households. *Journal of Asthma, 59*(5), 946–955.

Klepeis, N. N. W., & Ott, W. (2001). The National Human Activity Pattern Survey (NHAPS): A resource for assessing exposure to environmental pollutants. *Journal of Exposure Analysis and Environmental Epidemiology, 11*(3), 231–252.

Kurnitski, J., Eskola, L., Palonen, J., & Seppänen, O. (2007). Use of mechanical ventilation in Finnish houses. Proceedings of 2nd European BlowerDoor Symposium, Kassel, Germany, 152–161.

Laden, F., Schwartz, J., Speizer, F. E., & Dockery, D. W. (2006). Reduction in fine particulate air pollution and mortality: Extended follow-up of the Harvard Six Cities study. *American Journal of Respiratory and Critical Care Medicine, 173*(6), 667–672.

Langer, S., Ramalho, O., Le Ponner, E., Derbez, M., Kirchner, S., & Mandin, C. (2017). Perceived indoor air quality and its relationship to air pollutants in French dwellings. *Indoor Air, 27*(6), 1168–1176.

Logue, J. M., Price, P. N., Sherman, M. H., & Singer, B. C. (2012). A method to estimate the chronic health impact of air pollutants in U.S. residences. *Environmental Health Perspectives, 120*(2), 216–222.

Maestas, M. M., Brook, R. D., Ziemba, R. A., Li, F., Crane, R. C., Klaver, Z. M., & Morishita, M. (2019). Reduction of personal PM2.5 exposure via indoor air filtration systems in Detroit: An intervention study. *Journal of Exposure Science and Environmental Epidemiology, 29*(4), 484–490.

McNamara, M. L., Thornburg, J., Semmens, E. O., Ward, T. J., & Noonan, C. W. (2017). Reducing indoor air pollutants with air filtration units in wood stove homes. *Science of the Total Environment, 592*, 488–494.

Novoselac, A., & Siegel, J. A. (2009). Impact of placement of portable air cleaning devices in multizone residential environments. *Building and Environment, 44*(12), 2348–2356.

Ostro, B., & Rothschild, S. (1989). Air pollution and acute respiratory morbidity: An observational study of multiple pollutants. *Environmental Research, 50*, 238–247.

Park, H. K., Cheng, K. C., Tetteh, A. O., Hildemann, L. M., & Nadeau, K. C. (2017). Effectiveness of air purifier on health outcomes and indoor particles in homes of children with allergic diseases in Fresno, California: A pilot study. *Journal of Asthma, 54*(4), 341–346.

Pei, J., Dong, C., & Liu, J. (2019). Operating behavior and corresponding performance of portable air cleaners in residential buildings, China. *Building and Environment, 147*, 473–481.

Piazza, T., Lee, R. H., & Hayes, J. (2006). *Survey of the use of ozone-generating air cleaners by the California public.*

Pope, C. A., 3rd, & Dockery, D. W. (2006). Health effects of fine particulate air pollution: Lines that connect. *Journal of the Air & Waste Management Association, 56*(6), 709–742.

Pope, C. A., Burnett, R., Thun, M., Calle, E., Krewski, D., Ito, K., & Thurston, G. (2002). Lung cancer, cardiopulmonary mortality, and long-term exposure to fine particulate air pollution. *JAMA, 287*, 1132–1141.

Pope, C. A., Coleman, N., Pond, Z. A., & Burnett, R. T. (2020). Fine particulate air pollution and human mortality: 25+ years of cohort studies. *Environmental Research, 183*, 108924.

R Core Team. (2018). R: A language and environment for statistical computing. R Foundation for Statistical Computing. Vienna, Austria. Retrieved from https://www.R-project.org/

Rijal, H. B., Tuohy, P., Humphreys, M. A., Nicol, J. F., Samuel, A., Raja, I. A., & Clarke, J. (2008). Development of adaptive algorithms for the operation of windows, fans, and doors to predict thermal comfort and energy use in Pakistani buildings. *American Society of Heating Refrigerating and Air Conditioning Engineers (ASHRAE) Transactions, 114*(2), 555–573.

Rotko, T., Oglesby, L., Kunzli, N., Carrer, P., Nieuwenhuijsen, M., & Jantunen, M. (2002). Determinants of perceived air pollution annoyance and association between annoyance scores and air pollution ($PM_{2.5}$, NO_2) concentrations in the European EXPOLIS study. *Atmospheric Environment, 36*, 4593–4602.

Samet, J. (1993). Indoor air pollution: A public health perspective. *Indoor Air, 3*, 219–226.

Schwartz, J., Slater, D., Larson, T., Pierson, L., & Koenig, J. (1993). Particulate air pollution and hospital emergency room visits for asthma in Seattle. *American Review of Respiratory Disease, 147*, 826–831.

Schweiker, M., Ampatzi, E., Andargie, M. S., Andersen, R. K., Azar, E., Barthelmes, V. M., & Zhang, S. (2020). Review of multi-domain approaches to indoor environmental perception and behaviour. *Building and Environment, 176*.

Shao, D. Q., Du, Y. P., Liu, S., Brunekreef, B., Meliefste, K., Zhao, Q., & Huang, W. (2017). Cardiorespiratory responses of air filtration: A randomized crossover intervention trial in seniors living in Beijing Beijing Indoor Air Purifier StudY, BIAPSY. *Science of the Total Environment, 603*, 541–549.

Shaughnessy, R. J., & Sextro, R. G. (2006). What is an effective portable air cleaning device? A review. *Journal of Occupational and Environmental Hygiene, 3*(4), 169–181.

Shrubsole, C., MacMillan, A., Davies, M., & May, N. (2014). 100 unintended consequences of policies to improve energy efficiency of the UK housing stock. *Indoor and Built Environment, 23*(3), 340–352.

Spilak, M. P., Karottki, G. D., Kolarik, B., Frederiksen, M., Loft, S., & Gunnarsen, L. (2014). Evaluation of building characteristics in 27 dwellings in Denmark and the effect of using particle filtration units on PM2.5 concentrations. *Building and Environment, 73*, 55–63.

van der Wal, J., Moons, A., & Cornelissen, H. (1991). Indoor air quality in renovated Dutch homes. *Indoor Air, 4*, 621–633.

Vyas, S., Srivastav, N., & Spears, D. (2016). An experiment with air purifiers in Delhi during winter 2015–2016. *PLoS One, 11*(12).

Weichenthal, S., Mallach, G., Kulka, R., Black, A., Wheeler, A., You, H., & Sharp, D. (2013). A randomized double-blind crossover study of indoor air filtration and acute changes in cardiorespiratory health in a First Nations community. *Indoor Air, 23*(3), 175–184.

Weisel, C. P., Zhang, J., Turpin, B. J., Morandi, M. T., Colome, S., Stock, T. H., & Shendell, D. (2005). Relationship of Indoor, Outdoor and Personal Air (RIOPA) study: Study design, methods and quality assurance/control results. *Journal of Exposure Analysis and Environmental Epidemiology, 15*(2), 123–137.

Whitby, K. T. A., Anderson, G. R., & Rubow, K. L. (1983). Dynamic model for evaluating room-sized air cleaners. *ASHRAE Transactions, 89–2A*, 172–182.

WHO. (2006). *Air quality guidelines: Global update 2005: Particulate matter, ozone, nitrogen dioxide, and sulfur dioxide.* World Health Organization.

WHO (2013). *Health effects of particulate matter: Policy implications for countries in eastern Europe, Caucasus and central Asia.* Retrieved from Denmark: www.euro. who.int›pdf_file›Health-effects-of-particulate-matter-final-Eng

WHO. (2019). Global burden of disease. Retrieved from https://www.who.int/data/gho/data/themes/mortality-and-global-health-estimates

Zhan, Y., Johnson, K., Norris, C., Shafer, M. M., Bergin, M. H., Zhang, Y., & Schauer, J. J. (2018). The influence of air cleaners on indoor particulate matter components and oxidative potential in residential households in Beijing. *Science of the Total Environment*, *626*, 507–518.

4 Hospitalised patients' adaptation strategies and how they influence their indoor environmental comfort

Sara Willems, Dirk Saelens, and Ann Heylighen

Introduction

Hospitals are one of the building types for which the improvement of comfort through the indoor environment is important for patients. Hospitals rated with a high indoor environmental quality (IEQ) have been found to enhance patients' healing (Nimlyat & Kandar, 2015). For example, when patients experience the indoor environment as satisfactory, the length of their hospital stay was found to reduce (Choi et al., 2012; Nimlyat & Kandar, 2015). Moreover, patients' length of stay was related to the window orientation, view on nature, and illuminance level in studies by Benedetti et al. (2001), Choi et al. (2012), and Ulrich (1984). Mortality was affected by, for example, window orientation, the direction of air flow, and the filtration of air in studies performed by Beauchemin and Hays (1998), Leaf et al. (2010), Shirani et al. (1986), and Passweg et al. (1998). In this chapter, the focus is on patient rooms because hospitalised patients spend most of their time there.

The indoor environment and people interrelate in different ways. The design of indoor environments can have an impact on people's emotions, and these emotions, in turn, can affect their experienced indoor environmental comfort (Ortiz et al., 2017). Supporting indoor environmental comfort through positive emotions can also have a positive impact on health. For example, positive emotions have been associated with lower blood pressure levels, reduced inflammatory processes and neuroendocrine, cardiovascular, and immune strengthening; while negative emotions can cause stress, anxiety, depression, and eventually damaging changes in the cardiovascular system (Ortiz et al., 2017). The indoor environment also impacts health independently from comfort. Indoor conditions can limit physical stressors causing infirmity, disease, and potentially shorten life expectancy (Rohde et al., 2020). Furthermore, positive emotions can impact wellbeing (Rohde et al., 2020; Steemers & Manchanda, 2010).

People are not passively exposed to the indoor environment. Emotional responses to the indoor environment are related to adaptation (Ortiz et al., 2017). Adaptation refers to people's reaction to restore their comfort

DOI: 10.1201/9781003344711-5

when a change occurs that causes discomfort (Nicol & Humphreys, 2002). People can adapt in different ways. Based on the literature, de Dear and Brager (1998) distinguished between behavioural, physiological, and psychological adaptation.

To ensure that the indoor environment is comfortable in buildings someresearchers have attempted to understand what a comfortable indoor environment is (Andrade & Devlin, 2015; Fanger, 1970). Others have focused on understanding how people behave in a specific setting (Stazi et al., 2017). Influenced by differences in the research objective(s), these studies have applied different research approaches to realise their aims. Researchers adopt ontological (i.e., assumptions about the nature of reality) and epistemological positions (i.e., assumptions about the origin, limits, and nature of knowledge), which connect with researchers' theoretical lens, methodology, and methods (Creswell & Plano Clark, 2018).

Despite the wide variety of studies, it is not yet well understood what a comfortable indoor environment is. For example, it is not completely understood what roles the built environment plays in experiences (RBEE). Understanding these roles in depth is the objective of RBEE research. One setting focused upon is healthcare (Annemans et al., 2018a, 2018b; Anåker et al., 2019; Douglas & Douglas, 2004; Jellema et al., 2020; Nielsen & Overgaard, 2020). One of the factors that requires further research are the roles that perceived control and adaptation play in patients' comfort and wellbeing. According to Ulrich (1991), patients' lack of control is a major problem in healthcare settings. Ulrich's theory of supportive design advances three properties of healthcare settings that support patients' wellbeing: positive distractions, social support, but also perceived control over the material and social environment. However, in a study with orthopaedic patients, the respondents' stress was predicted not by how much control they perceived over the lighting, temperature, windows, and refrigerator, but by positive distraction and social support (Andrade et al., 2017). Andrade et al. (2017) argued that the expected positive effect on the stress level of patients with a high desire for control may be cancelled out by the absence of an effect for patients with a low desire.

To improve this understanding, we see potential in integrating RBEE research with research that has the objective to set up models for comfort predictions (MCP). MCP research includes studies on the threshold values for IEQ indicators and IEQ parameters in current standards and guidelines (Bureau for Standardisation, 2003, 2005; Berglund et al., 1999), as well as follow-up research on them (e.g., Parkinson et al., 2020 for the adaptive thermal comfort model). IEQ indicators are measurable quantities of indoor environmental conditions such as sound, light, temperature, humidity, and CO_2 levels. IEQ parameters are constructs such as thermal, visual, and acoustic comfort and indoor air quality. They can be assessed by people or estimated based on one or more IEQ indicators. It is observed in MCP research that perceived control over indoor conditions improves people's experience of them as it supports adaptation. This positive influence is observed in offices (Boerstra et al., 2013; Brackley et al., 2021; Sakellaris et al., 2019), in schools (Yun, 2018), and in residential buildings (Brown & Gorgolewski, 2014; Luo et al., 2014; Xu & Li, 2021). However, in MCP research, the roles of perceived control and adaptation in experience are not yet completely understood.

By integrating we mean bringing together and comparing results that can be associated with RBEE and MCP research, and interpreting the combined results (Creswell & Plano Clark, 2018, pp. 221–234). In this way, a synergy may be created between these two types of research. Integrating MCP research's sensor measurements with MPC and RBEE research's questionnaires, and with RBEE research's interviews may be needed to improve the understanding of roles of perceived control and adaptation in experience. Following this approach, the aims of the research presented in this chapter were to investigate (1) which adaptation strategies patients adopt, and (2) how these adaptation strategies influence their experience of indoor conditions.

Conceptual background

Before explaining the methodology, the understanding of some concepts needs to be clarified. Comfort, health, and wellbeing are understood differently across studies. Comfort is defined in MCP research as the "condition of mind that expresses satisfaction with the environment and is assessed by subjective evaluation" (de Dear & Brager, 2002). In healthcare literature, it is understood as a concept with two dimensions (Ortiz et al., 2017). One consists of three states required to be comfortable: relief, ease, and transcendence. The other deals with the context of comfort focused upon: the physical (bodily sensations), psychospiritual (the inner self), social (interpersonal, family, or cultural relationships), or environmental (light, noise, temperature, ambiance, colour, and natural versus synthetic elements) (Kolcaba, 1994; Ortiz et al., 2017). Despite differences in its definition, comfort relates across disciplines to subjective experiences, affected by various parameters (e.g., physical, physiological, psychological) that result from the interrelation between people and their environment (de Looze et al., 2003; Ortiz et al., 2017; Vink, 2005). The latter definition is adopted in this chapter.

Comfort partly overlaps with health. The Constitution of the World Health Organisation (WHO) has defined health as "a state of complete physical, mental, and social wellbeing not merely the absence of disease ..." (World Health Organization, 2020). To distinguish health from comfort, indoor environmental health can be understood as the indoor environmental conditions that limit physical stressors causing infirmity, disease and years of potential life loss (Rohde et al., 2020).

The term wellbeing lacks a clear definition in research, and there is no agreement yet on how it relates to other concepts such as comfort and health

(Pinto et al., 2017; Rohde et al., 2020; Watson, 2017). In literature on the indoor environment, wellbeing is used (1) as a synonym of comfort or health (Huisman et al., 2012; Xie et al., 2017), (2) to refer to the combination of comfort and health (Bluyssen, 2010; Ortiz et al., 2017; Rohde et al., 2020), (3) as a broader concept than comfort and health (Steemers & Manchanda, 2010), or (4) as a distinct concept from comfort and health (Rohde et al., 2020; Watson, 2017). In this chapter, we support the third view. We assume that comfort is not necessarily associated with a "feeling of neutrality", as is the case in the fourth view. This view supports how comfort is defined in healthcare literature. However, comfort is distinguished from happiness, in contrast to the second view. Some literature on happiness does not attend to the interrelation between people and their environment (Diener, 2009; Ryan & Deci, 2001). Furthermore, given our interest in the interrelation between the indoor environment and patients' subjective experience, we focus on comfort and its links with wellbeing.

Methods

Overview

Two mixed methods case studies were conducted, each at one or two hospital wards. Both quantitative and qualitative data were gathered, and they were analysed separately and in an integrated way. The research design of the two mixed methods case studies is reported in detail in Willems et al. (2022b). Based on the integrated analysis, a hypothesis was formulated about how perceived control and adaptation influence experience. This hypothesis was tested based on the quantitative data of case study 2. How the hypothesis is tested is reported in detail in Willems et al. (2022a). For conciseness some detail of the research has had to be removed. Additional detail can be found in Willems et al. (2022a, 2022b).

Cases

The case studies were conducted in Belgium. In consultation with hospital staff, we chose surgical wards as the patients on those wards were expected to be able to participate and stay for several days. Case 1 concerns a traumatology ward in a hospital building originating from 1984 and re-furbished in 2010. Indoor conditions in patient rooms are regulated by mechanical ventilation (70 m³/h in all rooms, supply temperature at out-door air temperature during data collection), windows operable by occupants, indoor and outdoor shading devices operable by occupants (except for north-east oriented windows), individual fans, radiators with a ther-mostatic valve, and artificial lighting without dimmers. Case 2 consists of two wards in a building originating from 2018: one for abdominal surgery, urology, and gynecological surgery and another for neurosurgery, plastic surgery and ear, nose, and throat diseases. Patient rooms are equipped with mechanical ventilation (100 m³/h per patient, supply temperature at 21 °C), operable windows which are locked, a fixed external sun shading, radiators with a thermostatic valve, and artificial lighting with dimmers. Neither of the case studies had a cooling system in the patient rooms. Figure 4.1 shows the floor plans and the layout of a double room.

Data collection

A self-reported questionnaire quantitatively gauged patients' assessments of their indoor environment, causes of (dis)comfort, perceived control and, for case 2, states of adaptable building characteristics. The questionnaire was inspired by the CBE questionnaire (ASHRAE PMP, 2010; Hyojin, 2012; Peretti & Schiavon, 2011) and adapted to hospitals based on insights from evidence-based design research in this context (Huisman et al., 2012; Ulrich et al., 2008). For case study 2, the questionnaire was improved based on insights gleaned from case study 1. An overview of the type of questions, the questions asked, the response scales and percentages of missing values per question can be found in Willems et al. (2022b, 2022a). Within the wards, simple random sampling was adopted. One or two days a week randomly selected (case 1) or all patients (case 2) were invited to participate. In total, 84 (case 1) and 238 (case 2) agreed, provided informed consent, and responded.

To gain an in-depth understanding of patients' experience, perceived control and adaptation, we used semi-structured interviews, and, for case 1, a probe, which is a form of self-documentation that invites participants to express their experiences and actions they might not think of during an interview (Gaver et al., 2004). The interviews addressed how interviewees experienced their hospital stay, especially related to their indoor environmental comfort and adaptation. In between the interviews, interviewees could complete the questionnaire or probe. The probe consisted of a timeline or booklet for taking notes. Convenience sampling was applied. Interviewees were selected by nurses based on the patients' ability and willingness to participate. They were interviewed until saturation in data collection was reached (i.e., new data repeat what was expressed in previous data; Saunders et al., 2018). Interviews were conducted with 12 respondents and four others for case 1, and 15 respondents and four others for case 2. The probe was completed by 8 interviewees. All participants provided informed consent. All participants of case 1 and ten of case 2 were interviewed twice, with about three to four days in between.

Sensors were used to measure IEQ indicators to understand which indoor conditions patients were experiencing, assessing, and adapting. Figure 4.1 shows the rooms of interviewees where measurements took place during their hospital stay for case study 1, as well as fixed sensor locations in patient rooms for case 2. For case 1, we picked out eligible patients who stayed in different room types (i.e., single versus double room and different window

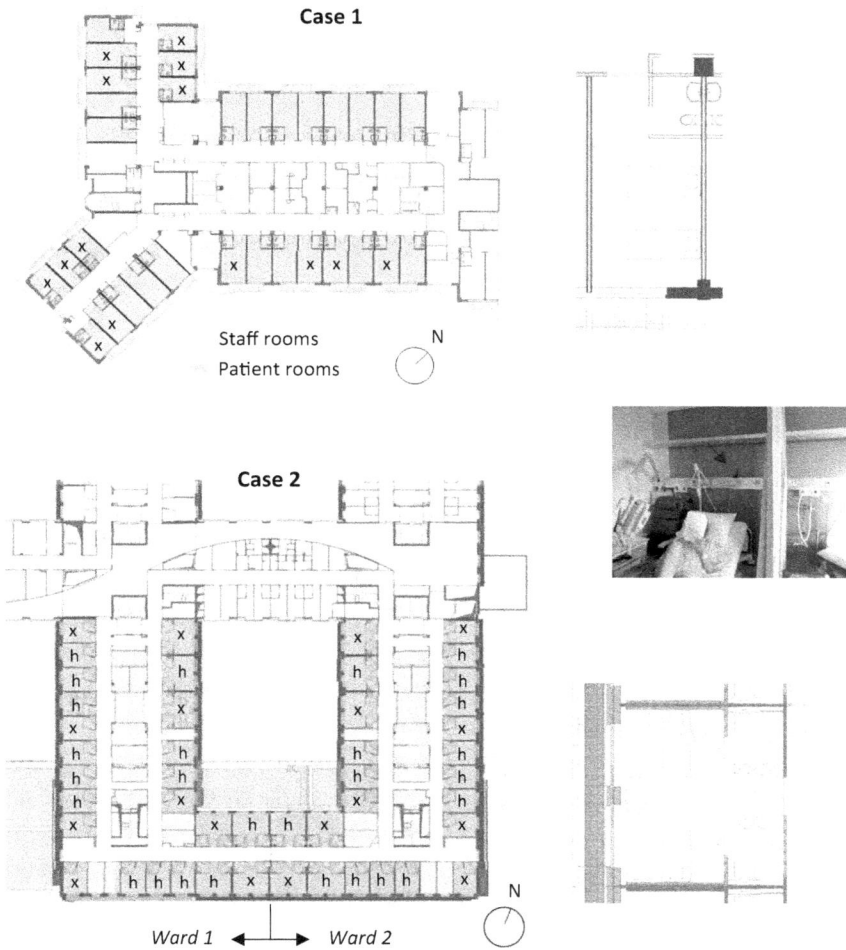

Figure 4.1 Floor plans of the wards where research was conducted for case 1 (top) and case 2 (bottom), and a picture of a respondent within the background a VersaSense Wireless Device (middle). The "x" on floor plans indicates rooms where a temperature and relative humidity probe as well as ambient illuminance and sound level probes were located during interviewees' hospital stay in case 1 (top) and permanently during case study 2 (bottom); "h" indicates those with only a temperature and relative humidity probe. (Plans case 1: based on the plan of the hospital's infrastructure planning department; plans case 2: based on the design of VK Architects & Engineers).

orientation) to maximise variety in measurement locations. Case 2 measurement locations were chosen to obtain an even spread of locations in both single and double rooms at each of the window orientations. Sensors were calibrated to ensure reliable measurements.

Data analysis

Patients' adaptation strategies were identified based on an integrated analysis of the quantitative and qualitative data. Based on the results of this integrated analysis, a hypothesis was formulated about how the different adaptation strategies influence experience. This hypothesis was tested based on the quantitative data of case study 2.

Identifying patients' adaptation strategies

Data were grouped according to differences in characteristics related to the setting (e.g., single versus double room). For two opposing groups, we then compared experiences, causes of (dis)comfort, perceived control, satisfaction votes, and measured values of IEQ indicators.

The different types of data were first analysed separately. Mann–Whitney U tests and Kruskal Wallis tests allowed comparing satisfaction votes between groups. The significance level (α) was taken equal to 0.1 because of the limited number of respondents per group for case study 1. The extent to which multiple-choice options were chosen was compared between groups via percentages. We only considered the options chosen by at least 10% of the respondents in one of both groups, and with a difference between both groups of at least 5%. Measured values of the IEQ indicators were grouped and their distributions (mean, 1st quartile, 3rd quartile, 5th percentile, and 95th percentile) compared. Unless mentioned otherwise, measurements during a heat wave (case study 1) were excluded from the groups, as this situation influenced the values considerably and was unevenly distributed over groups. The impact of differences in window orientations and seasons was considered during data interpretation. Threshold values of standards and guidelines gave an indication of how differences in measured values were expected to be experienced.

Interviews were audio-recorded and transcribed. Transcriptions were analysed qualitatively, together with the data of the self-documentation, questionnaires and sensor measurements, roughly following the Qualitative Analysis Guide of Leuven (Dierckx de Casterlé et al., 2012) and using NVivo software (NVivo, 2021). Interviews were analysed per interviewee and per group.

The integrated analysis was conducted iteratively with follow-up quantitative and qualitative analyses. For each of the compared groups, findings of the separate quantitative and qualitative analyses were merged via a joint display to draw out new insights beyond those gained from the separate analyses. During the integrated analysis, attention was given to whether findings of the quantitative and qualitative data were congruent (i.e., correspond), complementary (i.e., clarify, explain, or more fully elaborate each other), or discrepant (i.e., contradict each other) (Creswell & Plano Clark, 2018; Fetters et al., 2013; O'Cathain et al., 2010; Sandelowski, 2000). When silence (i.e., a concept is present in one data set but not in another one (O'Cathain et al., 2010; Uprichard & Dawney, 2019)) seemed to occur, a follow-up quantitative or qualitative analysis was conducted to check that the concept was not overlooked. If the concept could be identified, the integrated analysis was repeated.

Testing whether the different adaptation strategies influence experience differently

Once patients' adaptation strategies had been identified, it was hypothesised that different adaptation strategies influence experience differently. This hypothesis was tested in three steps. To start with, we linked the measured values of IEQ indicators in respondents' room to their sensation, preference, and satisfaction votes, the control they perceived over adaptable building characteristics and the state of these characteristics when they completed the questionnaire. To link questionnaire responses with measured values of IEQ indicators, we used mean values of the indoor air temperatures and illuminance levels measured in respondents' rooms during the hour before they started completing the questionnaire; and the background sound level measured during the 24 hours before the start. The background sound level and a period of 24 hours were used to exclude peaks in the sound level that result from own activities in the room from the analysis. The 1st quartile of the sound measurements, expressed in percentages, showed to be representative for the background sound level. This assumption could be made by comparing the value of the 1st quartile with the values of the continuous measurements.

In a second step, respondents were grouped according to the adaptation strategy they adopted. The grouping was based on respondents' questionnaire responses about their preferences, perceived control, and the state of adaptable building characteristics.

In a third step, we analysed by IEQ parameter whether tendencies could be noted in how each adaptation strategy related to how indoor conditions were experienced, how each adaptation strategy related to measured values of IEQ indicators, and how measured values of IEQ indicators related to experiences of indoor conditions. These tendencies were investigated in three ways. First, the tendencies were analysed for individual respondents by visually representing respondents' sensation, preference, and satisfaction votes and values of IEQ indicators measured in their room, and by interpreting this representation. Second, as the number of respondents per adaptation strategy is limited, we checked visually whether adaptation strategies differ in terms of how measured values and (sensation, preference and satisfaction) votes are distributed (i.e., mean, 1st and 3rd quartile, 5th and 95th percentile). Third, we analysed whether strategies differ significantly in terms of their distribution of measured values, and sensation and satisfaction votes. Neither measured values nor votes are normally distributed. Therefore, we performed Kruskal–Wallis tests ($\alpha = 0.1$) as well as pairwise Mann–Whitney U tests with Benjamini and Hochberg's (1995) adjustment method as post hoc pairwise test. We took the significance level alpha (α) equal to 0.1 as the number of respondents per adaptation strategy is limited.

Results

Patients' adaptation strategies and their relationship with comfort

This section describes the adaptation strategies that could be identified among patients and how they relate to patients' indoor environmental comfort. When participants had a wish for adaptation, they could either perceive control, i.e., be aware of possibilities to reduce the deviation between experienced and preferred indoor conditions, or not perceive such control. Four adaptation strategies were identified when patients perceived control (represented by the rectangles at the bottom right of Figure 4.2). They:

1 adapt indoor conditions in the room
2 adapt sensations or the experienced environmental information via physical means (e.g., changing clothing)
3 adapt their position by moving to more comfortable indoor conditions, or
4 adapt by choice to indoor conditions through choosing themselves to alter the attention given and meaning attributed to indoor conditions.

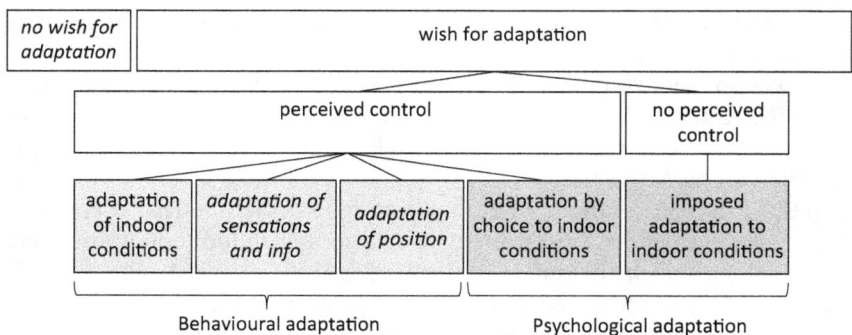

Figure 4.2 Patients' adaptation strategies and how they influence their indoor environmental comfort.

Adaptation by choice to indoor conditions occurs in two types of situations: when contextual parameters take priority over comfortable indoor conditions, or when some IEQ parameters take priority over others because the most comfortable condition of individual parameters cannot exist simultaneously.

When participants do not perceive control, they were
5   imposed to adapt to indoor conditions through altering the meaning and attention given to indoor conditions. This occurs in two types of situations: when actions taken to adapt indoor conditions do not suffice, or when the participant considers that no action can be taken.

The first three adaptation strategies are forms of behavioural adaptation. In this case, indoor conditions or sensations and the environmental information are adapted. The latter two strategies are forms of psychological adaptation. In these cases, the meaning given to indoor conditions is altered.

Comparing the findings from interviews, questionnaires, and sensor measurements indicates that the act of adapting, both behaviourally and psychologically, contributes to comfort. In addition, comfort is contributed to by the preferred experience of indoor conditions resulting from behavioural adaptation. A more extensive description of how the adaptation strategies were identified, and their influence on comfort can be found in Willems et al. (2022b).

Tendencies between patients' adaptation strategies and their experienced indoor environmental comfort

Based on the results reported in the previous section, it was hypothesised that the adaptation strategies influence the experience of indoor conditions differently psychologically. This section describes tendencies that could be identified between which adaptation strategy respondents apply and how they experience indoor conditions, between applied strategies and measured values of IEQ indicators, and between measured values of IEQ indicators and experiences of indoor conditions. These tendencies were analysed for three IEQ parameters: thermal, visual, and acoustic comfort. The analysis built on the adaptation strategies described in the previous section, but the ones considered differ slightly from it. We focused only on adaptation strategies that differ in how patients interact with indoor conditions via adaptable building characteristics. This choice was made because we mainly wanted to gain insights into the role that the built environment plays in adaptation and experiences of indoor conditions. To this end, we grouped respondents who have no wish for adaptation with those who adopt adaptation strategies that lead to indoor conditions they prefer and that do not involve adaptations of indoor conditions (i.e., adaptation of sensations and environmental information or of position) and refer to them as respondents who have "no wish to adapt indoor conditions". In Figure 4.2, this is visualised by the text in italics. Next to this, within the group of respondents who are imposed to adapt to indoor conditions, we distinguished those who are imposed to adapt after having already acted from those who did not. The former includes, for example, respondents whose lighting is on, and window curtains are open, who still prefer additional light, but who do not perceive a possibility to further increase illuminance levels. The latter include respondents who prefer additional light, but do not perceive control over available adaptable building characteristics to increase it. Measured values of IEQ indicators were expected to differ in both situations.

First, a tendency is noted between the adaptation strategy respondents and how they experience indoor conditions. Table 4.1 presents the percentage of dissatisfied per adaptation strategy. There is a slight indication that dissatisfaction, i.e., a satisfaction vote lower than neutral, is more common for visual and acoustic comfort when respondents choose or are imposed to adapt to indoor conditions compared to when they adapt indoor conditions or have no wish to do so. For thermal comfort, a similar tendency can be noted, but in this case several respondents are dissatisfied as well when having no wish to adapt indoor conditions. The first tendency could not only be observed for the extent to which dissatisfaction occurs but also for the distribution of the votes in general. Satisfaction votes are generally more distributed towards being satisfied (i.e., higher than neutral) when sensation votes are distributed more towards neutral (i.e., equal to zero) or the preference. This occurs more when respondents adapt indoor conditions or have no wish to do so. Furthermore, the mean ranks of acoustic and visual sensation votes as well as acoustic satisfaction votes differ significantly between adaptation strategies ($p < 0.001$; $p = 0.07$; $p < 0.001$). Pairwise comparisons between the strategies confirm the tendency described above.

Second, two opposite tendencies were noticed between the adaptation strategy adopted and measured values of IEQ indicators. On the one hand, adaptations of indoor conditions sometimes resulted in high or low values of IEQ indicators. In these situations, the adaptations of indoor conditions were

Table 4.1 Percentage of dissatisfied per adaptation strategy

Adaptation strategy	Percentage of dissatisfied		
	Thermal comfort	Visual comfort	Acoustic comfort
Adaptation of indoor conditions	0.01	0.009	0.02
No wish to adapt indoor conditions	0.09	0	0
Adaptation by choice to indoor conditions	0	0.06	0.55
Imposed adaptation with an action	0	0.06	0.31
Imposed adaptation without an action	0.13	0.1	0.41

reflected in (the distribution of) measured values. For example, higher indoor air temperatures and illuminance levels are measured when respondents increase the indoor temperature or the amount of light. On the other hand, actions seem to be taken to bring high or low values of IEQ indicators to a more "moderate" state, and adaptation strategies that involve psychological adaptation seem to be adopted to deal with situations in which IEQ indicators have a rather high or low value. In these situations, actions taken to adapt indoor conditions are not reflected in (the distribution of) measured values. For example, sound levels are similar in rooms of respondents who take actions that decrease the sound level compared to those where respondents have no wish to adapt them or prefer a lower sound level and adapt by choice or imposed to it without an action.

Third, across the adaptation strategies, no tendency could be identified between differences in the measured values of IEQ indicators and differences in how indoor conditions are experienced.

As differences in experience are not related to differences in measured values, the adaptation strategies seem to influence in a different psychological way how indoor conditions are experienced. These different psychological influences are indicated by the green and orange colour in Figure 4.2. A more extensive description of the identified tendencies between patients' adaptation strategies and their indoor environmental comfort can be found in Willems et al. (2022a).

Discussion

Contributions

The roles of perceived control in patients' comfort

The identified adaptation strategies and tendencies in how they impacted patient comfort improve the understanding of what role(s) perceived control plays in patient comfort. Rather than the difference between situations in which control is perceived and in which it is not, differences in experiences seem to relate to the difference between behavioural and psychological adaptation. First, having the ability to influence the experience of indoor conditions through adaptation contributes to comfort. This influence occurs through behavioural or psychological adaptation. Secondly, the indoor conditions that are experienced because of behavioural adaptation support comfort. The indoor conditions resulting from behavioural adaptation are preferable. Furthermore, patients' tendency to be less satisfied when they perceive control but adapt by choice – which is a form of psychological adaptation – helps to explain why perceived control did not predict patients' stress in studies by Andrade and Devlin (2015) and by Andrade et al. (2017). The positive influence that perceived control plays for some patients may be cancelled out by the absence or negative role it plays for other patients.

The roles of adaptation in patients' wellbeing

The two ways in which adaptation impacts comfort can be linked to the distinction that psychologists make between eudaimonic and hedonic wellbeing (Delle Fave et al., 2010; Hanc et al., 2019). Both perspectives on wellbeing focus on happiness. The former focusses on functioning well; the latter on people's subjective belief about whether their life is desirable, pleasant, and good (Diener, 2009). Eudaimonia is concerned with living in a way, and within an environment, that aligns with one's daemon or true self (i.e., congruent with deeply held values), and that encourages expressing one's full potential (Ryan & Deci, 2001; Ryff & Singer, 2008; Waterman, 1993). From this perspective, not all pleasure producing desires would yield wellbeing when fulfilled, as some outcomes may harm people (Ryan & Deci, 2001). Similarities are seen between how the perceived ability to influence the experience of indoor conditions through adaptation contributes to comfort and how eudaimonic wellbeing is defined. When patients could influence their experience through adaptation, this can give them the feeling that they are functioning well. Furthermore, similarities are seen between the preferable indoor conditions that are obtained through behavioural adaptation, and how Diener (2009) understands hedonic wellbeing. The preferable indoor conditions that result from behavioural adaptation can support people's subjective belief about whether their life is desirable, pleasant, and good.

Linking the distinction psychologists make between hedonic and eudaimonic wellbeing to the two ways in which adaptation influences comfort also may help explain why we observed a tendency towards more neutral or preferable sensations and higher satisfactions when patients adapt behaviourally or have no wish for adaptation compared to when they adapt psychologically. Both behavioural and psychological adaptation can support eudaimonic wellbeing, while only behavioural adaptation supports hedonic wellbeing.

In addition, the built environment influences adaptation, as reported in Willems et al. (2022b). Understanding how adaptation influences wellbeing and how the built environment influences adaptation therefore also improves the understanding of the roles that the built environment plays in wellbeing. These roles are not well understood yet (Altomonte et al., 2020; Hanc et al., 2019).

Limitations

The research was explorative in character, and it enabled an improved understanding of how perceived control and adaptation influence indoor environmental comfort in patient rooms. There are, however, several limitations that need to be discussed.

Limited dataset in terms of the number of participating patients and variation in patients' experience

The results cannot be generalised. First, while sufficient qualitative data were collected, this was not the case with respect to the quantitative data. More quantitative data would allow excluding the questionnaire responses of interviewees in the statistical analyses. Their responses may have been influenced by the interview they participated in prior to the questionnaire. This, in our view, poses a risk of bias. However, asking patients to complete the questionnaire prior to the interview can influence responses during the interview. In this case it is no longer possible to start with open questions and find out what interviewees start talking about themselves. Moreover, answers were already influenced by the multiple-choice options from the questionnaire. Furthermore, the effects of multiple confounders could often not be checked during data analysis. Including such confounders would provide more certainty about the internal validity of the results. It would also improve the credibility of the qualitative data's interpretation. After all, this credibility is enhanced via triangulation by findings based on the quantitative data.

Secondly, within the dataset of case study 2, there was little variation in participants' experience due to the case chosen. Indoor conditions only hindered or supported positive experiences to a limited extent. Regarding the qualitative data, attention to indoor conditions was therefore only present in participants' description of their experiences. Regarding the quantitative data, few participants were dissatisfied. When indoor air temperatures are within threshold values, only 5% of the are dissatisfied, which is lower than the predicted maximum of 10% (Lazarov & Stranger, 2017); and when illuminance levels are within threshold values, 3%. When they are outside the thresholds, only 0% and 3% are dissatisfied, respectively. When the A-weighted equivalent continuous sound level (LAeq) and the maximum instantaneous A-weighted sound pressure level, measured on fast response (LAmax, fast), in interviewees' room are used only 11% of the interviewees are dissatisfied with the acoustic comfort. In none of the rooms did the measured values comply with threshold values. A focus on buildings with more variable indoor conditions and higher dissatisfactions, and/or participants between whom there is more variability, could be a valuable approach in future research. This is likely to yield more variability in people's experience. Due to this higher variability, the roles of perceived control and adaptation in patients' comfort and wellbeing may become clearer.

Absence of a substantive focus in data collection

The research started by looking for ways in which RBEE and MCP research could be integrated. The choice to focus on how perceived control and adaptation influence experience evolved from the research. This resulted in a lack of a substantive focus in the data collection methods and some limitations resulting from it.

The questionnaire lacked some relevant questions, and they were, in hindsight, a little too broad. The questions about patients' wellbeing were based on the World Health Organisation's Quality of Life Questionnaire (WHOQOL-BREF) (De Vries & Van Heck, 1996). Questions could also specifically address hedonic and eudaimonic wellbeing. Questionnaires for both perspectives have been developed (Diener et al., 1985; Diener, 2009; Ryff & Keyes, 1995; Watson et al., 1988). These questionnaires can be adapted to focus specifically on indoor environmental comfort or the corresponding adaptation. Moreover, our research indicates that in future research questions should be added that enable identifying respondents who have no wish for adaptation, who adapt sensations and environmental information, and who adapt their position.

Because of these limitations, sequential mixed methods research designs are recommended for future research.

Shortcomings in the diversity of patients in the sample

The diversity of patients in the sample can be improved. Several patients with low cognitive competences, or who did not feel well, refused or were unable to participate in this research. Selecting those participants for (short) interviews or interviewing them together with an assistant (e.g., a nurse or guardian) could be a direction for the future.

The lack of attention for patients' health status

One characteristic that relates to the patients and that should be given more attention is their health status. Health status is expected to influence their indoor environmental comfort and adaptation because, as described earlier, health and comfort are interrelated. Health status is not expected to strongly influence the identified adaptation strategies; however, it may influence the observed tendencies. For example, if a patient adapts by choice or is imposed to, and is not feeling well at the time, it may strengthen dissatisfaction. We did check this and did not find this tendency; however, it is worthy of attention in future research.

Future research

Theoretical framework

In this chapter, results were linked to the distinction psychologists make between hedonic and eudaimonic wellbeing. The results suggest that this distinction can also be made with respect to comfort, but further research is needed in this regard.

Furthermore, the theories related to hedonic and eudaimonic wellbeing focus on happiness. These support understanding how different adaptation strategies influence comfort differently psychologically. If future research wants to gain more insight into when which adaptation strategy is applied, other theories seem interesting. Gibson's (1968) theory about affordances and further elaborations of it by other authors (Baggs & Chemero, 2021) are suggested. These theories point to the interrelationship between an occupant and the occupant's environment. According to Gibson (1979, 1968), the fundamental constituents of the environment when studied from the point of view of "behaving" people are "affordances". Affordances, in their original meaning, are the possible facilitations or hindrances provided by the substances, surfaces, objects, and other living creatures surrounding people in the immediate context of their current activity (Gibson, 1979, 1968; Ingold, 2011). Rietveld et al. (2018) defined it more recently as "relations between (a) aspects of the socio-material environment in flux and (b) abilities available in a 'form of life'". Affordances are properties of the environment taken with reference to a person, but not properties of the person's experience exclusive of the environment. Such interrelationships came up in the research (Willems et al., 2022b). It was observed that participants' competences influence whether they can use adaptable building characteristics to adapt indoor conditions. For example, some patients are physically not competent to leave their bed to open a door, or cognitively not competent to use complex lighting systems. Conversely, it can be stated that adaptable building characteristics should be aligned with patients' diverse competences. The latter is what designers need to consider. Presumably, existing insights into affordances can support the understanding of how patient room design can influence patients' comfort through its impact on their adaptation of, and to, indoor conditions via their perceived control.

Valorising improved insights into indoor environmental comfort and adaptation through scenario-based design techniques

Future research can valorise insights into the adaptation strategies that patients apply through scenario-based design techniques. Scenario-based design techniques enable researchers to explore potential use situations explicitly and iteratively (Van der Linden et al., 2019). Scenarios are often used in conjuncture with personas. Personas are a technique to create vivid user profiles that are usually founded on research. The scenarios and personas offer various stakeholders of the design process a way to integrate information about users, settings, and their interactions into a coherent story. They enable making issues that may occur during the building's use and people's spatial experience tangible, negotiable, and applicable during design. Moreover, they can support creative and reflective thinking by considering the diversity and dynamics of use situations and offer a frame of reference to evaluate design decisions (van der Bijl-Brouwer & van der Voort, 2013; Van der Linden et al., 2019). In this way, they may support architects in designing human-centred environments (Van der Linden et al., 2019).

From improved insights into indoor environmental comfort and adaptation to improved predictions of them

Future research should investigate how predictions of indoor environmental comfort and adaptation can be improved based on the improved understanding of how adaptation and perceived control influence the experience of indoor conditions. The improved understanding may contribute to new ways to quantify and predict them. It may contribute as well to those that have already been applied. The latter include adjustments of Fanger's Predicted Mean Vote (PMV)/Predicted Percentage of Dissatisfied (PPD) model or Gagge's standard effective temperature (SET) model to include differences between adaptation strategies (Schweiker & Wagner, 2015).

In addition, some researchers have developed models to predict adaption of indoor conditions (see Carlucci et al. (2020) for an overview). It should be explored how to integrate models that predict indoor environmental comfort with models of with models that predict adaption of indoor conditions. This will help to inform designs for automated and optimised systems with respect for comfort and energy use. By integrating the models, a better trade-off may be made between supporting comfort and reducing the use of building systems that use energy.

Implications for design practice

Although tentative, the results of this research have implications for design practice. The results suggest that designers should not only think about how comfortable indoor conditions can best be provided, but also about how patients can adapt them. Raising awareness among healthcare designers to patient adaptation strategies, and how they influence indoor environmental comfort, is needed to help improve healthcare design.

Conclusion

Two mixed methods case studies, which focus on hospital wards, provided insight into which adaptation strategies surgical patients use and tendencies in how these adaptation strategies relate to different experiences of indoor conditions.

Strategies with perceived control were identified as adaptation (1) of indoor conditions, (2) of sensations or the environmental information, (3) of position, and (4) by choice to indoor conditions; and without perceived control: (5) imposed adaptation to indoor conditions. The former three strategies are forms of behavioural adaptation, the latter two of psychological adaptation. Furthermore, a tendency towards more neutral or preferable sensations and higher satisfactions is observed when participants adapt behaviourally or have no wish for adaptation than when they adapt psychologically.

The identified adaptation strategies and tendencies increase the understanding of roles of perceived control in patients' comfort. Rather than to the difference between situations in which control is perceived and in which it is not, differences in experiences seem to relate to the difference between behavioural and psychological adaptation. It is found that perceived control does not necessarily play a positive role in experience when patients adapt by choice, which is a form of psychological adaptation. It was therefore not confirmed in previous studies that perceived control plays a positive role in patients' experience. The positive role that it plays for patients who adapt behaviourally may have been cancelled out by the absence or negative role it plays for patients who adapt by choice.

Links were identified between how the adaptation strategies impact comfort and the distinction psychologists make between hedonic and eudaimonic wellbeing. The behavioural adaptation of the first three adaptation strategies reported above seems to contribute to both hedonic and eudaimonic wellbeing. The psychological adaptation of the fourth adaptation strategy seems to contribute only to eudaimonic wellbeing. For the latter strategy, patients can experience eudaimonic wellbeing as well, and this only if they can tolerate the imposed adaptation.

This study must be considered as pilot study. Future research should verify the results based on a larger dataset, and ideally more variation in participants' experience; with data collection methods that focus on the role of perceived control and adaptation in patients' experience; a more diverse sample; and more attention for how patients' health state influences their comfort and adaptation. If confirmed, the results imply for design practice that adaptive opportunities should be provided. Providing adaptive opportunities will support perceived control and adaptation, and is in this way expected to contribute to patients' comfort and wellbeing.

Acknowledgements

This work was supported by a PhD fellowship (11A7521N) of the Research Foundation Flanders. We thank Geert Molenbergs for his advice on the design of the questionnaire and for checking the appropriateness of applied statistical methods; and Edwin Reynders and Gerrit Vermeir for sharing their insights about acoustics in hospitals. We also thank Patricia Elsen and Geert Bauwens for their technical support with the sensors; and Jasper Vastiau for his support upon hospital acoustics and the use of sensors. We also thank the participants for sharing their time and insights and the hospital management and staff for their support to conduct the research.

References

Altomonte, S., Allen, J., Bluyssen, P. M., Brager, G., Heschong, L., Loder, A., Schiavon, S., Veitch, J. A., Wang, L., & Wargocki, P. (2020). Ten questions concerning wellbeing in the built environment. *Building and Environment, 180*, 106949.

American Society of Heating, Refrigerating and Air-Conditioning Engineers. (2010). *Performance measurement protocols for commercial buildings*. American Society of Heating, Refrigerating and Air-Conditioning Engineers, Inc.

Anåker, A., von Koch, L., Heylighen, A., & Elf, M. (2019). "It's lonely": Patients' experiences of the physical environment at a newly built stroke unit. *HERD*, *12*(3), 141–152.

Andrade, C. C., & Devlin, A. S. (2015). Stress reduction in the hospital room: Applying Ulrich's theory of supportive design. *Journal of Environmental Psychology*, *41*, 125–134.

Andrade, C. C., Devlin, A. S., Pereira, C. R., & Lima, M. L. (2017). Do the hospital rooms make a difference for patients' stress? A multilevel analysis of the role of perceived control, positive distraction, and social support. *Journal of Environmental Psychology*, *53*, 63–72.

Annemans, M., Van Audenhove, C., Vermolen, H., & Heylighen, A. (2018a). Inpatients' spatial experience: Interactions between material, social, and time-related aspects. *Space and Culture*, *21*(4), 495–511.

Annemans, M., Van Audenhove, C., Vermolen, H., & Heylighen, A. (2018b). The role of space in patients' experience of an emergency department: A qualitative study. *Journal of Emergency Nursing*, *44*(2), 139–145.

Baggs, E., & Chemero, A. (2021). Radical embodiment in two directions. *Synthese*, *198*(9), 2175–2190.

Beauchemin, K. M., & Hays, P. (1998). Dying in the dark: Sunshine, gender and outcomes in myocardial infarction. *Journal of the Royal Society of Medicine*, *91*(7), 352–354.

Benedetti, F., Colombo, C., Barbini, B., Campori, E., & Smeraldi, E. (2001). Morning sunlight reduces length of hospitalization in bipolar depression. *Journal of Affective Disorders*, *62*(3), 221–223.

Benjamini, Y., & Hochberg, Y. (1995). Controlling the false discovery rate. *Journal of the Royal Statistical Society Series B*, *57*, 289–300.

Berglund, B., Lindvall, T., Schwelaand, D. H., & Goh, T. K. (1999). Guidelines for community noise. In *Protection of the human environment*. World Health Organization.

Bluyssen, P. M. (2010). Towards new methods and ways to create healthy and comfortable buildings. *Building and Environment*, *45*(4), 808–818.

Boerstra, A., Beuker, T., Loomans, M., & Hensen, J. (2013). Impact of available and perceived control on comfort and health in European offices. *Architectural Science Review*, *56*(1), 30–41.

Brackley, C., O'Brien, W., Trudel, C., & Bursill, J. (2021). The in-situ implementation of a feature-rich thermostat: A building engineering and human factors approach to improve perceived control in offices. *Building and Environment*, *199*, 107884.

Brown, C., & Gorgolewski, M. (2014). Assessing occupant satisfaction and energy behaviours in Toronto's LEED gold high-rise residential buildings. *International Journal of Energy Sector Management*, *8*(4), 492–505.

Bureau for Standardisation. (2003). *Light and lighting – Lighting of work places – Part 1: Indoor work places* (NBN EN Standard 12464-1:2003).

Bureau for Standardisation. (2005). *Indoor environmental input parameters for design and assessment of energy performance of buildings addressing indoor air quality, thermal environment, lighting and acoustics* (NBN EN Standard 15251:2005).

Carlucci, S., De Simone, M., Firth, S. K., Kjærgaard, M. B., Markovic, R., Rahaman, M. S., Annaqeeb, M. K., Biandrate, S., Das, A., Dziedzic, J. W., Fajilla, G., Favero, M., Ferrando, M., Hahn, J., Han, M., Peng, Y., Salim, F., Schlüter, A., & van Treeck, C. (2020). Modeling occupant behavior in buildings. *Building and Environment, 174*, 106768.

Choi, J.-H., Beltran, L. O., & Kim, H.-S. (2012). Impacts of indoor daylight environments on patient average length of stay (ALOS) in a healthcare facility. *Building and Environment, 50*, 65–75.

Creswell, J. W., & Plano Clark, V. L. (2018). *Designing and conducting mixed methods research* (3rd ed.). Sage.

de Dear, R. J., & Brager, G. S. (1998). Developing an adaptive model of thermal comfort and preference. *ASHRAE Transactions, 104*, 145–167.

de Dear, R. J., & Brager, G. S. (2002). Thermal comfort in naturally ventilated buildings: Revisions to ASHRAE Standard 55. *Energy and Buildings, 34*(6), 549–561.

Delle Fave, A., Massimini, F., & Bassi, M. (2010). Hedonism and eudaimonism in positive psychology. In A. Delle Fave (Ed.), *Psychological selection and optimal experience across cultures* (pp. 3–18). Netherlands: Springer.

de Looze, M. P., Kuijt-evers, L. F., & van Dieën J. (2003). Sitting comfort and discomfort and the relationships with objective measures. *Ergonomics, 46*(10), 985–997.

De Vries, J., & Van Heck, G. L. (1996). *WHOQOL-Bref*. Universiteit van Tilburg.

Diener, E. (2009). *The science of wellbeing: The collected works of Ed Diener* (1st ed.). Netherlands: Springer.

Diener, E., Emmons, R. A., Larsen, R. J., & Griffin, S. (1985). The satisfaction with life scale. *Journal of Personality Assessment, 49*, 71–75.

Dierckx de Casterlé, B., Gastmans, C., Bryon, E., & Denier, Y. (2012). QUAGOL: A guide for qualitative data analysis. *International Journal of Nursing Studies, 49*(3), 360–371.

Douglas, C. H., & Douglas, M. R. (2004). Patient-friendly hospital environments: Exploring the patients' perspective. *Health Expect, 7*(1), 61–73.

Fanger, P. O. (1970). *Thermal comfort: Analysis and applications in environmental engineering*. MacGraw-Hill.

Fetters, M. D., Curry, L. A., & Creswell, J. W. (2013). Achieving integration in mixed methods designs-principles and practices. *Health Services Research, 48*(6pt2), 2134–2156.

Gaver, W., Boucher, A., Pennington, S., & Walker, B. (2004). Cultural probes and the value of uncertainty. *Interactions, 11*(5), 53–56.

Gibson, J. (1968). *The senses considered as perceptual systems*. Allen and Unwin.

Gibson, J. (1979). *The ecological approach to visual perception*. Houghton Mifflin.

Hanc, M., McAndrew, C., & Ucci, M. (2019). Conceptual approaches to wellbeing in buildings: A scoping review. *Building Research & Information, 47*(6), 767–783.

Huisman, E. R. C. M., Morales, E., van Hoof, J., & Kort, H. S. M. (2012). Healing environment: A review of the impact of physical environmental factors on users. *Building and Environment, 58*, 70–80.

Hyojin, K. (2012). *Methodology for rating a building's overall performance based on the ASHRAE/CIBSE/USGBC performance measurement protocols for commercial buildings*. Texas A&M University.

Ingold, T. (2011). *Being alive: essays on movement, knowledge and description.* Routledge.

Jellema, P. (2020). *Foregrounding the built environment in experiences of (cancer) care: Learning lessons for human-centred design,* PhD Thesis, KU Leuven.

Kolcaba, K. Y. (1994). A theory of holistic comfort for nursing. *Journal of Advanced Nursing, 19*(6), 1178–1184.

Lazarov, B., & Stranger, M. (2017). *Aanbevelingen voor fysische parameters in het Vlaams binnenmilieubesluit.* Vito NV.

Leaf, D. E., Homel, P., & Factor, P. H. (2010). Relationship between ICU design and mortality. *Chest, 137*(5), 1022–1027.

Luo, M., Cao, B., Zhou, X., Li, M., Zhang, J., Ouyang, Q., & Zhu, Y. (2014). Can personal control influence human thermal comfort? A field study in residential buildings in China in winter. *Energy and Buildings, 72,* 411–418.

Nicol, J. F., & Humphreys, M. A. (2002). Adaptive thermal comfort and sustainable thermal standards for buildings. *Energy and Buildings, 34*(6), 563–572.

Nielsen, J. H., & Overgaard, C. (2020). Healing architecture and Snoezelen in delivery room design: a qualitative study of women's birth experiences and patient-centeredness of care. *BMC Pregnancy & Childbirth, 20*(1), 283.

Nimlyat, P. S., & Kandar M. Z. (2015). Appraisal of indoor environmental quality (IEQ) in healthcare facilities: A literature review. *Sustainable Cities and Society, 17,* 61–68.

Nvivo. (2021). *Unlock insights in your data with powerful analysis.* Nvivo. https://www.qsrinternational.com/nvivoqualitative-data-analysis-software/home

O'Cathain, A., Murphy, E., & Nicholl, J. (2010). Three techniques for integrating data in mixed methods studies. *British Medical Journal, 341*(7783), c4587–c4587.

Ortiz, M. A., Kurvers, S. R., & Bluyssen, P. M. (2017). A review of comfort, health, and energy use: Understanding daily energy use and wellbeing for the development of a new approach to study comfort. *Energy and Buildings, 152,* 323–335.

Parkinson, T., de Dear, R., & Brager, G. (2020). Nudging the adaptive thermal comfort model. *Energy and Buildings, 206,* 109559.

Passweg, J. R., Rowlings, P. A., Atkinson, K. A., Barrett, A. J., Gale, R. P., Gratwohl, A., Jacobsen, N., Klein, J. P., Ljungman, P., Russel, J. A., Schäfer, U. W., Sobocinski, K. A., Vossen, J. M., Zhang, M. J., & Horowitz, M. M. (1998). Influence of protective isolation on outcome of allogeneic bone marrow transplantation for leukemia. *Bone Marrow Transplant, 21*(12), 1231–1238.

Peretti, C., & Schiavon, S. (2011). *Indoor environmental quality surveys. A brief literature review.* Center for the Built Environment.

Pinto, S., Fumincelli, L., Mazzo, A., Caldeira, S., & Martins, J. C. (2017). Comfort, wellbeing and quality of life: Discussion of the differences and similarities among the concepts. *Porto Biomedical Journal, 2*(1), 6–12.

Rietveld, E., Denys, D., & Van Westen, M. (2018). Ecological-enactive cognition as engaging with a field of relevant affordances: The Skilled Intentionality Framework (SIF). In L. De Bruin, A. Newen & S. Gallagher (Eds.), *The Oxford handbook of 4E cognition* (pp. 41–70). Oxford University Press.

Rohde, L., Larsen, T. S., Jensen, R. L., & Larsen, O. K. (2020). Framing holistic indoor environment: Definitions of comfort, health and wellbeing. *Indoor & Built Environment, 29*(8), 1118–1136.

Ryan, R. M., & Deci, E. L. (2001). On happiness and human potentials: A review of research on hedonic and eudaimonic wellbeing. *Annual Review of Psychology*, *52*(1), 141–166.

Ryff, C. D., & Keyes, C. L. M. (1995). The structure of psychological wellbeing revisited. *Journal of Personality and Social Psychology*, *69*(4), 719–727.

Ryff, C. D., & Singer, B. H. (2008). Know thyself and become what you are: A eudaimonic approach to psychological wellbeing. *Journal of Happiness Studies*, *9*(1), 13–39.

Sakellaris, I., Saraga, D., Mandin, C., de Kluizenaar, Y., Fossati, S., Spinazzè, A., & Bartzis, J. (2019). Personal control of the indoor environment in offices: Relations with building characteristics, influence on occupant perception and reported symptoms related to the building-the officair project. *Applied Sciences*, *9*(16), 3227.

Sandelowski, M. (2000). Combining qualitative and quantitative sampling, data collection, and analysis techniques in mixed-method studies. *Research in Nursing & Health*, *23*(3), 246–255.

Saunders, B., Sim, J., Kingstone, T., Baker, S., Waterfield, J., Bartlam, B., Burroughs H., & Jinks, C. (2018). Saturation in qualitative research: Exploring its conceptualization and operationalization. *Quality & Quantity*, *52*(4), 1893–1907.

Schweiker, M., & Wagner, A. (2015). A framework for an adaptive thermal heat balance model (ATHB). *Building and Environment*, *94*(P1), 252–262.

Shirani, K. Z., McManus, A. T., Vaughan, G. M., McManus, W. F., Pruitt, B. A., & Mason, A. D. (1986). Effects of environment on infection in burn patients. *Archives of Surgery*, *121*(1), 31–36.

Stazi, F., Naspi, F., & D'Orazio, M. (2017). A literature review on driving factors and contextual events influencing occupants' behaviours in buildings. *Building and Environment*, *118*, 40–66.

Steemers, K., & Manchanda, S. (2010). Energy efficient design and occupant wellbeing: Case studies in the UK and India. *Building and Environment*, *45*(2), 270–278.

Ulrich, R. S. (1984). View through a window may influence recovery from surgery. *Science*, *224*(4647), 420–421.

Ulrich, R. S. (1991). Effects of interior design on wellness. *Journal of Health Care Interior Design*, *3*(1), 97–109.

Ulrich, R. S., Zimring, C., Zhu, X., DuBose, J., Seo, H.-B., Choi, Y.-S., Quan, X., & Joseph, A. (2008). A review of the research literature on evidence-based healthcare design. *Health Environments Research & Design Journal*, *1*(3), 61–125.

Uprichard, E., & Dawney, L. (2019). Data diffraction: Challenging data integration in mixed methods research. *Journal of Mixed Methods Research*, *13*(1), 19–32.

van der Bijl-Brouwer, M., & van der Voort, M. C. (2013). Exploring future use: Scenario based design. In C. de Bont, E. den Ouden, H. N. J. Schifferstein, F. Smulders, & M. C. van der Voort (Eds.), *Advanced design methods for successful innovation* (pp. 56–77). Design United.

Van der Linden, V., Dong, H., & Heylighen, A. (2019). Tracing architects' fragile knowing about users in the socio-material environment of design practice. *Design Studies*, *63*, 65–91.

Vink, P. (2005). *Comfort and design*. CRC Press.

Waterman, A. S. (1993). Two conceptions of happiness: Contrasts of personal expressiveness (eudaimonia) and hedonic enjoyment. *Journal of Personality and Social Psychology*, *64*(4), 678–691.

Watson, D., Clark, L. A., & Tellegen, A. (1988). Development and validation of brief measures of positive and negative affect. *Journal of Personality and Social Psychology*, *54*(6), 1063–1070.

Watson, K. J. (2017). Developing wellbeing valuation practices in the built environment. *Professional Practices in the Built Environment*, University of Reading, 120.

Willems, S., Saelens, D., & Heylighen, A. (2022a). Discrepancies between predicted and actual indoor environmental (dis)comfort: The role of hospitalized patients' adaptation strategies. *Building Research & Information*, *50*(7), 792–809.

Willems, S., Saelens, D., & Heylighen, A. (2022b). Patient wellbeing, adaptation of and to indoor conditions, and hospital room design: Two mixed methods case studies. *Building Research & Information*, *50*(1-2), 105–133.

World Health Organization. (2020). *Basic documents* (49th ed.). https://apps.who.int/gb/bd/pdf_files/BD_49th-en.pdf

Xie, H., Clements-Croome, D., & Wang, Q. (2017). Move beyond green building: A focus on healthy, comfortable, sustainable and aesthetical architecture. *Intelligent Buildings International*, *9*(2), 88–96.

Xu, C., & Li, S. (2021). Influence of perceived control on thermal comfort in winter, a case study in hot summer and cold winter zone in China. *Journal of Building Engineering*, *40*, 102389.

Yun, G. Y. (2018). Influences of perceived control on thermal comfort and energy use in buildings. *Energy and Buildings*, *158*, 822–830.

5 Environmental qualities and features in mental and behavioural health environments

Mardelle McCuskey Shepley, Kati Peditto, Naomi A. Sachs, Y Pham, Ruth Barankevich, Gary Crouppen, and Karyn Dresser

Introduction

An increasing body of research, supported by the trend in evidence-based design (EBD; Hamilton & Watkins, 2008), indicates a relationship between the built environment and outcomes for mental and behavioural health (MBH) staff (Haines et al., 2017; Shattell et al., 2015), and patients (Pyrke et al., 2017; Ulrich et al., 2018). As suicide rates in the US continue to increase compared to decreases seen in other developed countries, and as community mental health facilities serve a demonstrated role in suicide prevention, it is important to know more about these facilities (Hedegaard et al., 2018; Hung et al., 2020; OECD, 2015).

Considering the many unique restrictions, vulnerabilities, and challenges that mental health patients face, studies involving MBH patient populations attempt to understand their perspectives and relationships with the environment (Ahern et al., 2016; Schröder et al., 2016; Jovanović et al., 2019). Expanded work within this area has bolstered the identification of features and qualities of the built environment that contribute to patient outcomes. Throughout this chapter, the term "patients" is used to refer to both inpatients and outpatients. The term "residents" refers to inpatients. The term "staff" refers to psychiatric clinical staff.

Design research on MBH facilities

An increasingly broad range of papers has been published on the topic of healthcare facility design research and a detailed summary is beyond the scope of this chapter. Multiple theories serve as the foundation guiding the design of MBH facilities including anthroposophy (Steiner, 2002), generative design (Ruga, 2008), Planetree (Orr, 1995), and salutogenic design (Antonovsky, 1996). Literature published prior to this study on the design of MBH facilities is also ample and includes research on personal space and density (Salerno et al., 2012), choice and control (Johansson et al., 2006), spatial clarity and organisation (Eklund & Hansson, 2001), comfortable and homelike settings (Carr, 2011), positive distraction (Brown et al., 2020;

DOI: 10.1201/9781003344711-6

Nanda et al., 2011; Sachs et al., 2020), social interaction (Gutkowski et al., 1992; Jovanović et al., 2019; Kidd et al. 2015; Smith & Jones, 2014; Southard et al., 2012; Ulrich et al., 2018), access to nature and daylight (Bakos et al., 1980; Kimball et al., 2018; Shattell et al., 2008, 2015; Van der Schaaf et al., 2013), safety (Salerno et al., 2012), supervision (Ulrich et al., 2012), autonomy (Ahern, 2016; Southard et al., 2012), deinstitutionalisation (Bayramzadeh, 2017; Brown et al., 2020; Kalagi et al., 2018; Seppänen et al., 2018; Smith & Jones, 2014; Ulrich et al., 2018), noise (Brown et al., 2020; Camuccio et al., 2019; Haines et al., 2017; Veale et al., 2020), light (Haines et al., 2017; Okkels et al., 2020; Sheaves et al., 2018; Veale et al., 2020), maintenance and cleanliness (Brunero et al., 2009; Cleary et al., 2009; Smith & Jones, 2014), and aesthetics (Wikström et al., 2012).

The research described in this chapter employed the PSED and PPED survey tools. In addition to using surveys (Chrysikou, 2022), researchers working within MBH facilities have also conducted interviews (De Ruysscher et al., 2020; Mabala et al., 2019; Pyrke et al., 2017; Ulrich et al., 2018; Veale et al., 2020), photovoice (Olausson et al., 2021) and focus groups (Rose et al., 2015; Seppänen et al., 2018). Pre- and post-assessments, used in comparing outcomes in a new building or renovation, primarily utilise survey tools (Haines et al., 2017; Southard et al., 2012) but can also incorporate focus groups (Carnemolla et al., 2021) observations or interviews (Ahern et al., 2016).

The role of importance and effectiveness in mental and behavioural settings

When evaluating environments, apart from identifying whether a specific design goal is achieved, researchers must also examine whether a design characteristic is important to occupants. Designers and project teams might approach a project with preconceived notions of what is critical for incorporation. Facility evaluations may demonstrate that their goals have been achieved, but these goals might not reflect user needs. While effectiveness, per Frøkjaer (2000), may be independent of usability, as a component leading to satisfaction (Belanche et al., 2012; Brambilla et al., 2019) it is, along with efficiency and user satisfaction/experience, linked to usability (Alexander, 2006). The study described here addressed the evaluation of four facilities by considering both importance and effectiveness.

Existing literature has found a complicated relationship between staff and patient outcomes and evaluations in MBH facilities, revealing agreement concerning some features and qualities, but discrepancies between others. Most existing work examining perspectives of patients and staff within MBH environments has focused on clinical and demographic factors, with no direct reference to the built environment (Schröder et al., 2016). Unfortunately, even when aspects of the built environment are documented (Sheehan et al., 2013), there is still a gap in literature that examines the relationship between prioritised and present environmental qualities and features (Hedegaard et al., 2018).

Developed to address this gap, the Psychiatric Staff Environmental Design (PSED) (Shepley et al., 2017) tool and the recently developed Psychiatric Patient Environmental Design (PPED) tool provide methods to evaluate the built environment in connection with patient and staff preferences and satisfaction. The current study explores resident and staff evaluations at four MBH facilities in the US with the use of the PSED and PPED. Particular attention is focused on (1) the degree to which environmental qualities and features are considered to be important and effectively provided and (2) the impact on staff and patients. In our previous study (Shepley et al., 2017), the comparison of importance and effectiveness was limited to staff. The research described here also includes the responses of the residents.

The aims of the current study are to (1) identify important environmental attributes and evaluate the effectiveness of these goals in existing facilities, (2) explore the similarities and differences between staff and resident views, and (3) make value-based recommendations for healthcare management, designers, researchers, and future influencers. We anticipated that there would be discrepancies between environmental attributes in MBH facilities that are perceived to be important and those that are presently available (Hypothesis #1). Additionally, we hypothesised that differences would emerge between resident and staff perceptions of the importance and effectiveness of features and qualities, suggesting a difference in priorities between residents and staff (Hypothesis #2).

Methodology

This study used an updated version of the previously developed PSED tool and a newly created PPED tool. To develop the original PSED tool, the researchers began with a literature review and summarised the elements that were commonly cited as being important factors in MBH design. These factors were then vetted through interviews with psychiatric health and design practitioners and revised for the purposes of generating a facility evaluation survey (Mabala et al., 2019). The intent of the survey tool was to explore both the importance and effectiveness of qualities and features of inpatient and outpatient psychiatric environments. Subsequently, the PSED tool was piloted with a pool of psychiatric nurses ($N = 132$) in the US, Canada, Australia, and the UK (Shepley et al., 2017). Based on their input, the PSED was further revised for staff. Additional adaptations were made for patients/residents as the PPED tool.

Settings

Four facilities served as sites for this study, three in California administered by a single healthcare entity (referred to here as CA1, CA2, and CA3), and one in New York (referred to here as NY1). These facilities were selected because they were either recently renovated or planning renovations and the owners expressed an interest in obtaining information on the effectiveness of the facilities. Staff members at all four facilities participated in the PSED, and facilities who allowed us to recruit patients also participated in the PPED (CA1 and CA2).

Built in 2013, CA1 is a short-term facility with 14 beds, integrating individual as well as group counselling, psychiatric services, and introduction to community resources for 18- to 25-year-old individuals facing a mental health crisis. Recovery-based services and interventions last up to 90 days and provide youth with mental and physical health evaluations and services.

CA2, a 16-bed facility, is located in a complex with CA1. It is the newer of the two facilities and built to resemble a single-family home. It was completed in 2017 and staffed with 45 providers, including doctors, nurses, and counsellors. CA2 provides up to 90 days of short-term acute psychiatric treatment to those aged 18–59 years. This recovery-oriented facility provides an opportunity to individuals who could otherwise face hospitalisation, either involuntary or voluntary, or even incarceration.

CA3 was built in 1996 and includes a secure 16-bed facility that provides acute care to help stabilise patients, offering services to individuals ranging from 11 to 17 years old. The programmes include comprehensive services, including physical and psychiatric evaluation and treatment. This facility focuses on those who have endured intense trauma or challenges that necessitate treatment within a secure environment. These three CA facilities reflect the average size of residential treatment facilities in California. As of 2016 (the most recent inventory of California psychiatric services), nearly 50% of residential psychiatric facilities had 15 or fewer clients (SAMHSA, 2017).

NY1, which was evaluated prior to a renovation and expansion of inpatient services, and currently includes 20 adult and six adolescent beds, provides assessment and evaluation to deliver comprehensive treatment including recreation therapy, individual and group therapy, and planning for care after discharge. NY1 reflects the size of typical New York residential treatment facility, as facilities in New York range from 14 to 56 beds (New York State Coalition for Children's Mental Health Services, 2013).

Survey tools

Researchers have developed tools for the evaluation of MBH facilities. Among the most recent are ASPECT (Department of Health, 2008), Satisfaction AT Questionnaire (Müller et al., 2002), Safety Risk Assessment Tool (Center for Health Design, 2015), AEDET (NHS Estates, 2013), and MHEOOC (Watts et al., 2012). The PSED, which was used in this study, was intended to serve as a more traditional practitioner focused occupancy evaluation tool.

The PSED was validated in a study of psychiatric nursing staff (Shepley et al., 2017), the data for which are used in this study as a means of comparing responses longitudinally. After being revised, the PSED was adapted to be used in parallel with patients (PPED). During development of the survey (via the literature review and the interviews), certain characteristics rose to the surface as being specifically pertinent to inpatient facilities and not pertinent to outpatient facilities. For the purposes of making the survey less complicated for the staff respondents (some of whom were not working in residential settings), the researchers created a separate section of the survey to address inpatient facilities that only those who worked in those environments would see. An abridged summary of the questions is provided in Table 5.1. Participants that were current residents or staff members at an inpatient facility were then asked about importance and effectiveness of these elements are incorporated in their *current* environment.

Environmental qualities are defined in this study as overarching conceptual design goals (i.e., well-maintained, access to outdoors, attractive, homelike, and orderly). *Environmental features* are defined as specific physical interventions (i.e., staff safety mechanisms, noise control, daylighting, and comfortable furniture). *Environmental characteristics* are aspects of the environment that contribute to the effectiveness of the previously mentioned environmental qualities (i.e., unrestricted access to kitchen, spaces for therapy animals, and board games). A significant calculated difference between ratings of importance and effectiveness is considered an *inadequacy* in the environment. The relationship between these variables is described in Figure 5.1. While the term "importance" was perceived to be readily understood, the term "effective" was less clear. An effective feature was defined as whether the feature was adequately present in the facility. Definitions for all these terms were integrated into the questionnaire.

Procedure

For CA1 and CA2, direct supervisors sent staff an email with a link to the survey. Clinical staff participated in the online survey during their work shift, being relieved of their resident duties by team members and/or supervisors to allow time to complete the survey. At CA3, staff were recruited for completion of the online version of the PSED with an all-staff email sent by the residential programme director. Follow-up emails were sent to encourage participation to all staff in the middle and towards the end of the recruitment period. In addition, reminders to staff were given about survey completion weekly during morning staff meetings and at departmental meetings. Staff responded to the PSED survey via an email link distributed by a unit administrator and were entered into a drawing for $50.

The PPED was completed by residents in a group environment at both CA1 and CA2. It was introduced to residents each day during group time called "individual goal setting". A group incentive was offered for completing

Table 5.1 Abridged summary of PPED/PSED questions

Environmental attributes	Question
All facilities	
Qualities	Please evaluate the following qualities (attractiveness, homelike, access to outdoors, orderliness and well-maintained) in terms of how *important* you feel they are to the support of patients, staff, and families in all MBH facilities.
	Please evaluate how effectively the following qualities (see above) are incorporated *in your current facility.*
Characteristics	Please rank the following characteristics in terms of the degree to which they can contribute to an *attractive and aesthetically pleasing* environment in *all* MBH facilities: abstract art, art depicting nature, colourful furniture/finishes, visually interesting but relatively orderly, well-designed electric lighting and adequate daylight, and window views of the outdoors.
	Please rank the following characteristics in terms of the degree to which they can contribute to a deinstitutionalised environment in all MBH facilities: furniture/finishes similar to apartment or house, furniture/finishes similar to hotel, physical environments that allow for choice and control, spaces that support privacy, spaces that are comfortable and cozy, spaces that convey respect towards residents and/or facility's mission, accommodating entry space, and artwork or décor.
	Please rank the following characteristics in terms of the degree to which they can contribute to *access to nature and the outdoors* in *all* MBH facilities: outdoor spaces that support patient/resident safety and security, outdoor vegetable or flower gardens for patient/resident gardening, outdoor plants, trees, bird feeders, fountains, and flowers, pleasant outdoor spaces for group activities, pleasant outdoor spaces for one-on-one conversations, pleasant outdoor spaces for sitting alone, and unrestricted access to outdoor spaces.
	Please rank the following characteristics in terms of the degree to which they can contribute to an *orderly and organised environment* in *all* MBH facilities: absence of clutter, all equipment has designated storage area, navigable and readably layout and visually cohesive or matching furniture and finishes.
	Please rank the following characteristics in terms of the degree to which they can contribute to a *well-maintained environment* in *all* MBH facilities: clean floors, walls, and other surfaces, furniture and finishes in good condition, properly operating electrical fixtures and heating/cooling systems, and properly operating equipment.

(Continued)

Table 5.1 (Continued)

Environmental attributes	Question
Features	Please evaluate the following features (attractive furniture, comfortable furniture, damage resistant furniture, acoustics, daylight, electric lighting, staff safety, staff respite) in terms of how *important* you feel they are to the support of patients, staff, and families in all MBH facilities. Please evaluate how *effectively* the following features (see above) are incorporated *in your current facility.*
Inpatient facilities	
Qualities	Please evaluate the following qualities (autonomy, distraction, interaction, respite, suicide resistance) in terms of how important you feel they are to the support of patients, staff, and families in *all inpatient* MBH facilities. Please evaluate how *effectively* the following qualities (see above) are incorporated *in your current facility.*
Characteristics	Please rank the following characteristics in terms of their contributions to *autonomy and spontaneity* in an *inpatient* MVH facility: unrestricted access to exercise area, unrestricted access to outdoor spaces, unrestricted access to snack areas or kitchens, and unrestricted access to technology/entertainment. Please rank the following characteristics in terms of their contribution to *positive distraction* in an *inpatient* MBH facility: board games, playing cards, etc., books, magazines, newspapers, facilities and equipment for exercise, music systems, television, spaces for therapy animals, video game systems, indoor plants and/or decorative water features, and artwork. Please rank the following characteristics in terms of their positive contribution to *social interaction and community* in an *inpatient* MBH facility: group therapy rooms, group activity rooms, dining spaces, and outdoor spaces.
Features	Please evaluate the following features (therapy, observation, seating, smoking, counselling, enclosed/open nurse station, bathrooms) in terms of importance in *inpatient* MBH facilities. Please evaluate how *effectively* the following features (see above) are incorporated *in your current facility.*

the surveys to encourage high levels of participation, which entailed a pizza party that was given the week after survey completion. During the group time that was available for completion of the surveys at both programmes, the lead therapists reviewed the instructions that are included on the first page of the survey and assisted patients with understanding the meaning of words and with questions/items that needed clarification. The lead therapists

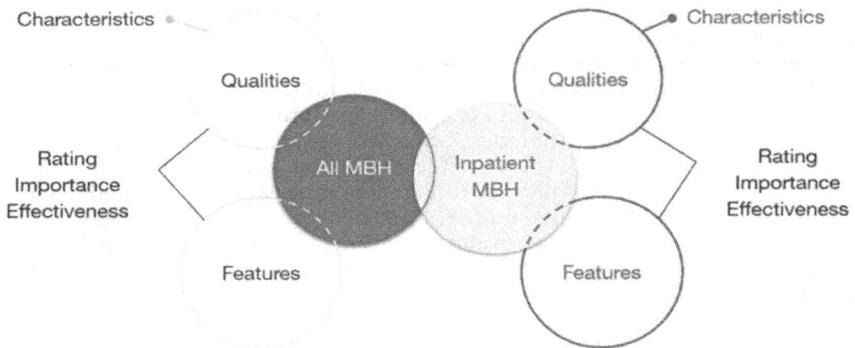

Figure 5.1 PPED/PSED framework.

assembled the surveys in envelopes at the end of the administration week and forwarded the envelopes to the administrator who oversees both programmes. The administrator scanned the completed patient surveys which were then securely emailed to the researchers. Residents in NY did not complete the survey due to hospital restrictions.

Participant demographics

One-hundred and fifty-eight participants completed the PSED, including 34 staff members at CA1, 32 staff members at CA2, 50 staff members at CA3, and 32 staff members at NY1 (Table 5.2). Ten respondents did not indicate a facility name, so their results were excluded from any facility-specific analysis. Most respondents selected "Psychiatric Nurse" ($n = 23$) or "Programme Staff" ($n = 23$) as their job title, although respondents included a wide range of staff positions, including administrative, clinical, and counselling staff. Many respondents had at least one year of experience in MBH (85.7%), with MBH experience ranging from less than one year to over 30 years. Similarly, most respondents had worked in their current facility for at least one year (67.9%). As the sample size was relatively small, other demographic data were not gathered as demographic analyses would be underpowered.

Twenty-four residents completed the PPED, including 12 residents at CA1 and 12 residents at CA2 (Table 5.3). Only CA1 and CA2 facilities provided both resident and staff surveys. All residents at CA3 and some at NY1 were adolescents and thus not eligible for participation in this study. The NY1 facility opted not to allow access to their residents. Most residents were between the ages of 20–24 ($n = 12$), with participants from 20 to 50+ years of age. Length of stay at current facility ranged from six days to 83 days ($M = 33$ days, $SD = 23$). As the sample size was relatively small, other demographic data were not gathered and demographic analyses would be underpowered.

Table 5.2 Frequency statistics by demographic variables: staff

Characteristic: staff (PSED)	n	%
Site		
CA1	34	22.9
CA2	32	21.6
CA3	50	33.7
NY1	32	21.6
Job Title		
Psychiatric nurse	23	15.5
Program staff	23	15.5
Psychiatric technician	8	5.4
Administrator	5	3.3
Educator	4	2.7
Psychiatric social worker	2	1.3
Other	47	31.8
Experience in MBH		
<1 year	16	10.8
1–5 years	49	33.1
6–10 years	18	12.2
11–15 years	15	10.1
16–20 years	6	4.1
21–30 years	6	4.1
>30 years	2	1.3
Experience at current facility		
<1 year	36	24.3
1–5 years	50	33.8
6–10 years	13	8.8
11–15 years	7	4.7
16–20 years	6	4.1

Analytical methods

PSED and PPED participants were first asked to rate the importance of environmental qualities and features across all MBH facilities, followed by a rating of the effectiveness of these elements in their current facility. To test Hypothesis #1, four sets of paired *t*-tests between importance and effectiveness were performed:

1 Staff: Difference between ratings of importance and effectiveness of elements in all MBH facilities.
2 Residents: Difference between ratings of importance and effectiveness of elements in all MBH facilities.
3 Staff: Difference between importance and effectiveness in current inpatient facility.
4 Residents: Difference between importance and effectiveness in current inpatient facility.

Table 5.3 Frequency statistics by demographic variables: resident

Characteristic: patient (PPED)	n	%
Site		
CA1	12	50.0
CA2	12	50.0
Age at time of questionnaire		
20–24	12	50.0
25–30	2	8.3
31–40	4	16.6
41–50	4	16.6
>50	2	8.3
Current length of stay		
<3 days	0	0
3–5 days	0	0
5–10 days	3	12.5
11–20 days	5	20.8
21–30 days	5	2.08
31–50 days	4	16.6
>50 days	6	25.0

Although Wilcoxon's signed-rank test (a non-parametric approach) is often recommended for Likert-style ordinal data, *t*-tests can reduce Type II error in Likert data, even with small sample sizes when assumptions have been violated. To protect from Type I error (a false positive when incorrectly rejecting a true null hypothesis) when conducting multiple comparisons, we used a more conservative alpha-value corrected with the Bonferroni statistical method.

To test Hypothesis #2, participants' difference scores between importance and effectiveness for all 15 inpatient environmental qualities and features were averaged to create a single "inadequacy" score for everyone. Inadequacy was calculated as *importance* minus *effectiveness* for each resident and each feature. Mean inadequacy of a facility was also calculated as the average inadequacy scores of residents within a facility. Two sets of independent samples *t*-tests were performed on these adequacy scores:

1 Difference in inadequacy scores between residents and staff at CA1.
2 Difference in inadequacy scores between residents and staff at CA2.

Only scores from CA1 and CA2 were included in the resident analysis because resident responses were not collected from CA3 or NY1.

Apart from the hypotheses described above we were interested in comparing the results from the 2017 study with psychiatric nurses to see whether there were consistencies in the responses.

Results

Importance and effectiveness

When comparing most and least important characteristics, there are some consistencies between the 2017 PSED study and the current PSED study (Figures 5.2 and 5.3). Staff safety and security in all settings and suicide resistance (design which reduces the opportunity for self-harm, such as features

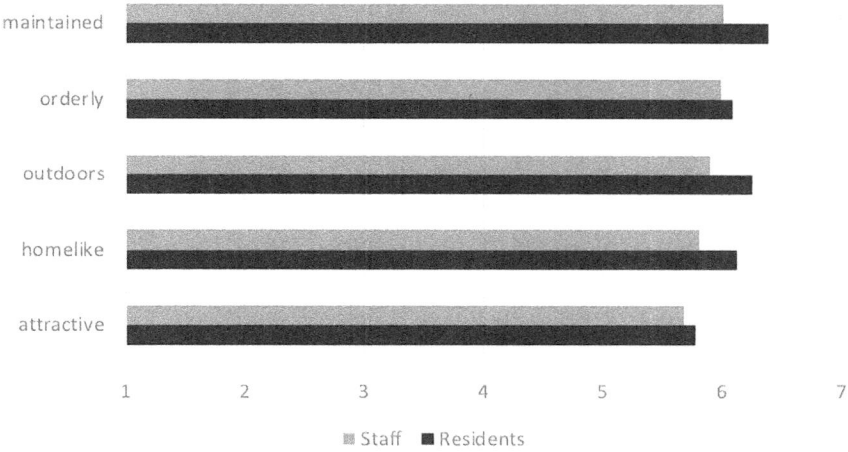

Figure 5.2 Importance of environmental qualities (Likert scale, 1–7).

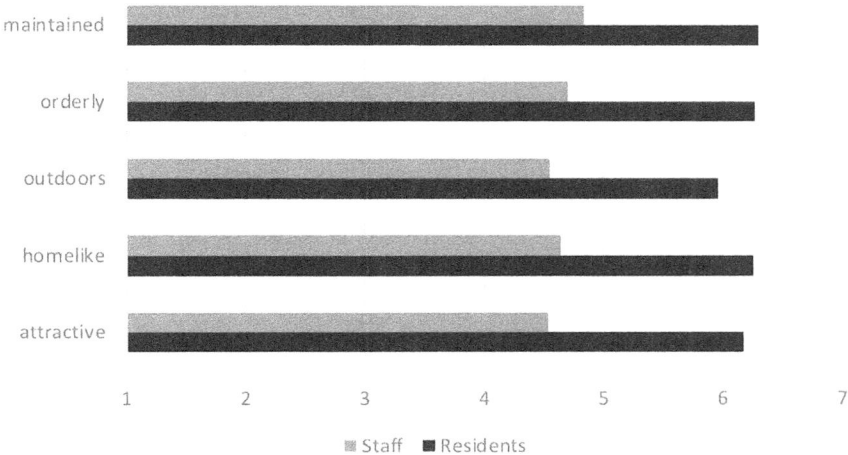

Figure 5.3 Effectiveness of environmental qualities (Likert scale, 1–7).

that avoid the opportunity for ligature) within inpatient settings (M_{2020} = 6.41; M_{2017} = 6.71) received the highest scores. Within all MBH settings, acoustical control and daylighting were also ranked highly in both studies. Attractive furniture was rated lowest in both studies (M_{2020} = 5.13; M_{2017} = 5.53), with deinstitutionalised/homelike environments receiving similarly lower ratings (M_{2020} = 5.81; M_{2017} = 5.88), although these ratings are still high compared to inpatient settings, where the lowest feature was rated significantly less important (smoking = 3.23).

Adequacy of all MBH environments

Overall, the facilities received relatively high ratings, particularly the CA units, in most categories on a 7-point Likert scale; however, the strength of the support varied across topics. Figures 5.2 and 5.3 summarise the staff and resident responses to the qualities of all MBH environments. The first section of the survey asked residents and staff to provide ratings based on their experience across *all* MBH facilities. When considering qualities that support staff, residents, and families across all facilities, there was a significant difference between staff ratings of importance and effectiveness across all five general qualities, $t(140) \geq 6.80$, $p < 0.0001$, where $\alpha_{adj} = (0.05/5) = 0.01$. In contrast, resident evaluations did not reveal any significant inadequacies (Table 5.4).

Adequacy of inpatient facilities

Of the 23 inpatient qualities and features evaluated by staff, there were significant inadequacies among 17 elements, where $\alpha_{adj} = (0.05/23) = 0.002$ (Table 5.4). Residents, however, did not report any inadequacies. In many cases, resident ratings of effectiveness exceeded ratings of importance.

To further investigate inadequacies reported by staff, participants were divided based on their parent organisation, creating two groups: (1) CA1, CA2, and CA3 and (2) NY1. A one-way ANOVA (a statistical tool to analyze differences in variance between samples) revealed no significant difference between the three CA facilities, but a significant difference between CA facilities and NY1 in evaluations of all five environmental qualities (attractive, homelike, outdoor access, orderly, and well-maintained). Staff at NY1 reported significantly greater inadequacies across all five qualities compared to staff across CA facilities.

Comparison of staff and patient evaluations

When comparing CA1 and CA2, staff reported inadequacies (M = 0.43, SD = 0.87) while residents did not (M = −0.15, SD = 0.50), where a higher number indicates larger inadequacy scores (Figure 5.4). A two-way ANOVA suggests a significant difference between staff and resident ratings, $F(1,77) = 9.01$, $p = 0.004$.

Table 5.4 Differences in importance and effectiveness between residents and staff

	Residents			Staff		
	M (SD) *Importance*	*Effectiveness*	t	M (SD) *Importance*	*Effectiveness*	t
General qualities						
Attractive/aesthetic space	5.78 (1.24)	6.17 (0.98)	−1.62	5.68 (1.33)	4.53 (1.73)	6.80*
Deinstitutional/homelike space	6.13 (0.69)	6.26 (0.62)	−1.00	5.81 (1.31)	4.64 (1.74)	7.68*
Outdoor spaces and views of nature	6.26 (0.81)	5.96 (0.88)	1.67	5.90 (1.39)	4.55 (1.81)	7.31*
Orderly space	6.09 (0.92)	6.27 (0.88)	−0.85	5.99 (1.30)	4.70 (1.65)	8.50*
Well-maintained	6.39 (0.50)	6.30 (0.93)	0.46	6.01 (1.48)	4.84 (1.63)	7.69*
Inpatient qualities and features						
Autonomy/spontaneity	5.96 (1.22)	6.00 (1.09)	−0.16	5.64 (1.09)	4.98 (1.30)	5.00*
Positive distraction	6.30 (0.64)	6.39 (0.66)	−1.00	6.13 (0.86)	5.10 (1.24)	8.38*
Social interaction	6.26 (0.75)	6.39 (0.66)	−1.00	6.21 (1.01)	5.57 (1.11)	5.75*
Staff respite	6.36 (0.73)	6.09 (1.02)	1.55	6.22 (0.88)	4.55 (1.88)	8.62*
Suicide resistance	6.57 (0.51)	6.57 (0.51)	0.00	6.41 (1.09)	5.79 (1.16)	6.22*
Indoor therapy (PT, OT, music, etc.)	6.13 (0.92)	6.09 (0.79)	0.21	6.16 (0.89)	5.49 (1.36)	5.39*
Direct observation	6.04 (0.93)	6.17 (0.89)	−0.59	6.28 (1.05)	5.56 (1.37)	5.52*
Mix of seating	6.05 (0.85)	6.21 (0.71)	−1.37	5.40 (1.28)	5.10 (1.45)	2.21
Smoking	4.05 (2.24)	4.68 (1.67)	−1.23	3.23 (1.97)	3.86 (2.01)	−2.97
Staff-patient consulting	6.14 (0.77)	6.00 (0.93)	0.77	6.08 (1.06)	5.23 (1.57)	5.46*
Enclosed nurse station	5.73 (1.67)	6.14 (0.89)	−1.34	5.51 (1.49)	5.61 (1.30)	−0.75
Open nurse station	4.81 (2.04)	4.71 (2.03)	0.21	4.38 (1.88)	4.30 (1.71)	0.59

(*Continued*)

Table 5.4 (Continued)

	Residents			Staff		
	M (SD) Importance	Effectiveness	t	M (SD) Importance	Effectiveness	t
Small cluster of patients (1–12 per unit)	6.22 (1.17)	6.39 (0.66)	-0.75	5.78 (1.26)	5.01 (1.65)	4.42[*]
Private bedrooms	6.09 (1.13)	5.96 (0.98)	0.57	5.13 (1.56)	4.78 (1.66)	1.92
Private bathrooms	6.43 (0.59)	5.87 (1.14)	2.51	5.14 (1.53)	4.73 (1.67)	2.54[*]
Attractive furniture	5.30 (1.15)	6.17 (0.83)	-3.54	5.13 (1.16)	4.69 (1.51)	3.20[*]
Comfortable furniture	6.00 (0.95)	6.30 (0.82)	-2.08	5.93 (1.02)	4.87 (1.54)	7.20[*]
Damage-resistant furniture	5.87 (0.97)	5.91 (1.08)	-0.17	5.93 (1.17)	4.80 (1.57)	7.15[*]
Good acoustical control	5.90 (0.94)	6.29 (0.64)	-1.79	6.17 (0.99)	4.50 (1.43)	11.34[*]
Good daylight	6.18 (0.66)	6.23 (0.97)	-0.20	6.17 (0.99)	4.47 (1.87)	8.70[*]
Good electric lighting	6.32 (0.65)	6.32 (0.72)	0.00	6.02 (1.08)	4.80 (1.66)	7.85[*]
Staff safety and security	6.48 (0.59)	6.30 (0.93)	0.89	6.52 (1.24)	5.02 (1.69)	8.62[*]
Space for staff respite	6.14 (0.83)	5.91 (1.02)	1.05	6.25 (0.96)	4.45 (2.01)	9.10[*]

Note.
[*] A significant inadequacy, defined as the difference between importance and effectiveness (α adjusted with Bonferroni corrections).

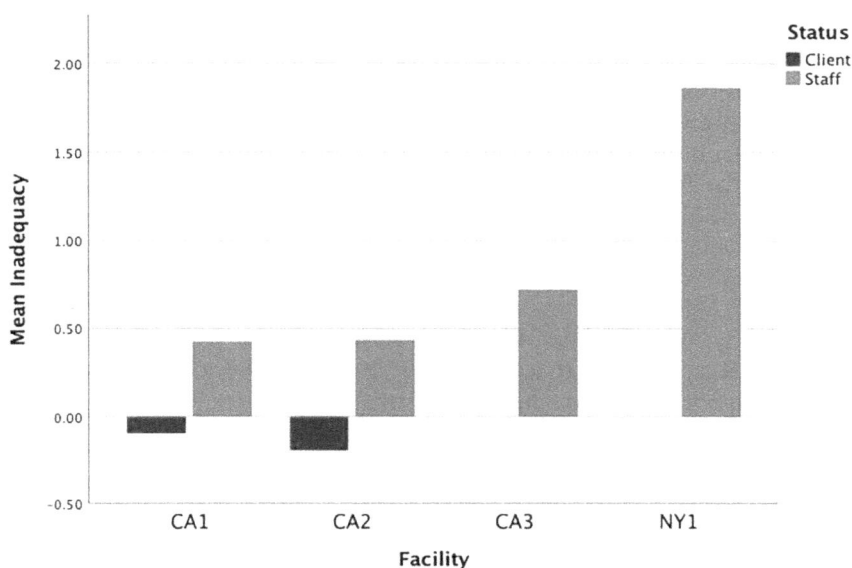

Figure 5.4 Mean inadequacy by facility.

Discussion

Importance and effectiveness

Hypothesis #1 was partially supported, as staff across all four facilities reported significant inadequacies in their environments. Residents, however, did not report the same inadequacies (Table 5.4, Hypothesis #2). Inadequacies may be the result of long-standing design trends and practices in MBH facilities, with only a recent interest in optimising these environments through patient-centred design and EBD. Since there is still a lack of rigorous research in this area, researchers have suggested the use of best practices to inform design decisions (Karlin & Zeiss, 2006), although further examination of existing evidence has revealed a deficiency in systematised guidelines for best practices (Shepley et al., 2016).

Considering the unique characteristics of MBH populations, special focus is often placed on safety components of patient/resident spaces and outcomes. While these measures are critical in determining the success of psychiatric facilities in preventing injury or harm to patients and staff, an examination of all contributing environmental components is vital and often missing. For example, many studies ask patients about their satisfaction with broad concepts like cleanliness and privacy (Brunero et al., 2009; Cleary et al., 2009). While some staff surveys include environmental components (Pink et al., 2020; Pyrke et al., 2017), they are often considered indirectly through the lens of staff safety (Jenkin et al., 2022), satisfaction, or well-being (Holmberg et al., 2016; Kelly et al. 2016).

Staff safety and security in all settings and suicide resistance within inpatient settings received the highest scores. These results are expected, as this population requires special consideration due to increased concerns of safety, both of patients and staff (Bayramzadeh, 2017). Suicide prevention is a mandate of the Joint Commission (JACHO) and a prominent consideration in the design of all psychiatric facilities. Rates of suicide per 100,000 inpatient years have risen in recent years and may be attributed to characteristics of the facility design (Walsh et al., 2015).

Across all MBH settings, acoustical control and daylighting were also ranked highly in importance. Previous research on the negative impact of noise in healthcare settings (Cunha & Silva, 2015) corroborates this finding as well as the importance of daylighting (Ulrich, 2012).

Comparing staff and resident perspectives

There is likely an inherent difference between what residents need for therapy and what staff need for work, although staff tend to appreciate environments that promote healing. Additionally, staff's greater familiarity with the building might make them more aware of the shortcomings. There was a significant difference between resident and staff ratings, supporting Hypothesis #2. Post-hoc tests revealed staff at NY1 reported significantly greater inadequacies compared to staff at CA1, CA3, and CA2. Because NY1 was the site of greatest inadequacy among staff, we may expect that NY1 residents would report similar concerns if they had been included in the study.

Within MBH environments, a comparison of assessments between staff and patient groups contains complexities. Evaluations of an MBH patient room and private bathroom mockup found that patients and staff agreed on the importance of safety, as well as deinstitutionalisation and homeyness, with access to daylight and control of lighting rated as the most positive characteristics (Sachs et al., 2020). Interviews discussing open-door wards with psychiatric nurses, psychiatrists, and patients revealed general agreement in their views of several strategies, including the importance of nature, the presence of seclusion rooms, and patient observation (Kalagi et al., 2018).

However, perhaps due to psychiatric patient characteristics and differing roles and responsibilities between staff and patients (Ulrich et al., 2012), other studies have revealed more pronounced differences in opinions (Rose et al., 2015; de Vries et al., 2016). In assessing different themes found within focus groups of both patients and staff, Rose et al. (2015) summarises that "the experiences of the two groups are characterised by different interpretations of the same themes" (p. 94).

When evaluating the ward climate of a secure facility, patient ratings of experienced safety and patient cohesion were higher than staff ratings, while staff evaluations were higher for the environment's ability to support therapy (de Vries et al., 2016). These findings for the safety and therapeutic environment dimensions were consistent with earlier ward climate studies (Dickens et al., 2014; de Vries et al., 2016). Other studies have found lower ratings by patients (De Ruysscher et al., 2020; Sachs et al., 2020). While consideration of individual variables revealed significant differences only for staff control, where patients had higher ratings than staff, results of the Ward Atmosphere Scale (WAS) showed consistently higher scores by staff than patients (Nicholls et al., 2015). A comparison of views after remodelling a nursing station into an open station revealed varied opinions between patients and staff (Southard et al., 2012). While nurses expressed concerns about increased work interruption, privacy, and confidentiality, patients felt liberated by the change and expressed a higher perception of safety due to increased supervision as well as connection to staff.

The results of this study show little agreement regarding the effectiveness of qualities (Figure 5.2) and more similarity regarding importance of these qualities (Figure 5.3) between residents and staff. There was some agreement on the importance of the following features: social interaction, indoor therapy, staff-patient consulting, open nurse stations, comfortable furniture, good daylight, and staff safety and security. Resident ratings were higher than staff ratings in this study, which could be explained by the nature of patient interactions with the ward environment. Specifically, resident exposure to the environment was short ($M = 33$ days), while most staff had worked at the site more than a year.

The ratings in this study are different than some previous MBH studies, where residents had lower ratings than staff (Cleary et al., 2009; Sachs et al., 2020). This could be a result of the lack of staff familiarity with the setting—one study was conducted two months after the move to a new facility, and the other used a mockup design.

Comparing evaluations between 2017 and 2020

When considering all settings, the 2017 and 2020 PSED studies had statistically similar ratings of all attributes. Additionally, there were consistently higher ratings of staff safety and security, good electric lighting, and well-maintained space and lower ratings of good acoustical control and staff respite. Several previous studies have highlighted a need for staff respite spaces (Shepley et al., 2016) and a lack of acoustical control, with the design of facilities contributing to noise levels (Brown et al., 2020; Veale et al., 2020). Similarly, an examination of inpatient settings revealed similarities on most attributes. Suicide resistance and social interaction received higher ratings in both studies, while space for staff respite and smoking received lower ratings.

Similar to ratings of importance, agreement on the effectiveness of certain attributes was mixed between the two studies (Table 5.5 and Figures 5.5 and 5.6). While ratings in the current study found staff safety and security, comfortable furniture, and well-maintained space as the most effective attributes in all settings, and suicide resistance, enclosed nursing stations, and

Table 5.5 Differences in importance and effectiveness (staff) between the 2020 and 2017 studies

		Importance			Effectiveness	
		M (SD)			M (SD)	
		2020	*2017*		*2020*	*2017*
All setting qualities and features						
Staff safety and security	1	6.52 (1.24)	6.60 (0.84)	1	5.02 (1.69)	5.12 (1.50)
Staff respite	2	6.22 (0.88)	5.87 (1.33)	10	4.55 (1.88)	4.11 (1.73)
Good acoustical control	3	6.17 (0.99)	6.38 (0.74)	12	4.50 (1.43)	3.81 (1.83)
Good daylight	4	6.17 (0.99)	6.33 (0.75)	13	4.47 (1.87)	4.79 (1.61)
Good electric lighting	5	6.02 (1.08)	6.09 (0.74)	4	4.80 (1.66)	5.21 (1.33)
Well-maintained	6	6.01 (1.48)	6.26 (0.69)	3	4.84 (1.63)	4.98 (1.46)
Orderly space	7	5.99 (1.30)	5.80 (0.96)	6	4.70 (1.65)	4.71 (1.42)
Comfortable furniture	8	5.93 (1.02)	6.11 (0.78)	2	4.87 (1.54)	4.55 (1.38)
Damage-resistant furniture	9	5.93 (1.17)	5.90 (1.15)	5	4.80 (1.57)	5.15 (1.31)
Outdoor spaces and views of nature	10	5.90 (1.39)	6.01 (0.80)	9	4.55 (1.81)	4.22 (1.77)
Deinstitutional/homelike space	11	5.81 (1.31)	5.88 (1.03)	8	4.64 (1.74)	4.29 (1.77)
Attractive/aesthetic space	12	5.68 (1.33)	5.92 (0.95)	11	4.53 (17.3)	4.43 (1.64)
Attractive furniture	13	5.13 (1.16)	5.53 (1.00)	7	4.69 (1.51)	4.55 (1.48)
Inpatient qualities and features						
Suicide resistance	1	6.41 (1.09)	6.71 (0.61)	1	5.79 (1.16)	5.78 (0.98)[*]
Direct observation	2	6.28 (1.05)	6.08 (1.18)	4	5.56 (1.37)	4.81 (1.75)
Space for staff respite	3	6.25 (0.96)	6.11 (0.86)	13	4.45 (2.01)	3.46 (1.60)
Social interaction	4	6.21 (1.01)	6.00 (0.68)	3	5.57 (1.11)	4.90 (1.18)
Indoor therapy (PT, OT, music, etc.)	5	6.16 (0.89)	6.46 (0.82)	5	5.49 (1.36)	5.03 (1.52)
Positive distraction	6	6.13 (0.86)	6.47 (0.61)	7	5.10 (1.24)	4.85 (1.25)
Staff-patient consulting	7	6.08 (1.06)	6.35 (0.87)	6	5.23 (1.57)	4.79 (1.63)
Small clusters of patients (1–12/unit)	8	5.78 (1.26)	6.13 (0.83)	9	5.01 (1.65)	[*]
Autonomy/spontaneity	9	5.64 (1.09)	5.84 (0.84)	10	4.98 (1.30)	3.92 (1.57)
Enclosed nurse station	10	5.51 (1.49)	3.68 (1.84)	2	5.61 (1.30)	3.57 (1.94)
Mix of seating	11	5.40 (1.28)	5.52 (1.19)	8	5.10 (1.45)	4.24 (1.68)
Private bathrooms	12	5.14 (1.53)	5.82 (1.07)	12	4.73 (1.67)	[*]
Private bedrooms	13	5.13 (1.56)	5.84 (0.95)	11	4.78 (1.66)	[*]
Open nurse station	14	4.38 (1.88)	5.27 (1.61)	14	4.30 (1.71)	4.62 (1.85)
Smoking	15	3.23 (1.97)	3.49 (2.39)	15	3.86 (2.01)	3.50 (2.14)

Notes

[*] *Small number of patients* was added in 2020. *Private bathrooms* and *private bedrooms* were characterised as *shared bathrooms* and *shared bedrooms* in 2017 and bundled under "suicide resistance" for 2017 ratings of importance and effectiveness.

social interaction receiving highest scores for the inpatient settings, these ratings were not wholly consistent the 2017 study results.

Ratings of the effectiveness of all settings reveal a broader range of scores in the 2017 study ($\Delta = 1.70$) than the current one ($\Delta = 0.55$). Similar trends occur for inpatient attributes, although less stark (2017: $\Delta = 2.32$; 2020: $\Delta = 1.93$). Discussion of similar rankings, therefore, does not always indicate similar scores between the two studies.

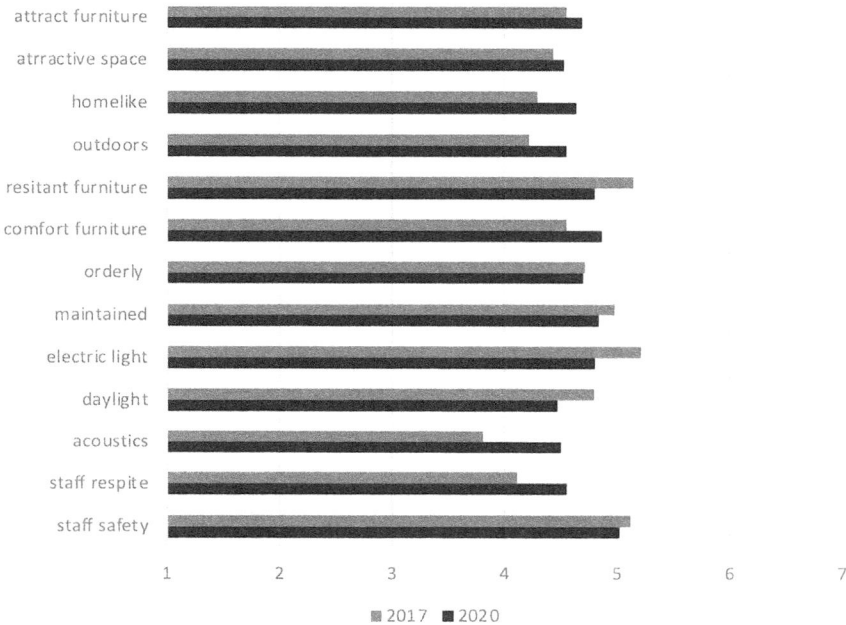

Figure 5.5 Staff rankings of importance differences between the 2020 and 2017 studies (Likert scale, 1–7).

Although there are many convergent findings among our studies (and others in the field), we were surprised by several results. When looking specifically at importance within residential MBH environments, there were some differences between the 2017 and 2020 studies. Although suicide resistance received the highest ratings in both 2017 and 2020, all other similarities were for the lowest-scoring attributes: private bathrooms, open nurse stations, and smoking. An examination of scores for private bathrooms, private bedrooms, and open nurse stations reveals a shift from higher scores in 2017 to lower scores in 2020 (Table 5.5), while a reverse pattern occurs for enclosed nursing stations.

Although most differences between survey years were not significant, enclosed nursing stations were viewed as significantly more important *and* effective in 2020 than 2017. For several years, health design literature has debated the influence of open versus enclosed nursing stations on both residents and staff. In MBH facilities, open nursing stations may improve communication and satisfaction (Shattell et al., 2015) without risking aggression or affecting the therapeutic milieu compared to enclosed stations (Southard et al., 2012). While recent literature on open nursing stations is promising, it is likely that design practices and occupant opinions do not reflect this evidence yet.

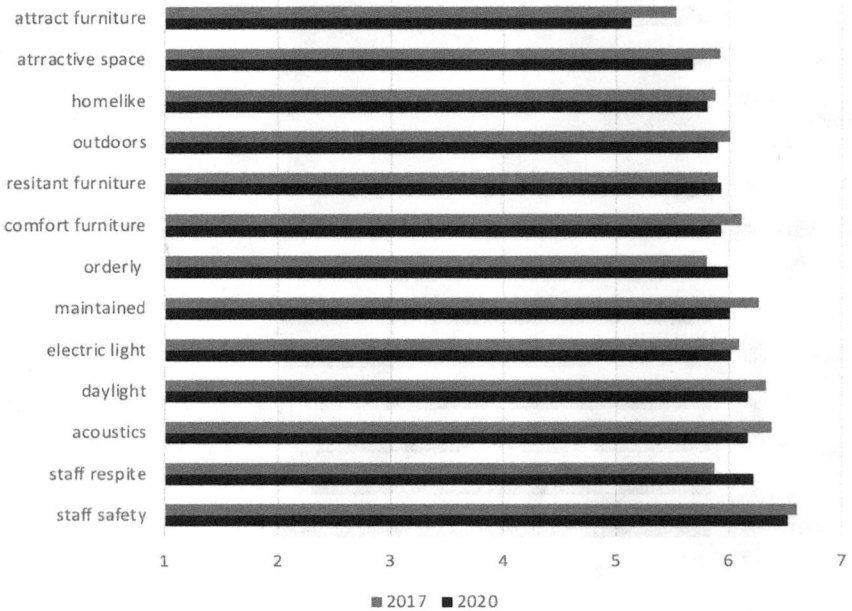

Figure 5.6 Staff rankings of effectiveness differences between the 2020 and 2017 studies (Likert scale, 1–7).

Across both the 2017 and 2020 studies, we also expected to see the importance of *deinstitutionalised/homelike environment* rated low compared to other qualities, given the importance placed on deinstitutionalisation in previous literature (Christensen, 2015; Sachs et al., 2020; Tapak, 2012). It is worth noting, however, that the average ratings ($M_{2020} = 5.81$; $M_{2017} = 5.88$) are still quite high on a 7-point Likert scale.

Limitations and future research

With only four facilities and two states represented, and with fewer resident participants than staff, we were limited in our ability to generalise the results to MBH facilities at large. Because two of the facilities were located on the same property, it is also possible that participants had experience in both facilities which could lead to non-independence of their evaluations. By comparing data from the current study and the previous study, we sought to increase the validity and generalisability of these results, despite sample size limitations.

Future studies using the PSED and PPED tools may be more generalisable if the number of participants was increased and included a more diverse population. A larger sample size and improved demographic information would enable researchers to address the impact of racial and social determinants on perceptions of MBH environments.

As the purpose of this study was to focus on perception of the physical environment, outcome measures such as length of stay or staff retention were not gathered. Subsequent studies might examine highly evaluated facilities (i.e., facilities where importance and effectiveness are comparable) to measure these variables.

Conclusions

We examined the importance of various environmental attributes, the differences between importance and how effectively these attributes were achieved, and the differences between psychiatric staff and resident responses. The most important qualities for residents were a well-maintained environment and suicide resistance. For staff they were staff safety, security, and suicide resistance. Rated across all facilities, staff reported significant differences between importance and effectiveness of environmental attributes ($p < 0.0001$), whereas residents did not report differences. Significant differences were found between staff and resident ratings of existing facilities ($p = 0.004$), with staff reporting more inadequacies than residents. Findings suggest a strong need for more supportive physical MBH environments, particularly from the perspective of staff.

Quantitative studies on the physical environment are almost exclusively correlational and often propose a "bundle" of changes, making it difficult to parse out which individual design components have impacts. Even when design changes are minimal and directed towards a certain component (Ulrich et al., 2018), changes to more than one feature or quality of the built environment is almost inevitable, requiring careful consideration and exploration of features and qualities to understand the contribution of each one. This quantitative study aimed to overcome these limitations by utilising the PSED and PPED tools to analyze specific qualities and features of MBH facilities.

Over the course of two studies, multiple years, and several different facilities in the US, MBH staff have reported significant differences between the importance and effectiveness of features in their environment, indicating design inadequacies. Additionally, staff have reported greater inadequacy in the environment than residents. These findings suggest a strong need for more appropriate physical MBH environments, particularly from the perspective of the staff who work in these spaces. While residents were less concerned about the quality of their facilities, staff, whose primary focus is to support their patients, were acutely aware of the need for improvement. Future research must consider the importance of quantitative and qualitative assessments from both patients and staff, to establish more effective EBD guidelines for MBH environments.

Regarding specific recommendations for the design of MBH environments, facilities that focus on resident suicide prevention and staff safety and respite are essential, regardless of budget limitations or international geographic location. Most facilities address the resident issues carefully by specifying ligature resistant hardware and fixtures and shatterproof materials (e.g., polycarbonate glazing) in resident areas. Regarding staff safety, spaces to which a staff member can quickly withdraw from patient aggression, and lounge spaces with access to nature are essential.

For the next level of environmental support, the selection of materials and room configuration and proportions to address acoustic control and good daylighting are essential. Materials should be sound absorptive but resilient to vandalism and rooms should be laid out to reduce sound reverberation by avoiding high ceilings. Daylighting can be achieved via windows, clerestories, and skylights, and when the site is limited daylight simulating lighting systems that reflect diurnal variation can be implemented. Likewise, when views of nature are minimal, the introduction of indoor plants and nature art can be supplemental. Preliminary research suggests that these features might contribute to reduced patient aggression and therefore increased safety for all (Ulrich et al., 2018). For specific recommendations to achieve these goals, designers might consult the guidelines outlined by Hunt et al. (2018).

Researchers note the incompatible requirements for mental health facilities, such as the need for a dense, efficient layout versus providing residents with sufficient space (Batrakova, 2021) and potential conflicts between a healing environment and a safe one (Lundin, 2021). Acknowledging these conflicts and based on the research generated from this study, it is difficult to judge the hierarchy of the environmental factors. Staff safety and security and suicide resistance were prioritised, but other environmental interventions such as acoustic control and daylighting were also valued. Whether these items can be considered as basic human rights (more so than other elements) raises an interesting discussion.

Design research on MBH environments is limited, although progress is being made to identify the components that should be considered, as new and re-modelled building projects are contemplated. The results of this study can be applied to the design of future environments. Two new mental healthcare environmental prototypes are being implemented and the PSED/PPED tools might be useful in exploring their effectiveness. These prototypes are the Emergency Psychiatric Assessment, Treatment, and Healing (EmPATH) model, which endeavours to support mental health emergency facilities by locating patients in a residential-like open space (Zeller, 2017, 2018; Zeller & Christensen, 2021), and community crisis centres that provide local access to triage and referral services. Initial research on EmPATH facilities has revealed reduced length of stay and increased emergency department revenue (Stamy et al., 2021), and a reduction in admissions for patients presenting with psychiatric ideation (Kim et al., 2022). The need to validate new design trends is critical. Simonsen and Duff (2021) found that efforts to create a transparent spatial experience in the nursing station design of a psychiatric facility had a negative impact on staff and patient relations due to implications of distance and uncertainty.

One of the lessons learned is that the goals of the project team might not reflect the desires of the facility users and they should be queried as part of the design process. In that context, we recommend designers address those components of the environment that have been found to be most important to residents in this study: suicide resistance, easily maintained, staff respite and safety, good electric lighting, and positive distraction; and those components most important to staff: suicide resistance, ability to directly observe residents, staff safety and security, and staff respite.

Acknowledgements

This research project was approved by the study sites under the ethical oversight of the Cornell University Institutional Review Board (#1802007752).

Disclosure statement: The authors have no financial interest or benefit arising from the direct applications of our research.

References

Ahern, C. C., Bieling, P., McKinnon, M. C., McNeely, H. E., & Langstaff, K. (2016). A recovery-oriented care approach: Weighing the pros and cons of a newly built mental health facility. *Journal of Psychosocial Nursing and Mental Health Services*, *54*(2), 39–48.

Alexander, K. (2006). The application of usability concepts in the built environment. *Journal of Facilities Management*, *4*(4), 262–270.

Antonovsky, A. (1996). The salutogenic model as a theory to guide health promotion. *Health Promotion International*, *11*(1), 11–18.

Bakos, M., Bozic, R., Chapin, D., & Neuman, S. (1980). Effects of environmental changes on elderly residents' behavior. *Psychiatric Services*, *31*(10), 677–682.

Batrakova, N. (2021). Design dilemmas in mental hospital architecture. In *ARCH19 June 12–13, 2019–Trondheim, Norway. Proceedings from the 4th Conference on Architecture Research Care & Health*. SINTEF Academic Press.

Bayramzadeh, S. (2017). An assessment of levels of safety in psychiatric units. *HERD: Health Environments Research & Design Journal*, *10*(2), 66–80.

Belanche, D., Casaló, L. V., & Guinalíu, M. (2012). Website usability, consumer satisfaction and the intention to use a website: The moderating effect of perceived risk. *Journal of Retailing and Consumer Services*, *19*(1), 124–132.

Brambilla, A., Rebecchi, A., & Capolongo, S. (2019). Evidence based hospital design: A literature review of the recent publications about the EBD impact of built environment on hospital occupants' and organizational outcomes. *Annali di Igiene: Medicina Preventiva e di Comunita*, *31*(2), 165–180.

Brown, S. D., Kanyeredzi, A., McGrath, L., Reavey, P., & Tucker, I. (2020). Organizing the sensory: Ear-work, panauralism and sonic agency on a forensic psychiatric unit. *Human Relations*, *73*(11), 1537–1562.

Brunero, S., Lamont, S., & Fairbrother, G. (2009). Using and understanding consumer satisfaction to effect an improvement in mental health service delivery. *Journal of Psychiatric and Mental Health Nursing*, *16*(3), 272–278.

Camuccio, C. A., Sanavia, M., Cutrone, F., Marella, I., Gregio, M., Cabbia, C., & Baldo, V. (2019). Noise levels in an acute psychiatric unit: An exploratory observational study. *Issues in Mental Health Nursing*, *40*(6), 493–502.

Carnemolla, P., Debono, D., Hourihan, F., Hor, S., Robertson, H., & Travaglia, J. (2021). The influence of the built environment in enacting a household model of residential aged care for people living with a mental health condition: A qualitative post-occupancy evaluation. *Health & Place*, *71*, 102624.

Carr, R. (2011). Psychiatric facility. *Whole building design guide*. Retrieved March 21, 2012, from http://www.wbdg.org/design/psychiatric.php

Center for Health Design. (2015). *A safety risk assessment for healthcare facility environments*. Concord, CA: Center for Health Design.

Christensen, R. D. (2015). *Transinstitutionalization: A case study of two residential care facilities in rural midwest North America* [Doctoral dissertation]. University of Missouri—Columbia].

Chrysikou, E. (2022). *Design for psychiatric patients: The complexities of therapeutic architecture decision-making*. SINTEF Academic Press.

Cleary, M., Hunt, G., & Walter, G. (2009). A comparison of patient and staff satisfaction with services after relocating to a new purpose-built mental health facility. *Australasian Psychiatry*, *17*(3), 212–217.

Cunha, M., & Silva, N. (2015). Hospital noise and patients' wellbeing. *Procedia-Social and Behavioral Sciences*, *171*, 246–251.

Department of Health Estates and Facilities. (2008). *A staff and patient collaboration toolkit (ASPECT)*. London, UK: Department of Health NHS.

De Ruysscher, C., Vandevelde, S., Tomlinson, P., & Vanheule, S. (2020). A qualitative exploration of service users' and staff members' perspectives on the roles of inpatient settings in mental health recovery. *International Journal of Mental Health Systems*, *14*(1), 1–13.

de Vries, M. G., Brazil, I. A., Tonkin, M., & Bulten, B. H. (2016). Ward climate within a high secure forensic psychiatric hospital: Perceptions of patients and nursing staff and the role of patient characteristics. *Archives of Psychiatric Nursing*, *30*(3), 342–349.

Dickens, G. L., Suesse, M., Snyman, P., & Picchioni, M. (2014). Associations between ward climate and patient characteristics in a secure forensic mental health service. *The Journal of Forensic Psychiatry & Psychology*, *25*(2), 195–211.

Eklund, M., & Hansson, L. (2001). Ward atmosphere, client satisfaction, and client motivation in a psychiatric work rehabilitation unit. *Community Mental Health Journal*, *37*(2), 169–177.

Frøkjær, E., Hertzum, M., & Hornbæk, K. (2000, April). Measuring usability: Are effectiveness, efficiency, and satisfaction really correlated? In *Proceedings of the SIGCHI conference on Human Factors in Computing Systems* (pp. 345–352).

Gutkowski, S., Ginath, Y., & Guttmann, F. (1992). Improving psychiatric environments through minimal architectural changes. *Hospital Community Psychiatry*, *43*, 920–923.

Haines, A., Brown, A., Mccabe, R., Rogerson, M., & Whittington, R. (2017). Factors impacting perceived safety among staff working on mental health wards. *BJPsych Open*. *3*, 204–211.

Hamilton, D. K., & Watkins, D. H. (2008). *Evidence-based design for multiple building types*. John Wiley & Sons.

Hedegaard H., Curtin S. C., & Warner M. (2018). Suicide mortality in the United States 1999-2017. *NCHS Data Brief.*

Holmberg, C., Sobis, I., & Carlström, E. (2016). Job satisfaction among Swedish mental health nursing staff: A cross-sectional survey. *International Journal of Public Administration, 39*(6), 429–436.

Hung, P., Busch, S. H., Shih, Y. W., McGregor, A. J., & Wang, S. (2020). Changes in community mental health services availability and suicide mortality in the US: A retrospective study. *BMC Psychiatry, 20,* 1–12.

Hunt, J. M., Sine, D. M., & McMurray, K. N. (2018). *Behavioral health design guide.* Behavioral Health Facility Consulting Inc.

Jenkin, G., Quigg, S., Paap, H., Cooney, E., Peterson, D., & Every-Palmer, S. (2022). Places of safety? Fear and violence in acute mental health facilities: a large qualitative study of staff and service user perspectives. *PloS One, 17*(5), e0266935.

Johansson, I., Skärsäter, I., & Kanielson, E. (2006). The health care environment on a locked psychiatric ward and its meaning to patients and staff members. *International Journal of Mental Health Nursing, 15,* 242–250.

Jovanović, N., Campbell, J., & Priebe, S. (2019). How to design psychiatric facilities to foster positive social interaction – A systematic review. *European Psychiatry, 60,* 49–62.

Kalagi, J., Otte, I., Vollmann, J., Juckel, G., & Gather, J. (2018). Requirements for the implementation of open door policies in acute psychiatry from a mental health professionals' and patients' view: A qualitative interview study. *BMC Psychiatry, 18*(1), 1–11.

Karlin, B. E., & Zeiss, R. A. (2006). Best practices: Environmental and therapeutic issues in psychiatric hospital design: Toward best practices. *Psychiatric Services, 57*(10), 1376–1378.

Kelly, E. L., Fenwick, K., Brekke, J. S., & Novaco, R. W. (2016). Well-being and safety among inpatient psychiatric staff: The impact of conflict, assault, and stress reactivity. *Administration and Policy in Mental Health and Mental Health Services Research, 43*(5), 703–716.

Kidd, S. A., Hasan, N., & Trapp, J. (2015). Exploring the use of digital picture frames on schizophrenia inpatient wards. *Psychiatric Services, 66*(3), 330.

Kim, A. K., Vakkalanka, J. P., Van Heukelom, P., Tate, J., & Lee, S. (2022). Emergency psychiatric assessment, treatment, and healing (EmPATH) unit decreases hospital admission for patients presenting with suicidal ideation in rural America. *Academic Emergency Medicine, 29*(2), 142–149.

Kimball, D., & Campbell S. (2018). Road to recovery: Person-centered design behavioral health - Trempealeau County Health Care Center. *AAH Academy Journal, 20,* 10–23.

Lundin, S. (2021). Can healing architecture increase safety in the design of psychiatric wards? *HERD: Health Environments Research & Design Journal, 14*(1), 106–117.

Mabala, J., van der Wath, A., & Moagi, M. (2019). Newly qualified nurses' perceptions of working at mental health facilities: A qualitative study. *Journal of Psychiatric and Mental Health Nursing, 26*(5–6), 175–184.

Müller, M. J., Schlösser, R., Kapp-Steen, G., Schanz, B., & Benkert, O. (2002). Patients' satisfaction with psychiatric treatment: Comparison between an open and a closed ward. *Psychiatric Quarterly, 73*(2), 93–107.

Nanda, U., Eisen, S., Zadeh, R. S., & Owen, D. (2011). Effect of visual art on patient anxiety and agitation in a mental health facility and implications for the business case. *Journal of Psychiatric and Mental Health Nursing, 18*(5), 386–393.

New York State Coalition for Children's Mental Health Services. (2013). Redesigning residential treatment facilities. https://cbhny.org/crm/wp-content/uploads/2015/12/CMH-ManattReport-Final.pdf

NHS Estates (2013). AEDET evolution design evaluation toolkit. Retrieved July 20, 2021, from http://www.wales.nhs.uk/sites3/documents/254/aedet_evolution_documentation_v100605.pdf

Nicholls, D., Kidd, K., Threader, J., & Hungerford, C. (2015). The value of purpose built mental health facilities: Use of the Ward Atmosphere Scale to gauge the link between milieu and physical environment. *International Journal of Mental Health Nursing, 24*(4), 286–294.

Okkels, N., Jensen, L. G., Skovshoved, L. C., Arendt, R., Blicher, A. B., Vieta, E., & Straszek, S. (2020). Lighting as an aid for recovery in hospitalized psychiatric patients: A randomized controlled effectiveness trial. *Nordic Journal of Psychiatry, 74*(2), 105–114.

Olausson, S., Wijk, H., Johansson Berglund, I., Pihlgren, A., & Danielson, E. (2021). Patients' experiences of place and space after a relocation to evidence-based designed forensic psychiatric hospitals. *International Journal of Mental Health Nursing, 30*(5), 1210–1220.

Organization for Economic Co-operation and Development (OECD). (2015). *OECD health statistics.* OECD Publishing.

Orr, R. (1995). The Planetree philosophy. In S. Marberry (Ed.), *Innovations in healthcare design* (pp. 77–87). New York, NY: Van Nostrand Reinhold.

Pink, S., Duque, M., Sumartojo, S., & Vaughan, L. (2020). Making spaces for staff breaks: A design anthropology approach. *HERD: Health Environments Research & Design Journal, 13*(2), 243–255.

Pyrke, R. J. L., Mckinnon, M. C., Mcneely, H. E., Ahern, C., Langstaff, K. L., Bieling, P. J. (2017). Evidence-based design features improve sleep quality among psychiatric inpatients. *HERD: Health Environments Research & Design Journal. 10*, 52–63.

Rose, D., Evans, J., Laker, C., & Wykes, T. (2015). Life in acute mental health settings: experiences and perceptions of service users and nurses. *Epidemiology and Psychiatric Sciences, 24*(1), 90–96.

Ruga, W. (2008). Your general practice environment can improve your community's health. *British Journal of General Practice, 58*(552), 460–462.

Sachs, N. A., Shepley, M. M., Peditto, K., Hankinson, M. T., Smith, K., Giebink, B., & Thompson, T. (2020). Evaluation of a mental and behavioral health patient room mockup at a VA facility. *HERD: Health Environments Research & Design Journal, 13*(2), 46–67.

Salerno, S., Forcella, L., Di Fabio, U., Figa Talamance, I., & Boscolo, P. (2012). Ergonomics in the psychiatric ward towards workers or patients? *Work, 41*, 1832–1835.

Schröder, A., Lorentzen, K., Riiskjaer, E., & Lundqvist, L. O. (2016). Patients' views of the quality of Danish forensic psychiatric inpatient care. *The Journal of Forensic Psychiatry & Psychology, 27*(4), 551–568.

Seppänen, A., Törmänen, I., Shaw, C., & Kennedy, H. (2018). Modern forensic psychiatric hospital design: Clinical, legal and structural aspects. *International Journal of Mental Health Systems, 12*(1), 1–12.

Shattell, M. M., Andes, M., & Thomas, S. P. (2008). How patients and nurses experience the acute care psychiatric environment. *Nursing Inquiry, 15*(3), 242–250.

Shattell, M., Bartlett, R., Beres, K., Southard, K., Bell, C., & Judge, C. A. (2015). How patients and nurses experience an open versus an enclosed nursing station on an inpatient psychiatric unit. *Journal of the American Psychiatric Nurses Association, 21*, 398–405.

Sheaves, B., Freeman, D., Isham, L., McInerney, J., Nickless, A., Yu, L. M., & Barrera, A. (2018). Stabilising sleep for patients admitted at acute crisis to a psychiatric hospital (OWLS): An assessor-blind pilot randomised controlled trial. *Psychological Medicine, 48*(10), 1694–1704.

Sheehan, B., Burton, E., Wood, S., Stride, C., Henderson, E., & Wearn, E. (2013). Evaluating the built environment in inpatient psychiatric wards. *Psychiatric Services, 64*(8), 789–795.

Shepley, M. M., Watson, A., Pitts, F., Garrity, A., Spelman, E., Fronsman, A., & Kelkar, J. (2017). Mental and behavioral health settings: Importance & effectiveness of environmental qualities & features as perceived by staff. *Journal of Environmental Psychology, 50*, 37–50.

Shepley, M. M., Watson, A., Pitts, F., Garrity, A., Spelman, E., Kelkar, J., & Fronsman, A. (2016). Mental and behavioral health environments: Critical considerations for facility design. *General Hospital Psychiatry, 42*, 15–21.

Simonsen, T. P., & Duff, C. (2021). Mutual visibility and interaction: Staff reactions to the 'healing architecture of psychiatric inpatient wards in Denmark. *BioSocieties, 16*(2), 249–269.

Smith, S., & Jones, J. (2014). Use of a sensory room on an intensive care unit. *Journal of Psychosocial Nursing and Mental Health Services, 52*(5), 22–30.

Southard, K., Jarrell, A., Shattell, M. M., McCoy, T. P., Bartlett, R., & Judge, C. A. (2012). Enclosed versus open nursing stations in adult acute care psychiatric settings: does the design affect the therapeutic milieu? *Journal of Psychosocial Nursing and Mental Health Services, 50*(5), 28–34.

Stamy, C., Shane, D. M., Kannedy, L., Van Heukelom, P., Mohr, N. M., Tate, J., & Lee, S. (2021). Economic evaluation of the emergency department after implementation of an Emergency Psychiatric Assessment, Treatment, and Healing Unit. *Academic Emergency Medicine, 28*(1), 82–91.

Steiner, R. (2002). *What is anthroposophy?: Three perspectives on self-knowledge.* SteinerBooks.

Substance Abuse and Mental Health Services Administration (SAMHSA). (2017). National Mental Health Services Survey (N-MHSS): 2016. Data on mental health treatment facilities. *BHSIS Series S-98, HHS Publication No. (SMA) 17-5049.*

Tapak, D. M. (2012). *Don't speak about us without us: Design considerations and recommendations for inpatient mental health environments for children and adolescents* [Unpublished master's thesis]. University of Manitoba, Winnipeg, Canada.

Ulrich, R. S., Bogren, L., & Lundin, S. (2012). Towards a design theory for reducing aggression in psychiatric facilities. In *ARCH12 Conference: International Conference ARCH12 and Forum Vårdbyggnad Nordic Conference 2012.* Chalmers Institute of Technology.

Ulrich, R. S., Bogren, L., Gardiner, S. K., & Lundin, S. (2018). Psychiatric ward design can reduce aggressive behavior. *Journal of Environmental Psychology, 57,* 53–66.

Van der Schaaf, P. S., Dusseldorp, E., Keuning, F. M., Janssen, W. A., & Noorthoorn, E. O. (2013). Impact of the physical environment of psychiatric wards on the use of seclusion. *The British Journal of Psychiatry, 202*(2), 142–149.

Veale, D., Ali, S., Papageorgiou, A., & Gournay, K. (2020). The psychiatric ward environment and nursing observations at night: A qualitative study. *Journal of Psychiatric and Mental Health Nursing, 27*(4), 342–351.

Walsh, G., Sara, G., Ryan, C. J., & Large, M. (2015). Meta-analysis of suicide rates among psychiatric in-patients. *Acta Psychiatrica Scandinavica, 131*(3), 174–184.

Watts, B. V., Young-Xu, Y., Mills, P. D., DeRosier, J. M., Kemp, J., Shiner, B., & Duncan, W. E. (2012). Examination of the effectiveness of the Mental Health Environment of Care Checklist in reducing suicide on inpatient mental health units. *Archives of General Psychiatry, 69*(6), 588–592.

Wikström, B-M., Westerlund, E., & Erkkilä, J. (2012). The healthcare environment— The importance of aesthetic surroundings: Health professionals' experiences from a surgical ward in Finland, *Open Journal of Nursing, 2*(3), 188–195.

Zeller, S. (2017). emPath units as a solution for ED psychiatric patient boarding. *Psychiatric Advisor.*

Zeller, S. (2018). What psychiatrists need to know: patients in the Emergency Department. *Psychiatric Times, 35*(8), 1–4.

Zeller, S. L., & Christensen, J. C. (2021). Delivery models of emergency psychiatric care. In *Behavioral Emergencies for Healthcare Providers* (pp. 451–463). Cham: Springer.

6 Mobility, independence, and spatial distance in rehabilitation centres for stroke

Maja Kevdzija and Gesine Marquardt

Introduction

Stroke is a sudden and devastating medical condition mainly affecting older adults (Kim et al., 2020) and causing the most complex disability compared to other conditions (Adamson et al., 2004). Furthermore, stroke is becoming more frequent in the younger adult population due to atypical cardiovascular risk factors (van Alebeek et al., 2018). People affected by stroke can, depending on the affected area of the brain, experience a variety of impairments, including, among others, motor impairments (Langhorne et al., 2009) and visuospatial deficits (Rowe et al., 2009). These common post-stroke impairments can often persist long after the stroke's onset and influence independence (Desrosiers et al., 2002) and quality of life (De Wit et al., 2017). As a result of these impairments, the relationship with the built environment also becomes altered for many stroke survivors, becoming a challenge to their usual way of life.

Due to complex post-stroke impairments, many stroke patients need rehabilitation after discharge from a hospital (Heuschmann et al., 2010). Rehabilitation involves a multidisciplinary approach, mainly focusing on physiotherapy and occupational therapy to regain the lost functions (Hempler et al., 2018). Other types of therapy include speech therapy and psychological counselling (Wallesch, 2015). The primary goals of rehabilitation are to regain independent mobility and skills in the activities of daily living (ADLs) (Luker et al., 2015). This process of recovering mobility and ADL autonomy occurs in therapies and through physical, cognitive, and social activities that patients engage in during their free time. When these functions are recovered or restored to an adequate status, rehabilitation goals extend to recovering skills needed to return to work (Wallesch, 2015). Stroke patients usually spend three to four weeks as inpatients in rehabilitation centres (Nikolaus et al., 2006; Bussmann et al., 2018), which can be extended by several months in some cases.

DOI: 10.1201/9781003344711-7

Rehabilitation environment and patients' needs

Much remains unknown about the spatial needs of stroke patients in rehabilitation and how the design of rehabilitation centres can better support the care processes. Because of the extended length of stay compared to other healthcare facilities such as hospitals, the physical environment of rehabilitation centres is likely to influence patients' behaviours and activities and its role in patient recovery deserves special attention. However, this research field is still in its early stages (Lipson-Smith et al., 2021). The research reported in this chapter aimed to examine the relationship between distance and patients' independent mobility in rehabilitation centres. The objectives were to investigate how much distance stroke patients cover each day during inpatient recovery and analyse how these distances impact patients' mobility independence. The findings will inform the actors involved in the process of designing and planning rehabilitation centres about the impact of distances resulting from different building layouts on stroke patients' daily lives during rehabilitation.

The built environment of rehabilitation centres usually consists of patient wards, therapy rooms, communal areas (such as a living room, a library, or a game room), a shared cafeteria, diagnostic facilities, administration offices, and other staff offices. Stroke inpatients stay on the wards and attend multiple therapies each day, sometimes in different parts of the building. The existing centres are often not purposely built for rehabilitation, and new centres are planned without sufficient evidence-based design knowledge (Lipson-Smith et al., 2020). These vastly different approaches in each facility's built environment design are unlikely always to be suitable for stroke patients' rehabilitation goals and recovery. At the same time, the size and spatial configuration of rehabilitation centres can create wayfinding challenges and other mobility barriers for patients (Kevdzija & Marquardt, 2018), who often experience navigation (Claessen et al., 2017) and motor (Langhorne et al., 2009) impairments after a stroke. Previous investigations in different settings for neurological rehabilitation indicate that their physical environment is hindering for stroke patients (Kevdzija & Marquardt, 2018; Anåker et al., 2017; Newall et al., 1997) and promotes loneliness (Anåker et al., 2019). Patients also describe the lack of places to meet others and the sterility and emptiness of the existing communal spaces in stroke unit wards (Anåker et al., 2019). Even though most rehabilitation facilities include a communal area for patients, their location in the building, distance from patient rooms, and design are not based on evidence-based knowledge about patients' spatial needs (Kevdzija & Marquardt, 2021). Furthermore, research studies on the effect of the enriched environment on patients' activity levels were inconclusive (Janssen et al., 2014b, 2021; Rosbergen et al., 2017), and the built environment was identified as a potential limiting factor to its implementation and the activity of patients (Janssen et al., 2021). Thus, there appears to be a discrepancy between how rehabilitation environments are designed and their intended purpose: to support stroke patients' recovery, activity, and mobility.

Distance as a mobility barrier

In our previous research (Kevdzija & Marquardt, 2018), we found that stroke patients and medical staff identified wayfinding as the most common mobility barrier in rehabilitation centres, followed by insufficient width of corridors and long distances. There is a lack of studies investigating the wayfinding of stroke patients in healthcare facilities, most likely due to the unique character of each facility and the logistical constraints (Ulrich et al., 2008, Kalantari & Snell, 2017). Wayfinding can also be a challenging topic to investigate since it is dependent on an interplay of various cognitive functions (Asselen et al., 2005) and the overall influence of post-stroke impairments on wayfinding ability is difficult to determine. Recent studies on wayfinding in healthcare facilities rely on virtual reality, which might not be comparable with patients' real-world experiences (Kalantari et al., 2021).

However, while wayfinding as a mobility barrier is complex and challenging to investigate, another related barrier in the built environment that deserves attention is the distance between spaces. Long distances are a common design issue in many healthcare facilities due to large and complex programmes, expansion over time, or adaptation from other functions. Because most studies on the relationship between the built environment and stroke patients focus on smaller settings such as stroke units or rehabilitation wards, it is unknown how much distance stroke patients cover daily in larger buildings of rehabilitation centres. Walking distance is an essential measurement in stroke recovery and is included in the Barthel Index (BI) scale, which assesses stroke patients' performance in daily activities (Mahoney & Barthel, 1965). According to this scale, the cut-off distance for determining the patients' mobility level is 50 yards (45.72 m). Although patients that can walk independently for 45 m are considered completely mobile (maximum of 15 points on the BI scale), the spatial distances they must cover in the centre frequently exceed 45 m. Because of the usually long distances between patient rooms and therapy rooms, rehabilitation centres often employ staff members who bring patients from their rooms to therapies, contributing to their feelings of dependence and loss of control. Therefore, spatial distances within the centre's building potentially affect the independent mobility of patients.

Even though spatial distance is likely to play a role in inpatients' rehabilitation experiences, research studies examining walking distance in healthcare facilities have been primarily focused on nursing staff in hospitals (Real et al., 2017; Seo et al., 2011; Welton et al., 2006). In most studies that measured patients' walking distances/activity, the research focused on walking ability and activity levels during various rehabilitation and therapeutic measures or activity levels following discharge (Killey & Watt, 2006;

Mansfield et al., 2015; Rand et al., 2009), rather than on distance covered. The main findings show that most participants did not meet the recommended physical activity levels (Rand et al., 2009), even for patients whose physiotherapists received feedback from their accelerometers (Mansfield et al., 2015); and that extra walking enhanced mobility and independence (Killey & Watt, 2006). The limited capacity to increase overall walking time could have been due to the "limited space or suboptimal environmental layout" (Mansfield et al., 2015, p. 853). Even though most studies use pedometers and step activity monitors that collect quantitative activity data, this approach lacks insight into how patients interact with the built environment, the mobility barriers they encounter, and the strategies they use to overcome them.

Distance was selected as the focus of this investigation since complex rehabilitation programmes require large multi-storey buildings, which creates long distances between spaces. Long distances are a common issue in healthcare facilities and one of the most challenging aspects of building design to alter once the building is completed since it results directly from the buildings' layout. So far, it is unclear how much distance patients cover during one day in large facilities such as rehabilitation centres and how the distances between crucial spaces (patient rooms and therapy areas) impact their mobility independence. Therefore, more knowledge is needed about how the building's spatial configuration and resulting distances affect stroke patients' activities in rehabilitation centres.

Methods

This study used patient shadowing as the primary research method combined with patient and staff surveys to examine the impact of distance on stroke patients' mobility in seven neurological rehabilitation centres in Germany. Ethical approval for the research was granted by the Ethical Committee at the Technische Universität Dresden. Neurological rehabilitation centres in Germany were contacted and asked if they wished to participate in the research. Eleven responded positively, invited the first author to visit (hereafter, the researcher), and were visited in the preliminary research phase. The initial assessment at each visited centre consisted of a tour of the facility given by a staff member and an informal interview with the centre's medical director. During conversations with medical directors, further information was obtained about the operational patterns of neurological centres, how patients were accommodated in the centres, and how their rehabilitation was organised.

Seven centres were selected for the study to ensure the inclusion of distinctive and different types of building layouts. This selection was made to assess a variety of spatial configurations and to analyse the travel distances resulting from them. The characteristics of each participating rehabilitation centre are shown in Figure 6.1. They were predominantly neurological

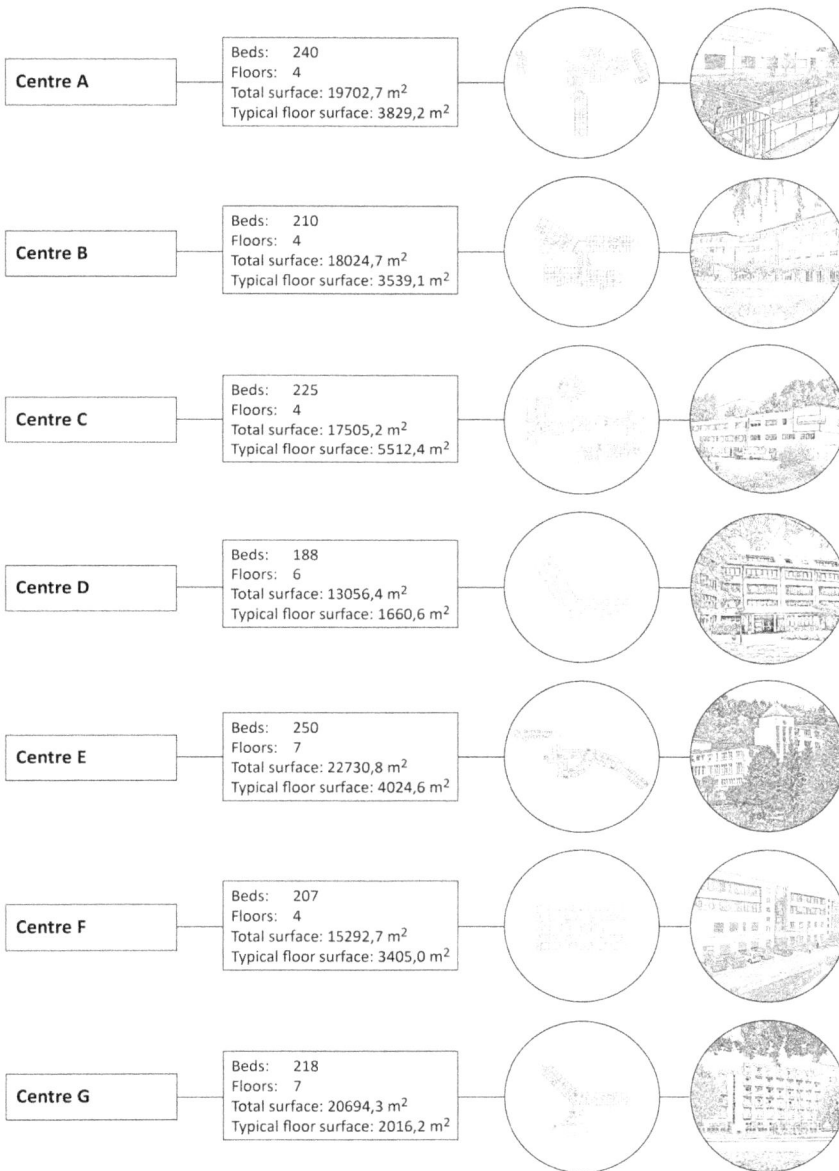

| Centre A | Beds: 240
Floors: 4
Total surface: 19702,7 m²
Typical floor surface: 3829,2 m² |

| Centre B | Beds: 210
Floors: 4
Total surface: 18024,7 m²
Typical floor surface: 3539,1 m² |

| Centre C | Beds: 225
Floors: 4
Total surface: 17505,2 m²
Typical floor surface: 5512,4 m² |

| Centre D | Beds: 188
Floors: 6
Total surface: 13056,4 m²
Typical floor surface: 1660,6 m² |

| Centre E | Beds: 250
Floors: 7
Total surface: 22730,8 m²
Typical floor surface: 4024,6 m² |

| Centre F | Beds: 207
Floors: 4
Total surface: 15292,7 m²
Typical floor surface: 3405,0 m² |

| Centre G | Beds: 218
Floors: 7
Total surface: 20694,3 m²
Typical floor surface: 2016,2 m² |

Figure 6.1 Characteristics of the participating centres with the typical floor plan and exterior view.

rehabilitation centres ranging from 188 to 250 beds. The physical environment accessible to patients consisted of their patient ward, therapy rooms (concentrated in one or various areas of the building depending on the centre), diagnostic facilities, the main cafeteria, and various communal areas (not present in every centre) such as a living room, a library or a café. These centres had different strategies for allocating patient wards, therapy rooms and other facilities. Some centres had a hotel-like configuration with patient wards and main therapy areas separated vertically. Others had patient rooms and therapy rooms combined on the same level. Several centres had a mix of the two: therapy rooms combined with patient rooms, and others separated vertically.

Inpatients undergoing rehabilitation in these centres were expected to attend meals and therapies independently, meaning that patients had to cover the distances between their patient rooms, various therapy rooms and the cafeteria multiple times per day. Aside from scheduled meals and therapy appointments, patients covered the additional distance to visit communal and other spaces in their free time.

Participant recruitment

The medical staff selected the potential participants in each centre based on the given inclusion and exclusion criteria, their health status and their psychological state (Table 6.1). The study included 70 patients of neurological rehabilitation centres that: (1) suffered a stroke, (2) were able to move independently in the centre (with or without the use of a wheelchair, walker or other equipment), and (3) gave their consent for the study. Patients diagnosed with dementia, severe communication and cognitive impairments, severe multi-morbidity (somatic, psychiatric, or psycho/geriatric), significant mobility impairment before the stroke, and/or orthopaedic, neurological, or other conditions of consequence for the study were excluded from

Table 6.1 Participants' characteristics

Characteristic	Participants (n = 70)
Age	≥60
Gender	
Female	32 (45.7%)
Male	38 (54.3%)
Mobility level	
Wheelchair	16 (22.9%)
Walker	23 (32.8%)
Independently walking	31 (44.3%)
Length of stay (days)	Median: 19.5
Range	3–139
Number of therapy appointments per day	Median: 4.36
Range	3–7

participation. All patients included in the analysis were over 60 years old due to the availability of participants during the observation weeks, as stroke is commonly a condition of advanced age.

Patients' mobility levels

Instead of using the BI for Mobility (from 0 = immobile to 15 = independent, but may use any aid; Mahoney & Barthel, 1965) or another assessment scale, the mobility aid was used to sort patients into mobility level categories. The participating patients were divided into three mobility level categories based on the mobility aid they used for mobility within the centres: using a wheelchair (level 1), using a walker (level 2), or independently walking (level 3). This decision was taken since it was observed that the mobility aid had a major impact on how patients moved and interacted with the built environment.

Following the explanation of the research study and the requirements to each potential participant by one of the centre's staff members, patients received a large-print information sheet to read and a large-print consent form to sign in case they wanted to participate. The patients were able to drop out of the study at any time. All 70 participants gave their written or verbal consent for the study.

Patient shadowing

Patient shadowing was used to gain insight into the daily life of stroke inpatients in rehabilitation centres and to examine the impact of distance on their mobility. Shadowing was chosen as a method for observing and recording a single individual's everyday activities (Mcdonald, 2005). Shadowing is a method that enables ethnographic observation of various stages and touchpoints in the care process (Gallan et al., 2021). Even though it is mainly a social science method, it has shown great potential in research studies in healthcare environments so far (Gualandi et al., 2019; van der Meide et al., 2015). During patient shadowing, an observer follows patients across various care experiences while recording information gathered through observations (Shaw et al., 2014). Building floor plans can also be used to map the locations of the observed activities/behaviours. Compared to the more commonly used purely quantitative method of behavioural mapping (observing from a distance), shadowing is neither truly qualitative nor truly quantitative (Mcdonald, 2005). When shadowing, the researcher navigates between the observation of events and behaviours from a distance and asking participants questions (van der Meide et al., 2015), which allows for different kinds of data to be collected – routes on the floor plans, specific locations of interest, patients' narratives, etc. This flexible method enables the inclusion of people who cannot express themselves verbally (van der Weele & Bredewold, 2021) due to the extended observation period, focusing on one individual at a time and emphasising non-verbal communication (van der Meide et al., 2015).

The shadowing method was used to record patients' daily covered distances and interactions with space. For this research study, an open attitude was adopted, aiming to record as much of what was observed as possible without using predetermined categories and behaviours. However, communication was considerably limited due to typical post-stroke speech impairments and a language barrier between the researcher and several the participants. For this reason, this chapter presents only the data from the observations without the patients' narrative data. Because of the nature of shadowing (an individual carefully following a subject for an extended period) and due to ethical considerations, the researcher could not remain a completely secret observer. Consequently, the Hawthorne effect (individuals changing their conduct in response to being observed) may have influenced the participants' behaviour. The study's goals were not disclosed to patients to minimise the Hawthorne effect. Patients were only told their usual daily routes in the centre were being observed.

Patients' routes in the centres were recorded on the previously prepared and then printed building floor plans with an extra sheet for the activity time log. This allowed for precise mapping of locations and the nature of patients' routes. One researcher observed patients in all corridors and communal areas (e.g., cafeteria, living room, dining room, library). Because the focus was on distances between spaces, it was decided not to follow patients inside the therapy rooms and their patient rooms to protect their privacy. Three complimentary types of notes were taken during the patient shadowing (Table 6.2).

Table 6.2 Types of notes recorded during patient shadowing

Routes on the floor plans	Time log of activities	Encounters with the built environment
Each patient route from place A to place B was drawn on the floor plans, using symbols and numbers to coordinate the corresponding activity time log on a separate sheet. These routes were later used to calculate the daily distances patients covered in the centres.	The time log sheet consisted of three columns to record the patient's position number, time and duration, and activity type in the form of textual description. All columns were empty prior to data collection; there were no predetermined activity categories on the sheets.	When the observed patient encountered a barrier in the built environment or unusually interacted with the environment, this was recorded in the form of a short textual note, sometimes followed by a sketch to additionally explain it.

Each patient was observed for 12 hours on a typical day in the centre, from 07:00 h to 19:00 h. The exact observation times differed somewhat among centres due to different meal times. The 12-hour observation usually began immediately before patients' breakfast and ended after dinner. Total observation time in all centres was 840 hours. Shadowing was supplemented with patient and staff surveys to gain additional insights into their spatial experiences. The observed patients (n = 60) and medical staff that cared for them (55 nurses and four physicians, n = 59) completed the surveys. Not all patients were able to complete the surveys due to post-stroke impairments. In the survey, patients were asked about the barriers they experienced in the built environment, while staff members were asked about the barriers they witnessed patients encountering.

Data analysis

As all data were collected on paper, patients' routes on floor plans and the time log sheets were digitalised after data collection. The travel distances were calculated using these digitally documented patient routes (digitalised with Autodesk AutoCAD). A route was defined as the distance a patient travelled to get from one location (point A) to another (point B). One of the 70 shadowed patients had to be excluded from the analysis because of the wandering syndrome. The total number of measured routes for all 69 included patients was n = 1,322. These were their usual daily routes (such as going from their room to therapy or the cafeteria) and were not a part of training supervised by a physical therapist or another healthcare professional.

Each route was categorised according to the patient's level of dependence with the help of the information recorded on time log sheets. One of the three possible codes was used for each route, signifying the levels of dependence and severity of the mobility issue the patient encountered. A route was categorised as "category A" if the patient faced no mobility barriers. "Type B" was defined as a route where the patient faced a mobility barrier but could overcome it without help. When a patient encountered a barrier and needed help on a route (verbal or physical, such as pushing a wheelchair), it was classed as "type C", the highest level of dependence. This research investigated the following types of mobility barriers: (1) issues with wayfinding, such as getting lost or not knowing which way to go, (2) issues with long distances, such as stopping to rest or asking for help, (3) insufficient width of corridors, (4) physical obstacles, and (5) floor slopes and surfaces. These mobility barrier categories emerged from shadowing data analysis. NVivo Pro 11 was used to analyse patient and medical staff open-ended survey responses. Their responses were translated from the German language to English before analysis. The results of patient shadowing are presented together with relevant patient and medical staff member quotations throughout the text.

148   *Maja Kevdzija and Gesine Marquardt*

Results

The daily distance covered by patients

The distance patients covered each day ranged from 912 m to 2108 m on average, depending on the centre (Table 6.3). The daily distances in centres likely varied due to differences in spatial configurations, zonal distribution of functions, such as patient rooms and treatment areas (Table 6.3), and amount of therapy appointments.

The centres with the shortest covered distances had compact layouts with a single central building containing all patient and therapy rooms. The exception is Centre D, where, despite the compact layout, the covered daily distance was longer. This is most likely owing to the complex layout of the basement level, which houses all therapy rooms and is shared with the orthopaedic centre. One patient of this centre noted that "long distances between therapies have to be covered", and another patient suggested that "therapies need to be more centralized". In terms of covered distance, the following functional layouts were the most efficient: patient rooms and therapy areas separated vertically (hotel-like configuration), and patient rooms and therapy rooms combined on the same level, with the additional therapy rooms separated vertically (mixed hotel-like configuration). Patients

Table 6.3 Average daily distance covered in each centre per patient

Centre	Functional configuration	Daily distance (m)	
		Mean	*Median*
Centre A	[P+T]-[P]-[P]-[P]-[T] / [T]	2108,0	2264,1
Centre B	[P+T] / [T]	960,3	989,3
Centre C	[P+T]-[P]-[T] / [T]	1201,9	1264,6
Centre D	[P] / [T]	1179,5	1158,9
Centre E	[P+T]-[P]-[T] / [T]	1562,2	1571,7
Centre F	[P+T] / [T]	970,1	910,9
Centre G	[P] / [T]	912,4	962,0

[P] patient wards; [T] therapy rooms; [P+T] mixed patient and therapy rooms

| vertical connection — horizontal connection.

in the centres with more complex functional configurations (mixed configurations) covered considerably longer distances during one day (Table 6.3).

"Since the rooms do not have a clear arrangement, the paths are unclear". This was an observation of a patient in Centre A, where the longest daily distance was recorded. As this centre expanded in stages and was not purposely built for rehabilitation, this resulted in large distances between some therapy areas. Hence, patients often had to travel from one end of the building to the next to reach the next therapy. One patient noticed this and stated, "you have to plan enough time to reach the therapies". Patients of Centre E shared similar experiences; they mentioned "very long paths, hard to read" and "distances too large with a walker, not enough seating opportunities to take a break" as barriers they encountered in the built environment. A staff member of this centre observed that "the house is large, there are many long hallways and levels. Also, several wards look similar", and another described the centre as "a large house with many corridors and passageways where patients become disoriented". A staff member of Centre A shared, "Since our patients are independent, there are only occasional orientation difficulties. They usually confuse the elevators at the main entrance and the therapy centre". Another staff member observed "dangerous uphill and downhill, very winding, many additions" as the main issues that patients might encounter in the built environment. The floor slopes resulted from adding new buildings (houses) to the existing structure over a long period. Similarly, staff members working in Centre C described it as "very labyrinthine". "There are always difficulties with good wayfinding of patients in our house". At the same time, another member of the staff explained that "this is why we have the patient transport service in the building, which transports the patients to the therapies, exercises". Therefore, patients often cannot cover these distances and find therapy rooms independently and must be brought there by staff transport service.

Impact of distance on patients' mobility and independence

Patients encountered one of the five previously identified mobility barriers (wayfinding issues, distance, dimensions, physical obstacles, and flooring) and/or needed help on 163 routes out of 1,322 routes (12.3%). There was a significant effect of distance on the number of all categories of mobility barriers that patients encountered in the built environment (Wilks' $\Lambda = 0.379$, $F(2.15) = 12.271$, $p = 0.01$). When all mobility barrier categories were observed in this sample, the longer distance was related to more barriers encountered and more help from medical staff needed (Figure 6.2). A total of 45 patients (65.2%) and their routes were included in the analysis with the General Linear Model (general multivariate regression model). Other 24 patients (34.8%) did not encounter any mobility barriers and did not need help on any of their routes during the observations.

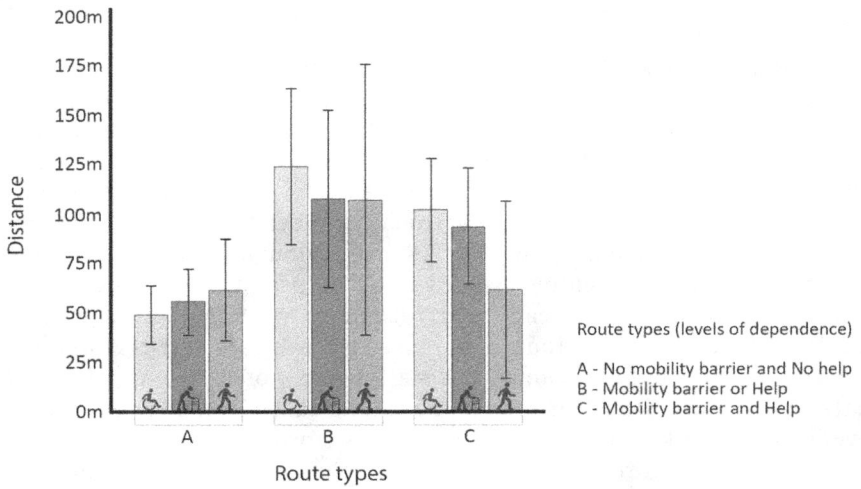

Figure 6.2 Effect of distance and mobility level on encountering barriers and/or needing help (General Linear Model).

There was no statistically significant effect of mobility level on encountering mobility barriers and needing help on longer distances in this sample (Wilks' Λ = 0.723, F (4.30) = 1.319, p = 0.286). The distance was related to an increased number of encountered mobility barriers in the built environment for all patients, with no significant difference between mobility levels (Figure 6.2). Longer distances increased the likelihood that a patient would encounter a mobility barrier or require help from staff to reach a specific location, independent of the patients' mobility level.

The overall number of routes where patients encountered a barrier and/or needed help varied greatly. Patients using wheelchairs experienced a mobility barrier and/or needed help more frequently than those using a walker or walking independently (Figure 6.3). Patients who could walk independently mainly encountered barriers related to wayfinding (20 out of 24 observed events), while patients using a wheelchair encountered all five categories of previously identified barriers (number of observed events: wayfinding = 10, distance = 13, dimensions = 11, physical obstacles = 5, flooring = 13). Therefore, patients using a wheelchair were generally more vulnerable to the barriers in the built environment and much more dependent on the staff members for help (Figure 6.3). This is also evident from the barriers patients described in their questionnaire responses. A patient of Centre B shared that long corridors were a barrier for him, "I am still weak and slow when driving the wheelchair". "There is a connecting corridor that is a slope. This can't be handled alone using a wheelchair" (patient of Centre D). A patient of Centre F also remarked that there is insufficient space in the corridors to park a wheelchair, and

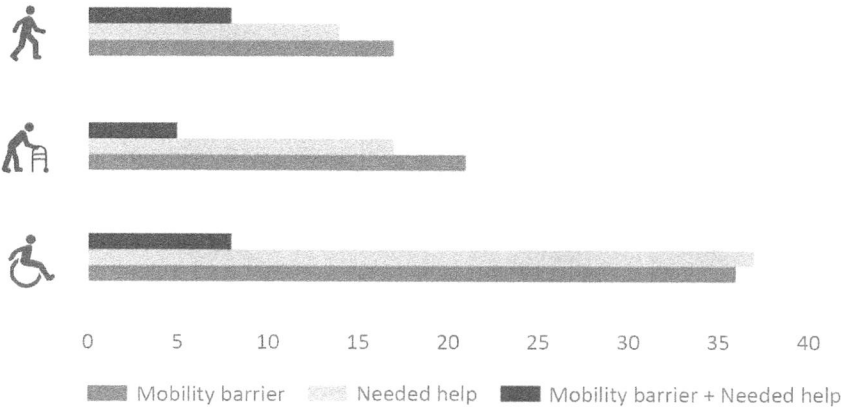

Figure 6.3 Comparison of numbers of routes with encountered barriers and/or help needed for each mobility level (n = 163).

patients of Centres B and D made a similar observation. "It is a bit too tight to pass with walkers or wheelchairs" (patient of Centre D). Other main barriers that patients mentioned were "too much stuff in the hallways" (Centre F), "mats in the entrance area", "uneven floor tiles", "carpet flooring stops movement" (Centre B), "exit to the garden not suitable for a person in a wheelchair" (Centre E) and "guidance system not clear" (Centre C).

The routes where patients did not encounter mobility barriers and did not need help were significantly shorter than those with barriers and/or needed help (Figure 6.4). Patients using a wheelchair could cover the

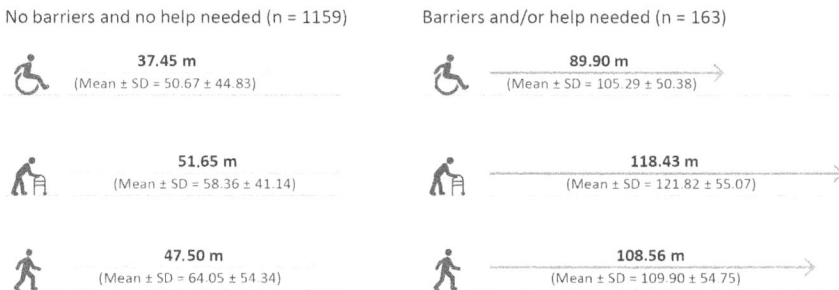

Figure 6.4 Median distances of routes that patients with different mobility levels could cover independently without encountering barriers and distances where they encountered barriers and/or needed help (total no. of routes = 1,322).

shortest distance without encountering any mobility barriers or needing help compared to patients using a wheelchair or independently walking. The patients' routes on which they encountered a mobility barrier or needed help were considerably shorter as well for patients using a wheelchair compared to the other two groups. Patients who could walk had shorter routes without barriers and help needed, as well as shorter routes with barriers and/or help needed compared to patients using a walker. As previously mentioned, wayfinding was the main mobility barrier for most of the more mobile patients.

We have already determined that patients' non-scheduled activity (free-time activities outside of planned therapies, appointments and meals) was much less frequent than scheduled activities and that there was a significant difference in the lengths of scheduled and non-scheduled routes (Kevdzija et al., 2022). Here, we investigated how much distance patients with different mobility levels travelled per day for scheduled and non-scheduled activities (Figure 6.5).

Even though patients' abilities in terms of mobility were different and patients using a wheelchair were the most dependent on staff and vulnerable to mobility barriers, there was no significant difference between these patients and the other two groups in terms of the median scheduled daily distance travelled per patient. In non-scheduled activities, patients using a wheelchair covered the longest daily distances in mean and median measured values (Figure 6.5). A great variation in the covered distance among patients was observed; 18 out of 70 patients did not engage in any non-scheduled activity on the observation day. These patients did not leave their rooms other than to attend scheduled therapies and meals. Distances that each patient group covered in a day were significantly different for scheduled and non-scheduled activities.

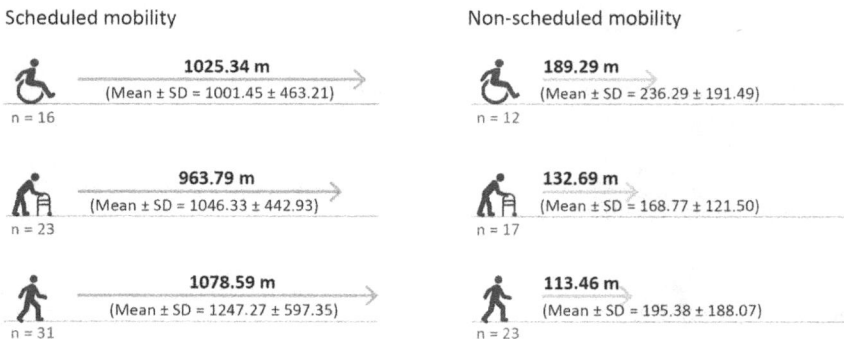

Scheduled mobility

1025.34 m
(Mean ± SD = 1001.45 ± 463.21)
n = 16

963.79 m
(Mean ± SD = 1046.33 ± 442.93)
n = 23

1078.59 m
(Mean ± SD = 1247.27 ± 597.35)
n = 31

Non-scheduled mobility

189.29 m
(Mean ± SD = 236.29 ± 191.49)
n = 12

132.69 m
(Mean ± SD = 168.77 ± 121.50)
n = 17

113.46 m
(Mean ± SD = 195.38 ± 188.07)
n = 23

Figure 6.5 Median scheduled and non-scheduled total daily covered distance per patient for each mobility level.

How individual patients experience distance and other mobility barriers

Many spatial features are intertwined and can influence each other and the patient's experience of space. The same is true for spatial distance. Multiple patients were observed to experience difficulties on long distances, such as being unable to find their way, needing to rest and relying on staff assistance. In some situations, it was also observed that patients' reliance on staff members and various forms of mobility aids varied across different distances in centres and even over the course of a single day. Several distinct situations are presented to illustrate this based on shadowing notes.

A patient of Centre A with hemiplegia on the left side of the body (paralysis of arm and leg) and using a wheelchair was observed to encounter many mobility barriers on just one route from the therapy room to his room. The patient's route between the therapy room and his room was 216.4-m long and spread over three building levels. The building of centre A is specific for its growth in phases where some parts are only connected on some building levels. The patient had to use two different and spatially separate elevators to reach his room on the third floor from the therapy room on the basement level. The mobility barriers this patient encountered on his way were wayfinding issues (he chose the wrong corridor upon exiting the elevator), problems with long distance (he stopped to rest in the corridor and asked the researcher to push his wheelchair) and losing control over the wheelchair (he hit the seating furniture on the side of the corridor).

In another example, a patient from Centre B with hemiparesis (muscle weakness) on the right side of her body and using a wheelchair struggled with the distance between her room and the therapy room. The patient's room was on the same floor as the therapy rooms, just across a wide corridor. This patient had to stop and rest many times on the route to therapies and back. On several occasions, she also used the handrail on the wall to pull herself forward. This patient had multiple therapies in the rooms accessed from the same therapy corridor. She showed the same mobility pattern each time she went to therapy and back. This patient was blocking traffic flow in the corridor since all patients from this centre accessed their therapies via this route. It was impossible for other patients using a wheelchair to pass through this corridor each time the observed patient stopped to rest. Therefore, this patient experienced difficulties with long distances and insufficient width of corridors. Another patient in Centre B was using a walker as a mobility aid during the whole day and could reach all spaces independently, but he switched to using a wheelchair at the end of the day. This patient stated that he was exhausted after a long day of therapy and that using a wheelchair allowed him to rest more while using less energy for mobility.

In centre C, a patient using a wheelchair encountered multiple mobility issues during one observation day. The ward where this patient was accommodated could be reached from both corridor ends via floor slopes. To reach the elevators on both ends of the ward, which was necessary to reach therapies, this patient had to cover either 42.38 and an uphill slope or 76.08 m and an uphill slope. The patient experienced difficulties controlling the wheelchair on these slopes, often going very slowly, and using only legs to "walk" in the wheelchair instead of rolling using arms. This led to blocking the traffic in the corridor on two occasions, once in front of the nurses' station. No other patient could reach the nurses while this patient was in the corridor due to its insufficient width.

In another case, a patient of Centre D using a wheelchair was brought to all therapies and appointments by staff during the observation day. She could independently visit only the communal room on the ward, which was around 38 m away from her room. All therapy areas and diagnostic facilities where she attended appointments were far from her room, ranging from 74.4 m to 136.75 m, and on another building level. Therefore, while this patient could be independent on short distances, she needed assistance to visit places farther away from her room.

In Centre E, a patient using a wheelchair encountered mobility difficulties due to carpet flooring in the ward's corridor. As the patient had to cross this carpeted area to reach his room, he experienced challenges each time, stopping to rest or losing control of the wheelchair and hitting the equipment left in the corridor. On two occasions, when going back to the room after therapy, this patient decided to take a much longer route through the building and reach his room using a different elevator to avoid a part of the corridor with the carpet. This way, the patient only had to cover 7.48 m of distance with carpet flooring instead of the usual 42.2 m to reach his room. Another patient in this centre was observed to change the direction and roll his wheelchair backwards on the carpet, sharing that it is easier to cover longer distances this way.

These examples provide a glimpse into the daily activities of stroke in-patients and how they interact with the built environment when going to and back from therapies. Distance is often combined with other barriers, which causes patients to get tired, must stop and rest, and sometimes even lose control of their wheelchairs. The interplay of barriers in the built environment differs for each patient, but their mobility needs and abilities can also change on different distances, as illustrated in several examples. It was observed that patients using a wheelchair were most vulnerable to all types of previously identified mobility barriers.

Discussion

Both staff and patients recognise spatial distance as a common challenge in rehabilitation centres. This was confirmed with patient shadowing; all patient groups were affected by longer distances, but patients using a wheelchair were the most vulnerable and most dependent on staff members.

Observing individual patients during their one typical day in rehabilitation revealed different information compared to studies using accelerometers to track patients' mobility (Mansfield et al., 2015; Rand et al., 2009) or behavioural mapping to record their activity levels (Janssen et al., 2014a; Kārkliņa et al., 2021; Anåker et al., 2017). The results suggest that barriers in the built environment are frequently intertwined, can influence each other, and can be difficult to separate when analysing how the built environment affects patient mobility. Additionally, patients using a wheelchair were the most impacted by long distances, experiencing them as a barrier and being brought to therapies by staff members.

As patients are encouraged to go to their therapies independently, their travels to therapies and their free time activities can also be an effective exercise and could contribute to their recovery (Cowdell & Garrett, 2003; Dixon et al., 2007). Patients' independence and walking ability have been found to improve with increased walking activity in addition to regular therapies (Killey & Watt, 2006). Medical staff members also reported independent mobility as exceptionally important during patients' recovery (Kevdzija & Marquardt, 2018). Thus, rehabilitation is not limited to scheduled therapy; any independent activity or mobility can potentially help improve patients' capabilities. If independence is not achieved at the end of the rehabilitation, the extensive burden falls on caregivers to care for the patient after a stroke (Rigby et al., 2009). In the event of high dependence and the absence of a caregiver, the patient needs to be admitted to a long-term care facility (Ween et al., 1996). As a result, independent mobility should be encouraged and promoted to decrease the dependence on others and feelings of loss of control.

Because of their importance, patient mobility, activity, and independence are becoming the focus of numerous studies in healthcare design research. Together with implementing the enriched environment (Janssen et al., 2014b, 2021; Rosbergen et al., 2017), creating opportunities for patients to be more independent and active requires a response in the built environment's design. Because of this, many aspects of the built environment should be thoroughly considered for impact on patient mobility and activity. Distance between crucial functional zones in a rehabilitation centre is one of the aspects that should be intentionally planned for enabling and supporting patients' independent mobility. Distance is also experienced differently by patients using different mobility aids. In this study, we found that patients using a wheelchair covered the same amount of daily distance as other patient groups, as they were all accommodated in the same way in the rehabilitation centres. As a result, patients using a wheelchair were often brought to therapy because of the long distance between their room and the therapy room, while patients who could walk would go independently. The physical environment should be designed to enable patients to participate in recovery-promoting activities in their free time to support their recovery (Lipson-Smith et al., 2019). Therefore, when not carefully designed, distance can become a significant

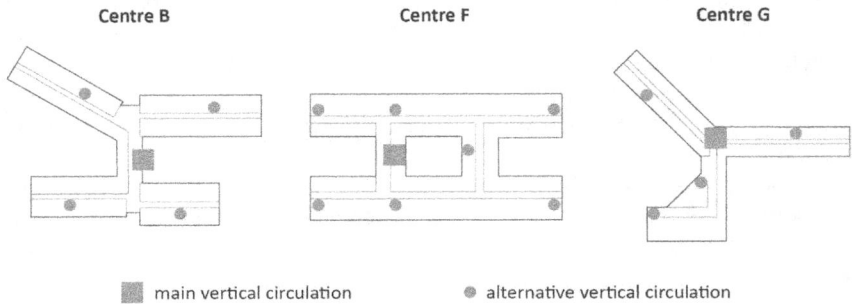

Centre B   Centre F   Centre G

■ main vertical circulation   ● alternative vertical circulation

Figure 6.6 Floor plan layouts of the centres with shortest daily covered distances.

mobility barrier for some patients, while creating a valuable training opportunity for others.

As the travel distance results from the building's configuration, it is essential to plan for different possibilities to reach spaces for different patient groups. For example, the most efficient building layouts identified in this research study were simple, compact layouts with a central vertical core (Figure 6.6). On the wards, these vertical circulation cores were complemented by stairs and/or elevators for alternate vertical circulation. This combination of one central vertical core and alternate vertical connections between floors provided patients with several options for reaching locations inside the centres while ensuring the shortest possible distances. As a result, when planning layouts that create the shortest spatial distances for both patients and staff members, simple and compact layouts with a central vertical core and additional alternative vertical connections should be considered. Patients needed to cover considerably longer distances in the centres with more complex configurations. Although this type of layout may reduce daily patient travel distance, it is unclear how it impacts wayfinding and patient traffic in centres.

Patient populations and their mobility abilities must be considered when designing patient wards and their connections to other centre areas. The main connection that should be carefully planned in terms of distance is between patient rooms and therapy rooms. These are routes that each patient travels multiple times per day, depending on the number of daily therapy appointments. In this research, we found that patients covered longer distances in centres where therapy rooms were scattered in different building areas. For patients using a wheelchair and experiencing severe motor impairments, shorter distances might offer an opportunity for autonomy in the centre. At the same time, patients in the advanced stages of rehabilitation who can already walk independently could benefit from long distances as a form of exercise. In this research, centres with the most efficient layouts in terms of distance also had a specific vertical distribution of functions – a hotel-like

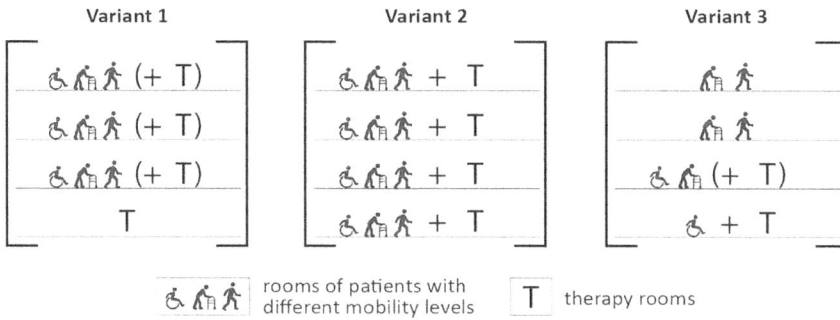

Figure 6.7 Schematic representation of building sections with different distributions of functions.

organisation. This organisation includes having patient rooms of all mobility levels on the upper floors and shared therapy rooms on the bottom floor (Variant 1, Figure 6.7). Sometimes, smaller therapy rooms can also be found on the same level where patient rooms are located (Centres B and F).

Another possibility to create the shortest distances between patient rooms and patient rooms would be to always place them on the same floor (Variant 2, Figure 6.7). This option is challenging to implement as rehabilitation clinics have several large therapy spaces, such as a therapy pool, a gym or a space for group sports therapy. Repeating these rooms on each floor would not be possible. This is why Variant 3 could be considered in the design of rehabilitation centres – having main shared therapy rooms on the same floor where the least mobile patients using a wheelchair are accommodated. Optional additional therapy rooms could be located on the floor that accommodates other patients with lower mobility levels, while most fairly mobile patients would need to travel farther to reach the therapies (Figure 6.7). In this way, less mobile patients would have more independence to reach therapies on their own and patients who are more mobile could have additional training complementing the scheduled therapies. For patients using mobility aids, rest places also need to be planned on the routes to therapies. These places might be small corridor widenings providing spaces for wheelchair users and seats with armrests.

The findings on how stroke patients experience spatial distance in rehabilitation centres may also inform design decisions at the patient ward level. Achieving patients' independence and improving their activity levels requires, among others, addressing the distance between spaces, not only wards and other areas outside but also spaces within the wards. Providing patients with a variety of opportunities to leave their rooms and independently engage in activities alone or with others may be vital to their rehabilitation process. Research so far suggests that distance plays a role and that patients more frequently visit communal spaces closer to their rooms

(Kevdzija & Marquardt, 2021). Therefore, wards should offer communal spaces close to patients' rooms in addition to the usual communal areas shared with the whole building (such as a library, café, etc.). Furthermore, as patients need to attend meals three times per day, a dining room is another space whose distance from patient rooms should be carefully planned. Most patients have meals in the main centre's cafeteria or smaller dining rooms on the wards. The location of these spaces is important, as bedside meals should be avoided, and patients should be enabled to reach the dining spaces independently. If all patients are expected to eat in the main cafeteria, patients using wheelchairs should be accommodated in the wards nearby to reach them independently. Otherwise, smaller dining rooms should be planned on the wards where patients with low mobility are accommodated, while the more mobile patients could eat in the main cafeteria and exercise their mobility. These smaller dining rooms can be separate spaces on the ward, but can also serve as communal living rooms or rooms for different kinds of free-time activities for patients outside of meal times.

According to the findings of this study, distance should be considered as one of the potential factors that limit patients' activity and mobility in studies looking at ways to improve patients' activity levels during rehabilitation. This is especially relevant for research studies attempting to increase their activity levels using interventions such as the enriched environment. Many design strategies to promote patient activity levels, such as attractive communal areas in rehabilitation centres (common room, library, gaming room, etc.), may not be sufficient if located far from patient rooms. Therefore, when designing ward environments, it is essential to take a more tailored approach to create environments for patients with varying mobility abilities rather than accommodating them all in the same way. To achieve this, many aspects other than distance need to be considered. This research suggests that barriers in the built environment are frequently intertwined, can influence each other, and can be difficult to separate when analysing how the built environment affects patients' mobility and activity. Even though it is a complex topic to investigate, further research focusing on distance is needed since it can impact patients' mobility independence and potentially contribute to their low activity levels during inpatient rehabilitation.

Strengths and limitations

The strength of this study is the use of the shadowing method on a large scale (70 patients, 840 hours of observations). This enabled insight into the daily routines, travelled distances and interactions with the built environment of individual stroke patients via direct observation. Although the shadowing method is the main strength of this study, this method choice also introduced certain limitations that need to be mentioned.

Since the participating centres have around 200 patients each, the sample size of ten patients per centre could be considered small. Due to the exploratory character of this study, the sample of 70 patients was enough to study the phenomenon in question more deeply. Further studies investigating the topic only quantitatively or using mixed methods would benefit from a larger representative sample of stroke patients. Moreover, excluding the younger patient from the analysis removed the representation of young patients' experiences, whose needs also require special attention. Additionally, the field research and data collection phase for this study were conducted pre-COVID-19, and the influence of the pandemic on everyday life in rehabilitation centres could not have been observed.

Conclusion

The spatial needs of stroke patients and their relationship with the built environment have yet to be sufficiently investigated to determine which design strategies are most beneficial to the patients, as this field is still in its early stages. The findings of the study indicate that decisions made during the early phases of building design concerning the layout of the facility and the distances between different areas might have a major influence on patients' mobility and independence. Shorter distances were identified as an aspect that, if carefully planned, could enable independent mobility for all patients, even those with limited mobility. This potential influence on patients' mobility and the impact of other mobility barriers needs to be further examined. Further research studies could examine how longer distances affect patients' free-time activities and visiting communal spaces within the centres. The relationship between distance and wayfinding in rehabilitation centres is another topic that has not been investigated before and should be addressed in future research. Another relevant direction to be further explored is patients' experiences with various barriers and facilitators in the built environment in a more qualitative way. Since the physical environment of rehabilitation can hinder patients' mobility and independence during rehabilitation, it is necessary to investigate further the impact of individual spatial features and their interactions. Consequently, rehabilitation centres' currently prevalent "same for all" design should be replaced with a more tailored approach to create the best possible environments for different patient groups and their changing spatial needs during recovery.

Acknowledgements

The research study was supported by the European Social Fund (ESF) and the Sächsische Aufbaubank (RL ESF Hochschule und Forschung 2014 bis 2020, scholarship agreement no. 100235479) and the Graduate Academy at the Technische Universität Dresden.

References

Adamson, J., Beswick, A., & Ebrahim, S. (2004). Is stroke the most common cause of disability? *Journal of Stroke and Cerebrovascular Diseases, 13*(4), 171–177.

Anåker, A., von Koch, L., Heylighen, A., & Elf, M. (2019). "It's lonely": Patients' experiences of the physical environment at a newly built stroke unit. *Health Environments Research and Design Journal, 12*(3), 141–152.

Anåker, A., Von Koch, L., Sjöstrand, C., Bernhardt, J., & Elf, M. (2017). A comparative study of patients' activities and interactions in a stroke unit before and after reconstruction - The significance of the built environment. *PLoS One, 12*(7), 1–12.

Asselen, M. Van, Kessels, R. P. C., Kappelle, L. J., Neggers, S. F. W., Frijns, C. J. M., & Postma, A. (2005). *Neural Correlates of Human Wayfinding in Stroke Patients, 7*, 1–10.

Bussmann, M., Neunzig, H., Gerber, J., Steinmetz, J., Jung, S., & Deck, R. (2018). Effects and quality of stroke rehabilitation of BAR phase D. *Neurology International Open, 02*(01), E16–E24.

Claessen, M., Visser-Meily, J., Meilinger, T., Postma, A., de Rooij, N. K., & van der Ham, I. (2017). A systematic investigation of navigation impairment in chronic stroke patients: Evidence for three distinct types. *Neuropsychologia, 103*, 154–161.

Cowdell, F., & Garrett, D. (2003). Recreation in stroke - Rehabilitation part two: Exploring patients' views. *International Journal of Therapy and Rehabilitation, 10*(10), 456–462.

Desrosiers, J., Noreau, L., Rochette, A., Bravo, G., & Boutin, C. (2002). Predictors of handicap situations following post-stroke rehabilitation. *Disability and Rehabilitation, 24*(15), 774–785.

De Wit, L., Theuns, P., Dejaeger, E., Devos, S., Gantenbein, A. R., Kerckhofs, E., Schuback, B., Schupp, W., & Putman, K. (2017). Long-term impact of stroke on patients' health-related quality of life. *Disability and Rehabilitation, 39*(14), 1435–1440.

Dixon, G., Thornton, E. W., & Young, C. A. (2007). Perceptions of self-efficacy and rehabilitation among neurologically disabled adults. *Clinical Rehabilitation, 21*, 230–240.

Gallan, A. S., Perlow, B., Shah, R., & Gravdal, J. (2021). The impact of patient shadowing on service design: Insights from a family medicine clinic. *Patient Experience Journal, 8*(1), 88–98.

Gualandi, R., Masella, C., Viglione, D., & Tartaglini, D. (2019). Exploring the hospital patient journey: What does the patient experience? *PLoS ONE, 14*(12), 1–15.

Hempler, I., Woitha, K., Thielhorn, U., & Farin, E. (2018). Post-stroke care after medical rehabilitation in Germany: A systematic literature review of the current provision of stroke patients. *BMC Health Services Research, 18*(1), 1–9.

Heuschmann, P., Busse, O., Wagner, M., Endres, M., Villringer, A., Röther, J., Kolominsky-Rabas, P., & Berger, K. (2010). Schlaganfallhäufigkeit und Versorgung von Schlaganfallpatienten in Deutschland. *Aktuelle Neurologie, 37*(07), 333–340.

Janssen, H., Ada, L., Bernhardt, J., McElduff, P., Pollack, M., Nilsson, M., & Spratt, N. (2014a). Physical, cognitive and social activity levels of stroke patients undergoing rehabilitation within a mixed rehabilitation unit. *Clinical Rehabilitation, 28*(1), 91–101.

Janssen, H., Ada, L., Bernhardt, J., McElduff, P., Pollack, M., Nilsson, M., & Spratt, N. J. (2014b). An enriched environment increases activity in stroke patients undergoing rehabilitation in a mixed rehabilitation unit: A pilot non-randomised controlled trial. *Disability and Rehabilitation*, 36(3), 255–262.

Janssen, H., Ada, L., Middleton, S., Pollack, M., Nilsson, M., Churilov, L., Blennerhassett, J., Faux, S., & New, P. (2021). *Altering the Rehabilitation Environment to Improve Stroke Survivor Activity: A Phase II trial*, 0(0), 1–9.

Kalantari, S., & Snell, R. (2017). Post-occupancy evaluation of a mental healthcare facility based on staff perceptions of design innovations. *HERD*, 10(4), 121–135.

Kalantari, S., Tripathi, V., Rounds, J. D., Mostafavi, A., Snell, R., & Cruz-Garza, J. G. (2021). Evaluating wayfinding designs in healthcare settings through EEG data and virtual response testing. bioRxiv.

Kārkliņa, A., Chen, E., Bērziņa, G., & Stibrant Sunnerhagen, K. (2021). Patients' physical activity in stroke units in Latvia and Sweden. *Brain and Behavior*, 11(5), 1–8.

Kevdzija, M., & Marquardt, G. (2018). Physical barriers to mobility of stroke patients in rehabilitation clinics. *Breaking Down Barriers*, 147–157.

Kevdzija, M., Bozovic-Stamenovic, R., & Marquardt, G. (2022). Stroke patients' free-time activities and spatial preferences during inpatient recovery in rehabilitation centers. *Health Environments Research & Design Journal*, 1–18.

Kevdzija, M., & Marquardt, G. (2021). Stroke patients' nonscheduled activity during inpatient rehabilitation and its relationship with the architectural layout: A multi-center shadowing study. *Topics in Stroke Rehabilitation*, 00(00), 1–7.

Killey, B., & Watt, E. (2006). The effect of extra walking on the mobility, independence and exercise self-efficacy of elderly hospital in-patients: A pilot study. *Contemporary Nurse: A Journal for the Australian Nursing Profession*, 22(1), 120–133.

Kim, J., Thayabaranathan, T., Donnan, G. A., Howard, G., Howard, V. J., Rothwell, P. M., Feigin, V., Norrving, B., Owolabi, M., Pandian, J., Liu, L., Cadilhac, D. A., & Thrift, A. G. (2020). Global Stroke Statistics 2019. *International Journal of Stroke*, 15(8), 819–838.

Langhorne, P., Coupar, F., & Pollock, A. (2009). Motor recovery after stroke: A systematic review. *The Lancet Neurology*, 8(8), 741–754.

Lipson-Smith, R., Churilov, L., Newton, C., Education, D., Zeeman, H., Hons, B., Neuro, M., Bernhardt, J., & Physio, B. (2019). *A Framework for Designing Inpatient Stroke Rehabilitation Facilities: A New Approach Using Interdisciplinary Value-Focused Thinking*, 12(4), 142–158.

Lipson-Smith, R., Pflaumer, L., Elf, M., Blaschke, S.-M., Davis, A., White, M., Zeeman, H., & Bernhardt, J. (2021). Built environments for inpatient stroke rehabilitation services and care: A systematic literature review. *BMJ Open*, 1–11.

Lipson-Smith, R., Zeeman, H., & Bernhardt, J. (2020). What's in a building? A descriptive survey of adult inpatient rehabilitation facility buildings in Victoria, Australia. *Archives of Rehabilitation Research and Clinical Translation*, 2(1), 100040.

Luker, J., Lynch, E., Bernhardsson, S., Bennett, L., & Bernhardt, J. (2015). Stroke survivors' experiences of physical rehabilitation: A systematic review of qualitative studies. *Archives of Physical Medicine and Rehabilitation*, 96(9), 1698–1708.e10.

Mahoney, F. I., & Barthel, D. W. (1965). Functional evaluation: The Barthel Index: A simple index of independence useful in scoring improvement in the rehabilitation of the chronically ill. *Maryland State Medical Journal*, 14, 61–65.

Mansfield, A., Wong, J. S., Bryce, J., Brunton, K., Inness, E. L., Knorr, S., Jones, S., Taati, B., & McIlroy, W. E. (2015). Use of accelerometer-based feedback of walking activity for appraising progress with walking-related goals in inpatient stroke rehabilitation: A randomised controlled trial. *Neurorehabilitation and Neural Repair, 29*(9), 847–857.

Mcdonald, S. (2005). Studying actions in context: A qualitative shadowing method for organisational research. *Qualitative Research, 5*(4), 455–473.

Newall, J. T., Wood, V. A., Hewer, R. L., & Tinson, D. J. (1997). Development of a neurological rehabilitation environment: An observational study. *Clinical Rehabilitation, 11*(2), 146–155.

Nikolaus, G., Zwingmann, C., & Jäckel, W. H. (2006). The system of rehabilitation in Germany. In J. Bengel, W. H. Jäckel, J. Herdt (Eds.), *Research in rehabilitation. Results from a research network in Southwest Germany* (pp. 3–19). Stuttgart: Schattauer.

Rand, D., Eng, J. J., Tang, P. F., Jeng, J. S., & Hung, C. (2009). How active are people with stroke?: Use of accelerometers to assess physical activity. *Stroke; a Journal of Cerebral Circulation, 40*(1), 163–168.

Real, K., Bardach, S. H., & Bardach, D. R. (2017). The role of the built environment: How decentralised nurse stations shape communication, patient care processes, and patient outcomes. *Health Communication, 32*(12), 1557–1570.

Rigby, H., Gubitz, G., & Phillips, S. (2009). A systematic review of caregiver burden following stroke. *International Journal of Stroke, 4*(4), 285–292.

Rosbergen, I. C., Grimley, R. S., Hayward, K. S., Walker, K. C., Rowley, D., Campbell, A. M., McGufficke, S., Robertson, S. T., Trinder, J., Janssen, H., & Brauer, S. G. (2017). Embedding an enriched environment in an acute stroke unit increases activity in people with stroke: a controlled before–after pilot study. *Clinical Rehabilitation, 31*(11), 1516–1528.

Rowe, F., Brand, D., Jackson, C. A., Price, A., Walker, L., Harrison, S., Eccleston, C., Scott, C., Akerman, N., Dodridge, C., Howard, C., Shipman, T., Sperring, U., Macdiarmid, S., & Freeman, C. (2009). Visual impairment following stroke: Do stroke patients require vision assessment? *Age and Ageing, 38*(2), 188–193.

Seo, H. B., Choi, Y. S., & Zimring, C. (2011). Impact of hospital unit design for patient-centered care on nurses' behavior. *Environment and Behavior, 43*(4), 443–468.

Shaw, J., Pemberton, S., Pratt, C., & Salter, L. (2014). Shadowing: A central component of patient and family-centred care. *Nursing Management, 21*(3), 20–23.

Ulrich, R. S., Zimring, C., Zhu, X., DuBose, J., Seo, H.-B., Choi, Y.-S., Quan, X., & Joseph, A. (2008). A review of the research literature on evidence-based healthcare design. Healthcare Leadership White Paper Series #5. *Health Environments Research & Design Journal, 1*(Part I), 101–165.

van Alebeek, M. E., Arntz, R. M., Ekker, M. S., Synhaeve, N. E., Maaijwee, N. A. M. M., Schoonderwaldt, H., van der Vlugt, M. J., van Dijk, E. J., Rutten-Jacobs, L. C. A., & de Leeuw, F. E. (2018). Risk factors and mechanisms of stroke in young adults: The FUTURE study. *Journal of Cerebral Blood Flow and Metabolism, 38*(9), 1631–1641.

van der Meide, H., Olthuis, G., & Leget, C. (2015). Participating in a world that is out of tune: shadowing an older hospital patient. *Medicine, Health Care and Philosophy, 18*(4), 577–585.

van der Weele, S., & Bredewold, F. (2021). Shadowing as a qualitative research method for intellectual disability research: Opportunities and challenges. *Journal of Intellectual & Developmental Disability*, *46*(4), 340–350.

Wallesch, C. W. (2015). Integrated stroke care. *Bundesgesundheitsblatt – Gesundheitsforschung – Gesundheitsschutz*, *58*(4–5), 393–397.

Ween, J. E., Alexander, M. P., D'Esposito, M., & Roberts, M. (1996). Factors predictive of stroke outcome in a rehabilitation setting. *Neurology*, *47*(May 1994), 388–392.

Welton, J. M., Decker, M., Adam, J., & Zone-Smith, L. (2006). How far do nurses walk? *Medsurg Nursing: Official Journal of the Academy of Medical-Surgical Nurses*, *15*(4), 213–216.

7 Outdoor activity-friendly environments for older adults with disabilities

A case study in China from a functioning perspective

Qing Xie and Xiaomei Yuan

Introduction

Populations are rapidly ageing worldwide, and ageing is often accompanied by a decline in mental, sensory, and movement functioning (Chatterji et al., 2015). Healthy ageing has been developed into a global strategy and is defined as "a process of maintaining functional ability to enable well-being in older age" (WHO, 2015b). There is growing evidence that the outdoor environment is beneficial for the health and wellbeing of older adults by promoting outdoor activities (Finlay et al., 2015; Orr et al., 2016; Sugiyama & Thompson, 2007b). Thus, an outdoor activity-friendly environment, which refers to an outdoor or semi-outdoor environment that promotes meaningful activities, is an important facet of healthy ageing. In China, like many countries, the combination of an ageing population and better awareness of healthy lifestyles is a driver for creating outdoor activity-friendly environments for older adults.

In this chapter, we explore the relationship between older adults with disabilities and outdoor activity-friendly environments. The case study is a long-term care facility (LTCF) for older people in China. The focus of the research is a functioning perspective based on the International Classification of Functioning, Disability, and Health (ICF). In China, LTCFs are usually places where older residents with disabilities live collectively and seldom leave, so outdoor activity-friendly environments are particularly important for the residents. The research objectives were to (1) explore how body functions and structures of older people, the outdoor environment, and outdoor activities interact with each other; (2) identify the environmental needs of older adults with disabilities; and (3) determine whether the outdoor environment of the studied LTCF was activity friendly.

Functioning and environment model

Some theoretical models in the field of rehabilitation and gerontology have explained the relationships among people, the environment and behaviour, providing an interdisciplinary theoretical basis for this physical environment

DOI: 10.1201/9781003344711-8

study. Nagi's disability model views disability as the gap between a person's capabilities and the demands created by the social and physical environments (Nagi, 1965). The environmental press model describes individual behaviour as the outcome of the transaction between individual competence and environmental demands (Lawton & Nahemow, 1973). The person-environment-occupation (PEO) model emphasises occupational performance as the outcome of PEO interactions (Law et al., 1996). More than a theoretical model, the ICF aims to provide a unified and standard language and framework for the description of health and health-related states and defines functioning and disability as the interaction of a health condition with environmental and personal factors (WHO, 2001). These theoretical models improve our understanding of functioning which is an essential component of health and well-being. They further inspire us to think about the relationship between functioning and the environment. However, the potential role of the physical environment and activities as health interventions remains under-emphasised in these models.

With reference to the existing theoretical models, especially the conceptualisation of functioning in the ICF, the functioning and environment model was developed to guide this research (Figure 7.1). Unifying the language with the ICF, body functions are physiological or psychological functions of body systems, and body structures are anatomical parts of the body. Impairments are problems in body function or structure. Functioning is used as an umbrella term for body functions and structures, activities, and participation, while disability similarly serves as an umbrella term encompassing impairments, activity limitations, and participation restrictions. The model suggests that in the context of outdoor activity-friendly environments for older adults with disabilities, functioning and disability are the health and

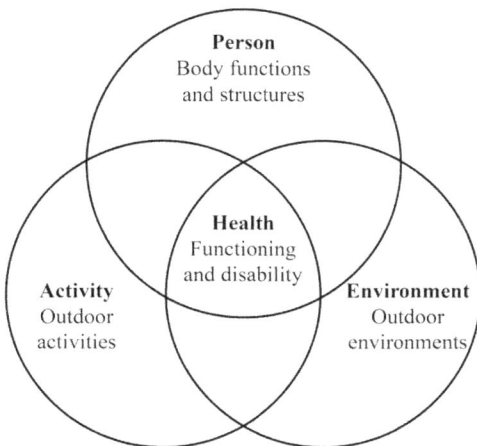

Figure 7.1 Functioning and environment model.

health-related outcomes of the interactions among the body functions and structures of an older adult, the outdoor activities engaged by the older adult, and the outdoor environment in which the older adult lives. In other words, not just focusing on the individual, the rehabilitation of the older adult, the programming of outdoor activities, and the design of the outdoor environment are equally important strategies for promoting healthy ageing. This is still a preliminary model and how these three aspects play their roles is explored in this research.

Evidence on outdoor activity-friendly environments for older adults with disabilities

Empirical research regarding age-friendly environments has examined specific outdoor activities rather than just getting outdoors. Sugiyama and Thompson (2007a, 2007b) suggested that outdoor environments contributed to older adults' health and wellbeing by providing places for contact with nature, physical activity, and social interaction. Bengtsson and Carlsson (2013) found that older residents appreciated outdoor areas for joyful and meaningful activities, including stationary, physical, social, and therapy activities. Pleson et al. (2014) recommended community green spaces to organise group activities and equip for age-friendly exercise. The need for various outdoor activity spaces has been proposed, but further research on the detailed environmental characteristics for older adults with disabilities is lacking.

A number of studies have revealed that neighbourhood environmental factors, such as land use mix, walkability, pleasing scenery, and access to parks/open spaces, positively influence older adults' physical activity (Barnett et al., 2017; Moran et al., 2014; Van Cauwenberg et al., 2018). Some studies further examined the environmental needs of older adults with mobility disabilities. Shumway-Cook et al. (2003, 2002) found that older adults with mobility disabilities reported fewer encounters with and greater avoidance of environmental challenges than those without mobility disabilities regarding temporal factors, physical load, terrain, and postural transitions. The physical activity of older adults with poor lower extremity function was negatively associated with a high variation in vegetation and poor perceived safety and positively associated with the presence of water; these associations were not found for those with intact function (Gong et al., 2014; Keskinen et al., 2018; Sakari et al., 2017).

Previous research has shown that the outdoor environment contributes to behaviour modification, sleep quality, emotional state, and quality of life in older adults with dementia (Gonzalez & Kirkevold, 2014; Motealleh et al., 2019; Whear et al., 2014). For dementia-friendly neighbourhoods, environmental characteristics such as clear street layout, flat paths, visible signage, meaningful landmarks, and reduction in disorienting stimuli were found to enhance the wayfinding of older adults (Gan et al., 2022; Mitchell & Burton, 2010). In memory care facilities, natural elements such as plants and water features were shown to provide sensory stimulation to improve cognitive function and reduce disruptive behaviour (Anderson et al., 2011; Gonzalez & Kirkevold, 2015).

Although mobility and cognitive disabilities have received attention, there is a lack of research on outdoor activity-friendly environment integrating environmental needs from older adults' mental, sensory, and movement functioning and disability. Many older adults have multiple disabilities and experience more outdoor environmental challenges than those without and with one disability (Barnett et al., 2016; Hovbrandt et al., 2007). Additionally, engaging in most types of outdoor activities requires the use of multiple types of body functions and structures.

A few garden and park practices have considered the outdoor activities and disabilities of older adults (Marcus & Sachs, 2013), but few of them have examined whether their design goals are achieved. Eight therapeutic gardens in a care facility were evaluated as achieving the design goals except for providing a place to maintain the hobby of gardening (Heath & Gifford, 2001). An enabling garden in a nursing home was evaluated as having positive effects on meaningful activities and functional competency (Raske, 2010). An exercise intervention using a senior exercise park improved the balance and physical functions of older adults with mild fall risk (Sales et al., 2017). However, both the practice and evaluation of outdoor age-friendly environments are lacking in China.

Influenced by theory, research, and practice, physical environmental assessment tools such as Housing Enabler (Iwarsson et al., 2012), EVOLVE (Lewis et al., 2010), and the Universal Design Assessment Protocol (Sanford, 2012) were developed from the perspective of functioning and disability. Nevertheless, they still focus on removing physical barriers rather than promoting outdoor activities. The seniors' outdoor survey (SOS) has included "walking and outdoor activities" as one domain (Rodiek et al., 2016), but its consideration for specific outdoor activities and disabilities is still insufficient.

In summary, it is critical to consider disabilities and outdoor activities in research and practice related to outdoor environments for older adults. Although healing gardens and neighbourhood environments for older adults with mobility or cognitive disabilities have been increasingly studied, evidence on outdoor activity-friendly environments for older adults with disabilities is still weak. Furthermore, previous studies were mostly conducted in Western countries, and findings from China add to this body of knowledge.

Methods

The functioning and environment model (Figure 7.1) was used as the underlying model for this research. The qualitative case study collected data regarding body functions and structures, outdoor environments, and outdoor activities at one typical Chinese LTCF. Research methods included demographic and health surveys, interviews, and behavioural observations. Older adults and staff were included as participants to provide individual experiences and professional views, respectively. The research was approved by the ethical committee of the Second Affiliated Hospital of South China University of Technology (K-2019-057-01). Written or oral informed consent was obtained from all participants.

Setting

This study was carried out at a purposefully chosen LTCF, which is located on an 80,000 m^2 campus in the suburbs of Guangzhou, China, with a building area of 35,000 m^2, where approximately 950 older adults live. Guangzhou is a first-tier city located in southern China that has a warm and humid climate. The facility is managed by the local government and has been rated by the government as a five-star LTCF for older adults with high-quality physical environments, equipment, management, and services.

Older adults aged 60 or above can apply for admission to the facility, and those with disabilities and/or aged 80 or above have priority. Thus, most older residents in the facility have disabilities, which is in accordance with the target population of this study. The older adults are admitted to the independent living area, assisted living area, skilled nursing area, geriatric hospital (including the skilled nursing area), rehabilitation centre (including the assisted living area), and memory care area (an enclosed residential area for older adults with dementia) depending on their health conditions and willingness.

The facility was originally built in 1965, and after several reconstructions and expansions, the current layout was formed in 2015 (Figure 7.2). The central area of the site is the central garden and recreational centre, with residential and supporting areas in the north and south. Networked streets connect all buildings. The facility covers a variety of outdoor and semi-outdoor spaces, including the central garden, streets, courtyards, entrance squares, semi-outdoor spaces on the ground floor, and roof gardens, providing a diverse outdoor environment for this study. The central garden and its surrounding streets were the main outdoor activity spaces shared by older adults from different residential areas and contained diverse landscape features, such as trees, water features, paths, and pavilions.

Participants

Older adults

All older adults at the facility, except for the memory care area, were invited by staff members to participate in this study. Recruitment was based on their willingness to participate and the following inclusion criteria: (1) be at least 65 years old; (2) have at least one type of disability; (3) have no serious speech impairment or cognitive impairment; and (4) have stable vital signs. The screening information was collected via self-reports from the older adults and was confirmed by medical staff.

Ninety-five older adults were recruited to participate in the demographic and health survey and interviews (Table 7.1). There were more females

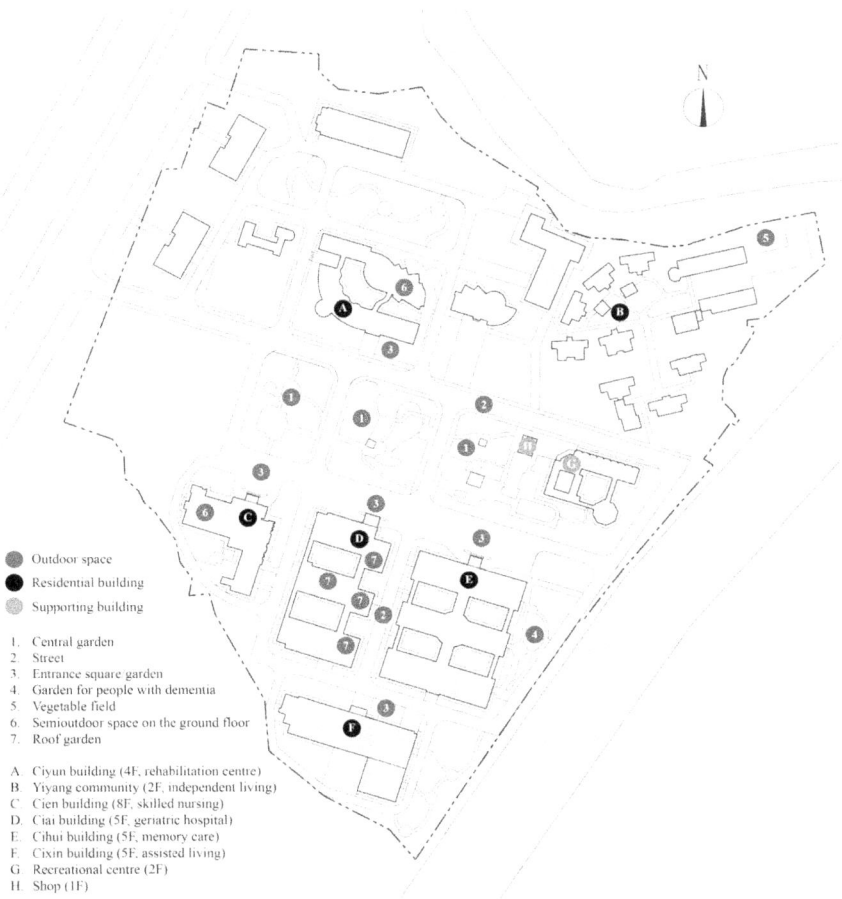

Legend:

- Outdoor space
- Residential building
- Supporting building

1. Central garden
2. Street
3. Entrance square garden
4. Garden for people with dementia
5. Vegetable field
6. Semioutdoor space on the ground floor
7. Roof garden

A. Ciyun building (4F, rehabilitation centre)
B. Yiyang community (2F, independent living)
C. Cien building (8F, skilled nursing)
D. Ciai building (5F, geriatric hospital)
E. Cihui building (5F, memory care)
F. Cixin building (5F, assisted living)
G. Recreational centre (2F)
H. Shop (1F)

Figure 7.2 Site plan of the long-term care facility.

(61.7%) than males (38.3%), with a mean age of 83.2 years. Some of them had private caregivers (30.6%). Two-thirds walked or moved outdoors with mobility aids. The common diseases reported by the older adults were hypertension (62.1%), orthopaedic diseases (30.5%), diabetes (28.4%), and ophthalmic diseases (28.4%). They usually had multiple impairments, with reduced lower extremity function (67.4%), poor stamina (66.3%), and poor balance (52.6%) reported most frequently.

According to the survey and interview data, 12 older adults were purposely selected from the interviewed older adults to represent different sexes, impairments, and residential areas and were further studied through behavioural observations. Most of the observed adults had poor balance ($N = 10$), poor stamina ($N = 8$), and reduced lower extremity function ($N = 7$).

Table 7.1 Characteristics of the interviewed older adults (N = 95)

Characteristic	N (%)
Age (years)	
Mean (SD)	83.2 (7.3)
Range	67–97
Sex	
Female	59 (62.1%)
Male	36 (37.9%)
Private caregiver	
No	66 (69.5%)
Yes, part time	5 (5.3%)
Yes, full time	24 (25.3%)
Mobility aid (outdoor)	
None	30 (31.6%)
Cane	9 (9.5%)
Walker with seat	2 (2.1%)
Wheelchair used as a walker	16 (16.8%)
Wheelchair pushed by others	36 (37.9%)
Electronic wheelchair	2 (2.1%)
Self-reported disease	
Hypertension	59 (62.1%)
Ophthalmic diseases	29 (30.5%)
Diabetes	27 (28.4%)
Orthopaedic diseases	27 (28.4%)
Heart disease	24 (25.3%)
Presbycusis	21 (22.1%)
Stroke	19 (20.0%)
Alzheimer's disease and other dementias	8 (8.4%)
Depression	4 (4.2%)
Parkinson's disease	3 (3.2%)
Chronic obstructive pulmonary disease (COPD)	3 (3.2%)
Chronic kidney diseases (CKD)	2 (2.1%)
Self-reported impairment	
Reduced lower extremity function	64 (67.4%)
Poor stamina	63 (66.3%)
Poor balance	51 (52.6%)
Reduced trunk function	36 (37.9%)
Visual impairment	29 (31.6%)
Poor coordination	28 (29.5%)
Respiratory impairment	27 (28.4%)
Hearing impairment	21 (21.1%)
Reduced upper extremity function	17 (17.9%)
Reduced fine motor skills	16 (16.8%)
Cognitive impairment	16 (16.8%)
Emotional impairment	14 (14.7%)
Reduced neck function	9 (9.5%)

Table 7.2 Characteristics of the interviewed
staff members (N = 28)

Characteristic	N (%)
Sex	
Female	21 (75.0%)
Male	7 (25.0%)
Occupation	
Administrator	6 (21.4%)
Social worker	3 (10.7%)
Doctor	2 (7.1%)
Nurse	2 (7.1%)
Physical therapist	2 (7.1%)
Occupational therapist	2 (7.1%)
Psychotherapist	1 (3.6%)
Caregiver	10 (35.7%)

Staff members

To achieve the diversity of staff occupations, a purposive sample of staff was recruited from all residential and supporting areas to participate in the interviews. The 28 interviewed staff covered the major occupations in the LTCF, including administrators, social workers, doctors, nurses, therapists, and caregivers, and most of them were female (75%; Table 7.2). They had been working at the facility from one to 20 years.

Data collection

Demographic and health survey

A survey was first conducted within a month to collect information regarding the demographic and health characteristics of the older adults, including their age, sex, caregiver status, mobility aid use, disease, and impairment. The older adults were asked to complete the survey questionnaires independently in their apartments. Researchers provided assistance to those who could not read or write. The research team developed a self-reported questionnaire checklist, based on the ICF and the Housing Enabler, which included 13 types of impairments related to outdoor environments (Table 7.1). The data on the presence of impairments helped to summarise the health condition of the older adults and were used to guide interviews and behavioural observations.

Interviews

Following the survey, semi-structured interviews were conducted with older adults over a two-month period to collect information about the older adults' experiences and requirements regarding the outdoor environment. The interviewers were required to be familiar with the participant's demographic and health information before each interview. During the interviews, one interviewer asked questions, and another interviewer recorded the information through field notes and audio recordings. Older adults' apartments were chosen as interview locations to provide a quiet, private, and relaxing environment. The time per interview was 30–60 minutes. The main questions were as follows: (1) Can you describe how your disabilities affect your outdoor activities? (2) What barriers and facilitators have you encountered when using the outdoor environment at the facility? (3) How do you hope to improve the outdoor environment?

Over the next two months, staff members were also interviewed by two interviewers in their offices or resting spaces to provide their work experiences and views regarding the facility and older adults (including groups excluded from older adult participants). Each interview lasted approximately 30 minutes and was recorded through field notes and audio recordings. The questions covered the following: (1) the measures the facility adopted and their own work related to the older adults' disabilities; (2) their opinions regarding functioning, outdoor activities, and outdoor environments; and (3) their suggestions regarding outdoor activity-friendly environments.

Behavioural observations

Behaviour tracking was conducted on selected older adults who had typical impairments to collect objective information about how they interacted with the outdoor environment (Ng, 2016; Zeisel, 2006). Because interviews revealed that the older adults' daily routines were regular, each participant was observed without interference by one observer for one day from 6:00 am to 8:00 pm in warm or cold weather. The times, routes, outdoor activities, and physical environmental barriers and facilitators encountered were recorded via maps, forms, and photographs. The record form provided, but was not limited to, examples of outdoor activities and environmental features.

Data analysis

Descriptive statistics were used to describe the demographic and health characteristics of participants. Qualitative data from interviews and behavioural observations were analysed together to verify and supplement each other following Braun and Clarke's (2006) guidelines for thematic analysis. The interviews were transcribed based on the field notes and audio recordings by interviewers, and the behavioural observations were preliminarily presented as behavioural maps and descriptions by observers. The qualitative data were coded at the semantic level, and themes were identified inductively and deductively. The inductive approach allowed the themes to emerge from the data, whereas the deductive approach based on the functioning and environment model helped to focus on the research objectives. The steps are described briefly as follows: (1) two authors read the field notes, transcripts, maps, and photographs to familiarise themselves with all the data; (2) the first author generated initial codes regarding body functions and structures (e.g., emotional function, vision function, and lower extremity function), outdoor environments (e.g., plant, path, and square), and outdoor activities (e.g., walking, exercise, and gardening) and discussed them with the second author to reach a consensus; (3) the first author coded all the data and collated codes into potential themes, and the second author reviewed all the codes and themes; (4) the two authors defined and named all the themes; and (5) the first author performed the analyses, and the second author reviewed the analyses to ensure their completeness and accuracy. The data were analysed in Chinese. The quotations used in the article were translated into English by the first author and reviewed by the interviewers to avoid distortions of the meaning.

Results

Five themes were identified through analysis of interactions among body functions and structures, the outdoor environment, and outdoor activities. These were as follows: (1) natural environments with positive sensory stimuli; (2) accessible and personalised gardening spaces; (3) safe and comfortable walking environments; (4) spaces and equipment for playful exercise; and (5) gathering spaces mixing diverse people. Additionally, three patterns of interactions regarding how the outdoor environment could benefit functioning in older adults were revealed. These were as follows: (1) the outdoor environment could facilitate outdoor activities by compensating for impairments; (2) the outdoor environment could facilitate outdoor activities by utilising remaining body functions and structures; and (3) the outdoor environment could improve body functions and structures by facilitating outdoor activities.

The findings showed that the mental, sensory, and movement functioning of older adults was related to multiple types of outdoor activity spaces. Mental functions were perceived to be improved by natural environments, gardening spaces, and gathering spaces (Themes 1, 2, and 5). Sensory impairments needed special consideration in natural environments and walking environments, and sensory functions were stimulated by natural environments (Themes 1 and 3). Reduced movement functions and structures required physical assistance from gardening spaces and walking environments, and movement functions and structures were used and were expected to be improved in gardening spaces, walking environments, and exercise spaces (Themes 2, 3, and 4).

Multiple outdoor activities in which older adults participated were identified and categorised as follows: (1) passive exposures, which involved viewing the landscape while sitting or standing in the outdoor environment, such as watching fish, smelling flowers, and listening to birdsong (Theme 1); (2) active engagements, which included physical activity and/or social interaction in the outdoor environment, such as walking, gardening, and

Functioning	Interactions	Themes	Environmental needs	Environmental evaluations
Mental functioning		Natural environments with positive sensory stimuli	Relaxing natural environments / Added positive natural stimuli and avoided negative natural stimuli / Natural environments supporting natural-based therapies	Mostly achieved
		Accessible and personalized gardening spaces	Accessible gardening spaces and age-friendly gardening tools / Personalized gardening spaces and plants	Slightly achieved
Sensory functioning		Safe and comfortable walking environments	Accessible and safe walking environments from indoor to outdoors / Sufficient rest spaces and nearby walking routes / Appropriate mobility aids	Somewhat achieved
		Spaces and equipment for playful exercise	Comfortable exercise spaces / Age-friendly and playful exercise equipment with varied difficulty levels / Specially designed outdoor therapy spaces	Somewhat achieved
Movement functioning		Gathering spaces mixing diverse people	Gathering spaces with organized group activities or necessary activities / Spacious and tidy spaces	Mostly achieved

→ Pattern 1: The outdoor environment facilitates outdoor activities by compensating for impairments.
→ Pattern 2: The outdoor environment facilitates outdoor activities by utilizing remaining body functions and structures.
--→ Pattern 3: The outdoor environment improves body functions and structures by facilitating outdoor activities.

Figure 7.3 Summary of findings according to the five themes.

chatting (Themes 2, 3, 4, and 5); and (3) rehabilitation interventions, which involved therapy or training with specific therapeutic goals in the outdoor environment, such as gait training, horticultural therapy, and animal-assisted therapy (Themes 1, 2, and 4). Passive exposures and active engagements were common in the setting, while outdoor rehabilitation interventions were desired but had not yet been implemented as regular rehabilitation programmes.

The specific interactions, environmental needs, and environmental evaluations were analysed according to the five themes and are summarised in Figure 7.3.

Natural environments with positive sensory stimuli

Theme 1 was revealed from the interactions among mental and sensory functions, natural environments, and sensory experiences. The natural environment facilitated the sensory experience of older adults by compensating for sensory impairments and utilising remaining sensory functions. Through sensory experience, the natural environment stimulated the sensory functions of older adults and was perceived to improve their emotional function. The staff considered that the natural environment had the potential to improve mental functions by supporting nature-based therapy.

The natural environment was the reason why many interviewed older adults chose to live in the facility. They believed that the natural environment with sunlight, fresh air, and greenery made them feel relaxed. Specifically, natural elements, such as "brightly coloured flowers", "glistening water", "scents of Osmanthus", and "crisp birdsong", were perceived to provide fascinating sensory experiences (Figure 7.4). For example, Xu (female, 87 years old), who has long suffered from leg pain, appreciated her experience near the fishpond in the central garden:

(a)

(b)

(c)

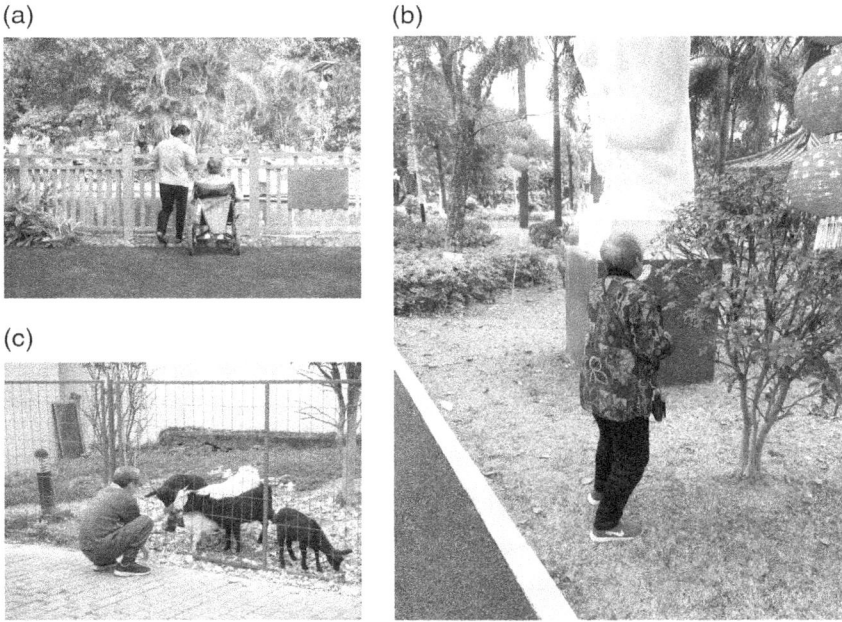

Figure 7.4 Natural sensory experience: (a) watching the pond; (b) smelling osmanthus; (c) feeding the sheep.

*I like to sit or stand near the fishpond, and sometimes feed the fish ...
Watching the water makes me feel relaxed, and the interaction with fish is
interesting. It helps me forget my pain.*

Due to sensory impairments and preference, increased sensory stimuli were
required by older adults. Some older adults provided detailed suggestions for
richer sensory stimulation from nature. Xu (female, 87 years old), who had
cataracts, suggested adding red, yellow, and pink seasonal flowers along the
streets. In addition to the visual experience, other sensory experiences
through sound, smell, and touch were also desired. For example, Jin (male,
85 years old) described his ideal garden with multiple sensory experiences:

*I prefer a dynamic landscape. Fish and fountains are important for a pond. If
there were music on the water, it would be better ... I also like scenes with
singing birds and fragrant flowers.*

In contrast, older adults argued that negative natural stimuli, such as frog
calls at night, plant pollen, and rotten leaves, should be controlled. Zhang
(male, 85 years old) with COPD was particularly sensitive to smells. He liked
to stay outdoors with fresh air instead of indoors with odours, but he had a

love-hate relationship with flowering trees: "The flowers are beautiful, but the fallen flowers, flocs, and leaves are everywhere. It is dirty".

Significantly, it was found that natural elements were particularly attractive to older adults with dementia. Several staff members pointed out that older adults in the memory care area liked to touch and feed the sheep in the enclosed garden (Figure 7.4(c)). A caregiver noticed that the older adult with dementia she took care of was very sensitive to natural elements:

I take my older adult to hang out outdoors every morning … She likes to touch the leaves, smell the flowers, and watch fish along the way.

Most of the staff talked about the health benefits of the natural environment for older adults, especially for those with depression or dementia. Encouraged by the popularity of the sheep, an occupational therapist was optimistic about the benefits of animal-assisted therapy for patients with dementia. Although outdoor psychotherapy was not offered as a regular programme at the facility, the psychological therapist sometimes took patients with depression to walk, view, and talk in the garden and appreciated the psychological benefits of nature.

In summary, environmental needs regarding "natural environments with positive sensory stimuli" were mostly achieved in the facility. The relaxing natural environment and varied sensory experiences were enjoyed by the older adults. Positive sensory stimuli from natural elements were desired to be richer, while negative stimuli were asked to be controlled. The natural environment has not been officially used for nature-based therapy.

Accessible and personalised gardening spaces

Theme 2 emerged from the interactions among mental and movement functions, gardening spaces, and gardening. The inaccessible gardening space and the lack of assistive technology hindered gardening of older adults due to the inability to compensate for reduced movement functions and structures. Spontaneous gardening spaces facilitated gardening by meeting older adults' psychological needs for personalisation. Gardening spaces were expected by the staff to improve mental and movement functions by supporting horticultural therapy.

The vegetable field in the independent living area was planned as a gardening space for the older adults but was not fully used due to its remote location and inaccessible design. Older adults, including those living independently, commonly had difficulties bending, kneeling and reaching with their arms and could barely accomplish tasks on the ground, overhead or requiring significant body movement. For example, Lu (male, 88 years old) explained why he did not participate in farming in the vegetable field:

As I know, the vegetable field is mainly taken care of by staff. I sometimes visit there … Vegetables are planted on the ground, but I can hardly bend or squat; so, farming is difficult for me.

In contrast to the underutilisation of the planned gardening space, some older adults spontaneously engaged in gardening on roof gardens, balconies, corridors, and green spaces around buildings. The spontaneous gardening spaces created and maintained by older adults themselves met their psychological needs for personalisation but encountered obstacles from unified management. Chen (female, 83 years old), who experienced the death of her husband and son, regarded gardening as her strategy for remaining optimistic and an important part of her daily life. She hoped to enjoy a personalised gardening space to maintain the habit of combining gardening with diet therapy:

> *Gardening helps me be happy … I grow edible and medicinal plants … The green space is managed by gardeners, and they always cut down my plants by mistake … I hope to have my own gardening space and grow my favourite plants.*

In addition to the lack of well-designed gardening spaces, the lack of age-friendly gardening tools was another hindering factor. According to the behavioural observations, unlike the widespread use of mobility aids and specifically designed tableware, assistive technology was rarely used in gardening. One of the few examples was Deng (female, 80 years old), who had both upper and lower extremity impairments but maintained the hobby of gardening. She kept a small shovel and a small watering pot in her wheelchair and went to the terrace to care for her plotted plants every day.

Furthermore, the staff's expectation of gardening spaces went beyond supporting leisure gardening. An occupational therapist appreciated the benefits of existing indoor horticultural therapy on mental and movement functions and hoped to utilise outdoor gardening spaces for horticultural therapy: "Outdoor gardening might be easier for older adults with the help of assistive technologies, such as raised beds and tools with longer handles and lighter weight".

As noted earlier, environmental needs regarding "accessible and personalized gardening spaces" were slightly achieved in the facility. The planned vegetable field was not used by the older adults because of inaccessibility, while spontaneous gardening spaces emerged but were limited. Outdoor gardening spaces had not been used for horticultural therapy.

Safe and comfortable walking environments

Theme 3 was derived from the interactions among movement and sensory functions, walking environments, and walking. Although the walking environment provided opportunities for older adults to maintain their walking ability, environmental barriers hindered walking due to harm to visual and movement functions. Sufficient rest spaces and nearby walking routes facilitated walking by compensating for reduced stamina. Mobility aids and caregivers also assisted the mobility of older adults.

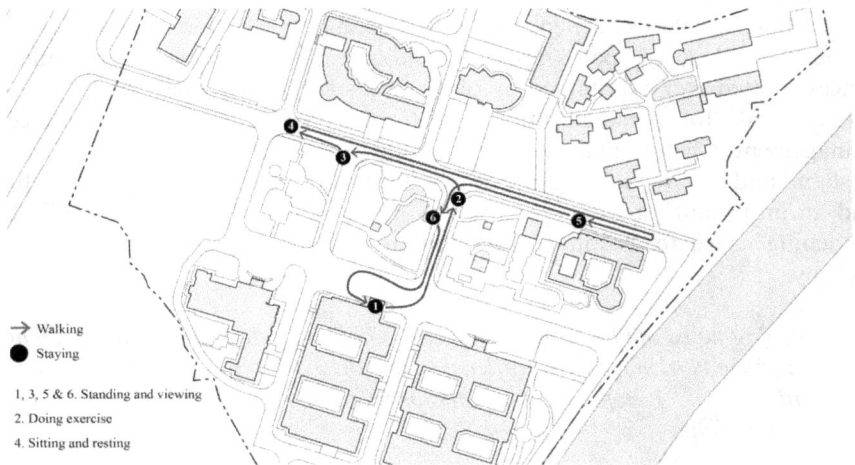

Figure 7.5 Walking route on the streets.

When talking about movement functions such as balance and coordination, many older adults shared their experiences with walking and falls. Although the staff and older adults mentioned that environmental modifications, including motor vehicle restrictions and pavement replacement, made the walking environment safer, the older adults still reported some environmental barriers, such as "steep wheelchair ramps", "uneven ground surfaces", and "sharp planter corners". To be safe, many older adults preferred to walk on wide and straight streets rather than narrow and curved paths. For example, Xie (male, 81 years old) was observed to walk back and forth along streets and hardly walk into the garden (Figure 7.5), which confirmed what he said:

> *I go out for a walk almost every day. I am used to walking along the street and enjoying the view of the garden … It is not convenient to push a wheelchair on the garden path.*

Rest spaces were an essential component of the walking environment, which was emphasised by older adults with reduced stamina. Liu (female, 81 years old) was observed to rest every time she walked a short distance. Her rest locations included chairs in the entrance hall, benches beside the sidewalk, and her own wheelchair in the shade. When the older adults described their favourite rest spaces, "comfortable benches", "tree shade", and "views of scenery" were frequently reported features. Walking routes near residential buildings were more accessible to frail older adults. Huang (female, 80 years old), who moved from Ciai Building to Cixin Building, complained that the central garden was too far away for a walk.

In addition to movement functions and structures, visual impairment was also related to mobility limitation in older adults. Older adults with low vision reported environmental barriers, such as "glare of the sun", "handrails with reflective material", and "vegetation blocking the vision along the path", which increased the safety risk of walking. For example, Xu (female, 87 years old), who had cataracts, recalled the reason for her fall:

> *I fell down at the entrance of the building because the sudden change in light made me feel dizzy.*

The staff said that they tried to train blind older adults with good movement functions and structures to walk around by themselves. However, the training was difficult to implement outdoors due to the lack of environmental support, such as "tactile paving", "continuous handrails", and "auditory cues". Liang (male, 67 years old), who had visual loss, was observed walking under the guidance of handrails indoors but did not go outdoors because there was no continuous handrail from indoor to outdoor.

In addition, mobility aids and caregivers influenced the mobility of older adults. According to the behavioural observations, the older adults pushed in their wheelchairs by caregivers had a large range of mobility, while the older adults in the wheelchair without caregivers could not go far away from their residential buildings. Most of them lacked training of lower-extremity function. Older adults who walked with mobility aids without caregivers had a moderate range of mobility and exercised their walking ability. Although the safety of using a wheelchair as a walker has been questioned, the approach was common in the facility. Xie (male, 81 years old) was observed to use his wheelchair in multiple ways, including walking, exercising, and sitting. He explained the advantages of wheelchairs:

> *I think wheelchairs are more stable than walkers and canes, so I use the wheelchair to keep my balance … When I feel tired, I can rest in the wheelchair.*

In short, environmental needs regarding "safe and comfortable walking environments" were somewhat achieved in the facility. The streets provided a safe and comfortable walking environment, while the garden paths and the entrances of buildings had environmental barriers for older adults with reduced movement or visual functions. Mobility aids were widely used in the facility, but the coordination between the walking environment and mobility aids still needed improvement.

Spaces and equipment for playful exercise

Theme 4 was revealed from the interactions among movement functions and structures, exercise spaces and equipment, and exercise. Large and comfortable spaces supported the group exercise of older adults, and land-scape features used as informal exercise equipment assisted their individual exercise, both of which utilised remaining movement functions and structures. In addition, outdoor spaces were expected by therapists to improve movement functions and structures by supporting physical and occupational therapy.

Group exercises, such as seated exercise and Tai Chi (a type of traditional Chinese exercise), organised in outdoor or semi-outdoor spaces were popular in the facility. Half of the observed older adults participated in group exercise in their residential areas or the recreational centre. Because the thermal comfort of exercise spaces was essential for frail older adults, the location of group exercise was adjusted according to the season and weather. Some interviewed older adults believed that the semi-outdoor space on the ground floor, which is common in warm and humid regions, was their preferred space for group exercise in warm weather because of the large space, flat ground, shelter, and breeze.

According to an administrator's explanation, outdoor exercise equipment was removed because of the safety risk: "General exercise equipment is dangerous for the older adults here". Several older adults with good movement functions and structures still proposed the need for exercise equipment. Fortunately, the lack of formal exercise equipment did not completely restrict the individual exercise of older adults and even made their exercise playful. The behavioural observations showed that some older adults exercised autonomously with the help of mobility aids, handrails, branches, benches, and children's slides (Figure 7.6). Xu (female, 70 years old) insisted on exercising every day and explained her preference for the fishpond:

I like the fishpond not only because of the fish but also because I can hold the handrails of the bridge to do exercise.

However, older adults with poor movement functions and structures could hardly exercise themselves effectively without professional spaces and equipment. The physical and occupational therapists suggested that it was necessary to provide outdoor therapy spaces for gait training and horticultural therapy. They also believed that it was a way to blur the boundary between leisure exercise and rehabilitation training to enhance the exercise initiative and autonomy of older adults with varied exercise abilities. A physical therapist shared his idea:

We have moved our therapy rooms to the ground floor. If the courtyard was modified into a therapy garden, we would provide physical therapy outdoors. It could better mimic real life.

In summary, environmental needs regarding "spaces and equipment for playful exercise" were somewhat achieved in the facility. Large and comfortable

(a)

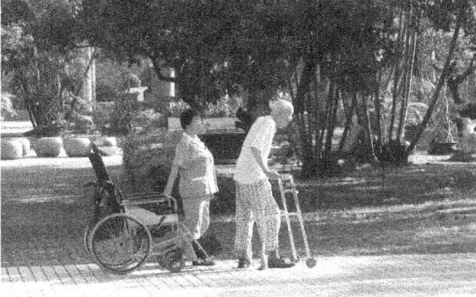

(b)

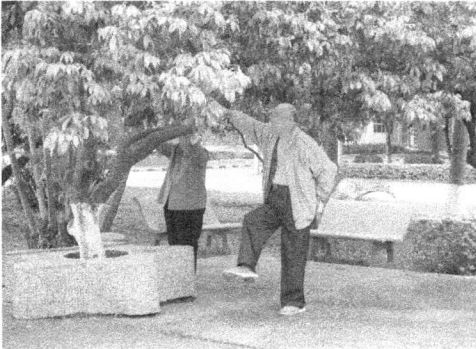

(c)

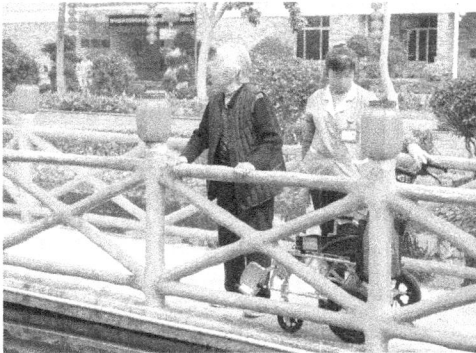

Figure 7.6 Autonomous exercise: (a) gait training with a walker; (b) exercising with branches; (c) exercising with handrails.

outdoor and semi-outdoor spaces provided good support for group exercise. Age-friendly and playful outdoor exercise equipment with varied difficulty levels was needed but lacking. The need for outdoor therapy spaces was proposed by therapists but was not achieved.

Gathering spaces mixing diverse people

Theme 5 emerged from the interactions among mental functions, gathering spaces, and social activities. Outdoor gathering spaces enabled older adults with different health conditions to participate in social activities together, which was perceived to improve their emotional and cognitive functions. The social activities started with organised group activities or necessary activities but were not limited to them.

Gathering spaces were found to be beneficial for older adults to overcome negative emotions. A few interviewed older adults believed that social activities helped them alleviate loneliness, boredom, and sadness caused by relocation, widowhood, and disease. For example, Guo (female, 84 years old) was happy to enjoy group activities in the gathering space:

The square near the residential building is where I mainly participate in activities, such as doing morning exercise, singing, and chatting. Traditional festivals are also celebrated there (Figure 7.7(a)) ... These activities make my life less boring.

It was revealed that the emotions of older adults were affected by the surrounding environment. According to the behavioural observations, some older adults seemed to be silent and depressed in dark indoor public spaces, while they tended to be lively and active in sunny outdoor gathering spaces. Several staff members reported that social workers, caregivers, and older adults with better health conditions would lead older adults with poor health conditions to participate in outdoor activities. A social worker explained the benefits of mixing diverse people in gathering spaces for older adults, especially for females:

Older adults with poor health conditions are likely to feel depressed if they always stay alone. Even just staying in the gathering space with an energetic atmosphere is beneficial for them ... Elderly women like these social activities more than men and play a more active role in them.

The courtyard of the recreational centre was a group activity location for older adults from different residential areas, including those with mild cognitive impairment (MCI) or dementia who did not live in the memory care area. For example, Xie (male, 80 years old), who had dementia and lived in Cixin Building, considered social interaction with others without dementia to be beneficial to his health. He was observed to follow his wife to participate in activities in the

(a)

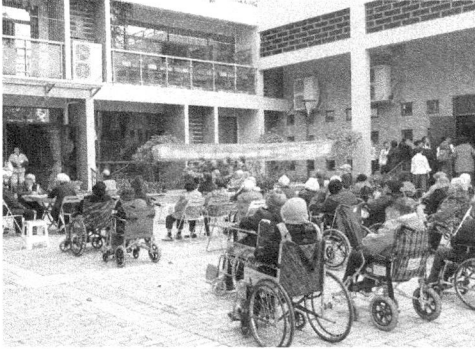

(b)

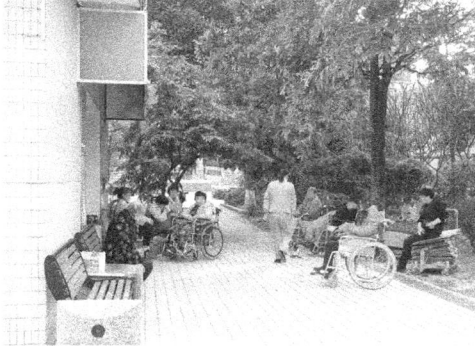

Figure 7.7 Social activities: (a) group activities near the residential building; (b) gathering near the shop.

courtyard of the recreational centre, such as performing morning exercise, chatting, and receiving gifts.

Different from the organised gathering spaces, the entrance square of the shop attracted older adults from different residential areas to gather and chat because of its shopping function (Figure 7.7(b)). As the only amenity in the LTCF, the shop contributed greatly to the sense of community. Half of the observed older adults visited the shop. They bought goods, chatted with shop clerks and other older adults, or just sat on benches watching other people. For example, Guan (female, 92 years old) was observed to select vegetables and talk with others in the shop entrance square and asked for a better physical environment:

I ask my caregiver to take me to the shop every day. The shop is small but busy, so sometimes goods are put outside the shop. I think the shop and its surrounding space should be more spacious and tidier.

In conclusion, environmental needs regarding "gathering space mixing diverse people" were mostly achieved in the facility. Outdoor spaces near residential buildings, the recreational centre, and the shop were used as gathering spaces, but the physical environment should be improved.

Discussion

The role of outdoor environments in functioning and disability

Existing theoretical models have regarded the environment as a critical factor in functioning and disability, and the ICF provides a list of natural and built environmental factors, but the specific patterns of how the environment influences functioning and disability have not been explained (Schneidert et al., 2003). The study confirms the importance of outdoor environments and provides evidence that outdoor environments may facilitate outdoor activities by compensating for impairments and utilising remaining body functions and structures, which could further improve body functions and structures. Although the outdoor environment is only part of the physical environment, the patterns revealed in this study validate and complement the theoretical assumptions of the functioning and environment model, providing a new perspective derived from the field of rehabilitation for age-friendly environmental studies.

Unlike most previous studies regarding older adults as one group (Bengtsson & Carlsson, 2013; Pleson et al., 2014) or focusing on one specific group with mobility or cognitive disability (Mitchell & Burton, 2010; Shumway-Cook et al., 2003), the present study addressed mental, sensory, and movement functioning and disability. The results showed that each type of functioning was related to multiple types of outdoor activity spaces. As shown in Figure 7.3, the relationships between mental, sensory, and movement functioning and natural environments, gardening spaces, walking environments, exercise spaces, and gathering spaces were preliminarily established, but further research is needed to examine these relationships.

To take advantage of the positive role of outdoor environments in functioning and disability, cooperation between medical and design fields is essential. This research was mainly conducted by researchers in landscape architecture and supported by professionals in rehabilitation medicine, which contributes to this study theoretically and operationally. The findings reported by Wagenfeld et al. (2017) and this study imply that environmental intervention is a benchmark for cooperation between medical and design fields, which can further promote the development of design projects, activity programmes, and care programmes. In addition, the research design of this study based on the functioning and environment model demonstrates the use of theory in interdisciplinary empirical research.

Outdoor activities

Most types of outdoor activities in this study have been identified in previous studies (Bengtsson & Carlsson, 2013; Pleson et al., 2014; Sugiyama &

Thompson, 2007a), including sensory experience, gardening, walking, exercise, group activities, and chatting. In contrast to studies conducted in Western countries, the outdoor activities identified in this study reflected Chinese culture, such as Tai chi, square dancing, traditional festival celebration, and planting preference for herbs, implying the importance of further research on outdoor environments supporting traditional Chinese exercises, festivals, and healthy habits.

The study showed that in addition to passive exposures and active engagements, rehabilitation interventions were also attempted outdoors, which is consistent with the increasing trend for outdoor space use to conduct physical and occupational therapy (Haering, 2016). A randomised controlled trial based on the findings of this study has shown that specially designed outdoor therapy spaces can enhance functioning in older adults (Zhou et al., 2020). Moreover, the boundary between leisure activities and rehabilitation therapies was considered to have the potential to be blurred, which confirms previous studies on the effectiveness of rehabilitation based on leisure activities (Kamioka et al., 2013). Although leisure activities contribute to preventing disabilities and rehabilitation therapies aim to foster recovery from disabilities, they have commonalities in activity forms and environmental features. In addition to the development of gardening into horticultural therapy (Wagenfeld & Atchison, 2014), it is worth modifying other types of leisure activities to serve as outdoor rehabilitation interventions.

Environmental needs and evaluations

By delving into disabilities and outdoor activities, the findings contribute to the knowledge regarding the environmental needs of older adults and further benefit the practice and evaluation of outdoor environments.

Many benefits that people receive from nature accrue through the five senses (Franco et al., 2017), but sensory impairments cause older adults to perceive and respond to the physical environment in different ways (Christenson, 1990). Theme 1 revealed the psychological benefits of the natural environment (Finlay et al., 2015; Rodiek, 2002) and highlighted the need for positive sensory stimuli from nature (Bengtsson & Carlsson, 2013; Orr et al., 2016). The attractiveness of natural elements to older adults with dementia implies that multisensory stimulation in a specially designed natural environment may be as beneficial as a Snoezelen room (Sánchez et al., 2013).

The study supports the finding of Brascamp and Kidd (2004) showing that active gardening is influenced more than passive natural exposure because of the physical limitations of older adults. Theme 2 further indicated that accessible spaces and assisted technology may be helpful to maintain the gardening ability of older adults with reduced movement functions and structures. Spontaneous gardening in informal spaces reflected not only the lack of well-designed gardening spaces but also the need for personalised gardening spaces. Community gardens can enhance social cohesion (Veen et al., 2016), while personalised gardening spaces can support the individual lifestyle of older adults. This result is in accordance with Wang and MacMillan's (2013) point that the benefits of gardening can be a way of life, extending beyond improving health and wellbeing.

Theme 3 has some commonalities with findings from neighbourhood studies that emphasise the influence of pedestrian infrastructure and rest areas on the physical activity of older adults (Moran et al., 2014). Regarding indoor-outdoor connections, although doorway problems examined by Rodiek et al. (2014) were not reported in this study, environmental barriers at the entrance of buildings, such as steep wheelchair ramps, sudden changes in light, and a lack of continuous handrails, were reported by older adults with reduced visual and movement functions. The findings support the notion that traditional barrier-free design is insufficient for age-friendly walking environments because this design is mainly for adult wheelchair users and ignores frail older adults, patients with dementia, visually impaired people, and people using varied mobility aids (Bigonnesse et al., 2018; Sanford, 2012; Steinfeld et al., 1979).

Theme 4 supports the previous finding that shade or shelter to protect older adults from uncomfortable weather is the main facilitator of outdoor exercise (Sales et al., 2018; Stride et al., 2017). In the warm and humid climate, this finding was emphasised by the popularity of semi-outdoor spaces on the ground floor for group exercise. Safety risk was the reason for removing outdoor exercise equipment in the facility, but it was not considered a critical issue in previous studies in which equipment was seldom used by older adults with disabilities (Chow, 2013; Cranney et al., 2016). The study showed that older adults differed in exercise ability, requiring different exercise forms and equipment, which has been considered in previous practice (Levinger et al., 2018). The landscape features used as informal exercise equipment imply that the integration of exercise equipment into landscape design may increase the entertainment of exercise compared with just placing equipment outdoors.

Theme 5 identified two types of gathering spaces, namely, outdoor spaces with organised group activities and outdoor spaces near amenities, which increased social interaction among older adults, including those with emotional or cognitive impairment. The older adults did not propose strict requirements for the physical environment of outdoor gathering spaces except for being spacious and clean. In addition to the shop in the facility, amenities such as cafes and restaurants can also increase the social interaction of older adults (Wen et al., 2018).

Although not reported as the main findings of this study, social factors, such as unified management, motor vehicle restriction, organisation of group activities, and presence of private caregivers, had a great impact on older adults' outdoor activities. Some of these social factors may be unique characteristics of Chinese LTCFs but support the notion that physical and social environments play crucial roles together in older adults' health and wellbeing (WHO, 2015a).

An informal environmental evaluation was conducted in accordance with the environmental needs identified in this study instead of using existing environmental assessment tools (Rodiek et al., 2016; Yuan et al., 2018). Although the studied setting meets some environmental needs of older adults with disabilities, it is still not adequately activity-friendly, especially with respect to gardening spaces, outdoor exercise equipment, and outdoor therapy spaces. To apply research evidence to practice, future research needs to carry out post-occupancy evaluations or experiments for intentionally designed projects. This also implies that age-friendly environmental assessment tools need to adopt evidence regarding various outdoor activity spaces.

Limitations

This case study focused on one LTCF in China, and although the facility could be seen as being typical of large-scale public facilities in China, the results may not be representative of similar facilities. We would expect to see a richer body of evidence in a larger study from the functioning perspective of the ICF; and we would also expect to see differences in other countries due to variations in culture, habits, and attitudes. The findings were also limited by the need to exclude some older adults who were unable to participate in interviews, a practical limitation inherent in this type of research. Furthermore, each adult was observed for only one day, which restricted the behavioural observation data, and we would expect a longer period of observation to reveal a greater degree of diversity. Another limitation is the self-reporting of diseases and impairments, which may not be sufficiently objective and accurate. Therefore, the findings are not generalizable to all regions, settings, and older adults with disabilities.

Conclusions

This study showed that the outdoor environment could facilitate outdoor activities, including passive exposures, active engagements, and rehabilitation interventions, by compensating for impairments and utilising remaining body functions and structures, which could further improve body functions and structures. Five themes emerged from specific interactions to derive environmental needs and conduct environmental evaluations. The outdoor environment of the studied LTCF was not adequately activity-friendly for older adults with disabilities.

This exploratory case study demonstrates some potential for future work to link theory, research, and practice: (1) theoretical models such as the ICF are worth further development to provide a theoretical basis for empirical research and a common language for interdisciplinary cooperation; (2) quantitative studies conducted in multiple settings around the world can yield strong evidence on the relationships among body functions and structures, outdoor environments, and outdoor activities in older adults; (3) outdoor spaces for specific types of outdoor activities and therapies, such as gardening, Tai Chi, and gait training, are worth studying; and (4) the development of outdoor activity-friendly environments for older adults should aim to improve functioning, and examinations of whether the design goals are achieved should be performed.

This study provides knowledge supporting the importance of outdoor activity-friendly environments for older adults with disabilities and enriches understanding of the relationship between functioning and the environment. It offers insights that are beneficial not only for the creation of environments for healthy ageing but also for interdisciplinary cooperation between medicine and design.

Acknowledgements

The authors thank Shunxi Zhang and Songbin Chen from Guangzhou First People's Hospital (Second Affiliated Hospital of the South China University of Technology) for their help with the development of the demographic and health survey and Tongyue Zhou, Yiman Li, and Jingjing Yan for their assistance with data collection. This research was supported by the National Key Research and Development Program of China (Grant Number 2017YFC0702905-03).

References

Anderson, K., Bird, M., MacPherson, S., McDonough, V., & Davis, T. (2011). Findings from a pilot investigation of the effectiveness of a snoezelen room in residential care: Should we be engaging with our residents more? *Geriatric Nursing*, *32*(3), 166–177.

Barnett, A., Cerin, E., Zhang, C. J. P., Sit, C. H. P., Johnston, J. M., Cheung, M. M. C., & Lee, R. S. Y. (2016). Associations between the neighbourhood environment characteristics and physical activity in older adults with specific types of chronic conditions: The ALECS cross-sectional study. *International Journal of Behavioral Nutrition and Physical Activity*, *13*, Article 53.

Barnett, D. W., Barnett, A., Nathan, A., Van Cauwenberg, J., Cerin, E., & Grp, C. O. A. W. (2017). Built environmental correlates of older adults' total physical activity and walking: A systematic review and meta-analysis. *International Journal of Behavioral Nutrition and Physical Activity*, *14*, Article 103.

Bengtsson, A., & Carlsson, G. (2013). Outdoor environments at three nursing homes- qualitative interviews with residents and next of kin. *Urban Forestry & Urban Greening*, *12*(3), 393–400.

Bigonnesse, C., Mahmood, A., Chaudhury, H., Mortenson, W. B., Miller, W. C., & Martin Ginis, K. A. (2018). The role of neighborhood physical environment on mobility and social participation among people using mobility assistive technology. *Disability & Society*, *33*(6), 866–893.

Brascamp, W., & Kidd, J. (2004). Contribution of plants to the well-being of retirement home residents. *Acta Horticulturae*, *639*, 145–150.

Braun, V., & Clarke, V. (2006). Using thematic analysis in psychology. *Qualitative research in psychology*, *3*(2), 77–101.

Chatterji, S., Byles, J., Cutler, D., Seeman, T., & Verdes, E. (2015). Health, functioning, and disability in older adults—Present status and future implications. *The lancet*, *385*(9967), 563–575.

Chow, H.-w. (2013). Outdoor fitness equipment in parks: A qualitative study from older adults' perceptions. *BMC Public Health*, *13*(1), 1–9.

Christenson, M. A. (1990). Adaptations of the physical environment to compensate for sensory changes. *Physical & Occupational Therapy in Geriatrics*, *8*(3-4), 3–30.

Cranney, L., Phongsavan, P., Kariuki, M., Stride, V., Scott, A., Hua, M., & Bauman, A. (2016). Impact of an outdoor gym on park users' physical activity: A natural experiment. *Health & Place*, *37*, 26–34.

Finlay, J., Franke, T., McKay, H., & Sims-Gould, J. (2015). Therapeutic landscapes and wellbeing in later life: Impacts of blue and green spaces for older adults. *Health & Place*, *34*, 97–106.

Franco, L. S., Shanahan, D. F., & Fuller, R. A. (2017). A review of the benefits of nature experiences: More than meets the eye. *International Journal of Environmental Research and Public Health*, *14*(8), Article 864.

Gan, D. R., Chaudhury, H., Mann, J., & Wister, A. V. (2022). Dementia-friendly neighborhood and the built environment: A scoping review. *The Gerontologist*, *62*(6), e340–e356.

Gong, Y., Gallacher, J., Palmer, S., & Fone, D. (2014). Neighbourhood green space, physical function and participation in physical activities among elderly men: The Caerphilly Prospective study. *International Journal of Behavioral Nutrition and Physical Activity*, *11*, Article 40.

Gonzalez, M. T., & Kirkevold, M. (2014). Benefits of sensory garden and horticultural activities in dementia care: A modified scoping review. *Journal of Clinical Nursing*, *23*(19-20), 2698–2715.

Gonzalez, M. T., & Kirkevold, M. (2015). Clinical use of sensory gardens and outdoor environments in Norwegian nursing homes: A cross-sectional E-mail survey. *Issues in Mental Health Nursing*, *36*(1), 35–43.

Haering, M. (2016). *The use of outdoor environments by occupational and physical therapy staff in the context of patient treatment in rehabilitation settings: An exploratory study* (Master's Thesis). Michigan State University, East Lansing, MI. Retrieved from https://d.lib.msu.edu/etd/3903. Available from MSU Libraries.

Heath, Y., & Gifford, R. (2001). Post-occupancy evaluation of therapeutic gardens in a multi-level care facility for the aged. *Activities, Adaptation & Aging*, *25*(2), 21–43.

Hovbrandt, P., Stahl, A., Iwarsson, S., Horstmann, V., & Carlsson, G. (2007). Very old people's use of the pedestrian environment: Functional limitations, frequency of activity and environmental demands. *European Journal of Ageing*, *4*(4), 201–211.

Iwarsson, S., Haak, M., & Slaug, B. (2012). Current developments of the Housing Enabler methodology. *British Journal of Occupational Therapy*, *75*(11), 517–521.

Kamioka, H., Tsutani, K., Yamada, M., Park, H., Okuizumi, H., Honda, T. & Handa, S. (2013). Effectiveness of rehabilitation based on recreational activities: A systematic review. *World Journal of Meta-Analysis*, *1*(1), 27–46.

Keskinen, K. E., Rantakokko, M., Suomi, K., Rantanen, T., & Portegijs, E. (2018). Nature as a facilitator for physical activity: Defining relationships between the objective and perceived environment and physical activity among community-dwelling older people. *Health & Place*, *49*, 111–119.

Law, M., Cooper, B., Strong, S., Stewart, D., Rigby, P., & Letts, L. (1996). The person-environment-occupation model: A transactive approach to occupational performance. *Canadian Journal of Occupational Therapy*, *63*(1), 9–23.

Lawton, M. P., & Nahemow, L. (1973). Ecology and the aging process. In C. Eisdorfer & M. P. Lawton (Eds.), *The psychology of adult development and aging* (pp. 619–674). Washington, DC: American Psychological Association.

Levinger, P., Sales, M., Polman, R., Haines, T., Dow, B., Biddle, S. J., Duque, G., & Hill, K. D. (2018). Outdoor physical activity for older people—The senior exercise park: Current research, challenges and future directions. *Health Promotion Journal of Australia*, *29*(3), 353–359.

Lewis, A., Torrington, J., Barnes, S., Dartan, R., Holder, J., McKee, K., ... Orrell, A. (2010). EVOLVE: A tool for evaluating the design of older people's housing. *Housing, Care and Support*, *13*(3), 36–41.

Marcus, C. C., & Sachs, N. A. (2013). *Therapeutic landscapes: An evidence-based approach to designing healing gardens and restorative outdoor spaces*. John Wiley & Sons.

Mitchell, L., & Burton, E. (2010). Designing dementia-friendly neighbourhoods: Helping people with dementia to get out and about. *Journal of Integrated Care*, *18*(6), 11–18.

Moran, M., Van Cauwenberg, J., Hercky-Linnewiel, R., Cerin, E., Deforche, B., & Plaut, P. (2014). Understanding the relationships between the physical environment and physical activity in older adults: A systematic review of qualitative studies. *International Journal of Behavioral Nutrition and Physical Activity*, *11*, Article 79.

Motealleh, P., Moyle, W., Jones, C., & Dupre, K. (2019). Creating a dementia-friendly environment through the use of outdoor natural landscape design intervention in long-term care facilities: A narrative review. *Health & Place*, *58*, Article 102148.

Nagi, S. Z. (1965). Some conceptual issues in disability and rehabilitation. In M. Sussman (Ed.), *Sociology and rehabilitation* (pp. 100–113). Washington, DC: American Sociological Association.

Ng, C. F. (2016). Behavioral mapping and tracking. In R. Gifford (Ed.), *Research methods for environmental psychology* (pp. 29–52): John Wiley & Sons, Ltd.

Orr, N., Wagstaffe, A., Briscoe, S., & Garside, R. (2016). How do older people describe their sensory experiences of the natural world? A systematic review of the qualitative evidence. *BMC Geriatrics*, *16*, Article 116.

Pleson, E., Nieuwendyk, L. M., Lee, K. K., Chaddah, A., Nykiforuk, C. I., & Schopflocher, D. (2014). Understanding older adults' usage of community green spaces in Taipei, Taiwan. *International Journal of Environmental Research and Public Health*, *11*(2), 1444–1464.

Raske, M. (2010). Nursing home quality of life: Study of an enabling garden. *Journal of Gerontological Social Work*, *53*(4), 336–351.

Rodiek, S. (2002). Influence of an outdoor garden on mood and stress in older persons. *Journal of Therapeutic Horticulture*, *13*, 13–21.

Rodiek, S., Lee, C., & Nejati, A. (2014). You can't get there from here: Reaching the outdoors in senior housing. *Journal of Housing for the Elderly*, *28*(1), 63–84.

Rodiek, S., Nejati, A., Bardenhagen, E., Lee, C., & Senes, G. (2016). The seniors' outdoor survey: An observational tool for assessing outdoor environments at long-term care settings. *The Gerontologist*, *56*(2), 222–233.

Sakari, R., Rantakokko, M., Portegijs, E., Iwarsson, S., Sipila, S., Viljanen, A., & Rantanen, T. (2017). Do associations between perceived environmental and individual characteristics and walking limitations depend on lower extremity performance level? *Journal of Aging and Health*, *29*(4), 640–656.

Sales, M., Polman, R., Hill, K., & Levinger, P. (2018). Older adults' perceptions of a novel outdoor exercise initiative: A qualitative analysis. *The Journal of Aging and Social Change*, *8*(1), 61–78.

Sales, M., Polman, R., Hill, K. D., & Levinger, P. (2017). A novel exercise initiative for seniors to improve balance and physical function. *Journal of Aging and Health*, *29*(8), 1424–1443.

Sánchez, A., Millán-Calenti, J. C., Lorenzo-López, L., & Maseda, A. (2013). Multisensory stimulation for people with dementia: A review of the literature. *American Journal of Alzheimer's Disease & Other Dementias®*, *28*(1), 7–14.

Sanford, J. A. (2012). *Universal design as a rehabilitation strategy: Design for the ages*. New York, NY: Springer Publishing Company.

Schneidert, M., Hurst, R., Miller, J., & Üstün, B. (2003). The role of environment in the International Classification of Functioning, Disability and Health (ICF). *Disability and Rehabilitation*, *25*(11–12), 588–595.

Shumway-Cook, A., Patla, A., Stewart, A., Ferrucci, L., Ciol, M. A., & Guralnik, J. M. (2003). Environmental components of mobility disability in community-living older persons. *Journal of the American Geriatrics Society*, *51*(3), 393–398.

Shumway-Cook, A., Patla, A. E., Stewart, A., Ferrucci, L., Ciol, M. A., & Guralnik, J. M. (2002). Environmental demands associated with community mobility in older adults with and without mobility disabilities. *Physical Therapy*, *82*(7), 670–681.

Steinfeld, E., Schroeder, S., Duncan, J., Faste, R., Chollet, D., & Bishop, M. (1979). The scope of barrier-free design. In E. Steinfeld (Ed.), *Access to the built environment: A review of the literature* (pp. 73–96). Washington, DC: Government Printing Office.

Stride, V., Cranney, L., Scott, A., & Hua, M. (2017). Outdoor gyms and older adults-acceptability, enablers and barriers: A survey of park users. *Health Promotion Journal of Australia: Official Journal of Australian Association of Health Promotion Professionals*, *28*(3), 243–246.

Sugiyama, T., & Thompson, C. W. (2007a). Older people's health, outdoor activity and supportiveness of neighbourhood environments. *Landscape and Urban Planning*, *83*(2-3), 168–175.

Sugiyama, T., & Thompson, C. W. (2007b). Outdoor environments, activity and the well-being of older people: Conceptualising environmental support. *Environment and Planning a-Economy and Space*, *39*(8), 1943–1960.

Van Cauwenberg, J., Nathan, A., Barnett, A., Barnett, D. W., & Cerin, E. (2018). Relationships between neighbourhood physical environmental attributes and older adults' leisure-time physical activity: A systematic review and meta-analysis. *Sports Medicine*, *48*(7), 1635–1660.

Veen, E. J., Bock, B. B., Van den Berg, W., Visser, A. J., & Wiskerke, J. S. C. (2016). Community gardening and social cohesion: Different designs, different motivations. *Local Environment*, *21*(10), 1271–1287.

Wagenfeld, A., & Atchison, B. (2014). "Putting the occupation back in occupational therapy:" A survey of occupational therapy practitioners' use of gardening as an intervention. *The Open Journal of Occupational Therapy*, *2*(4), Article 4.

Wagenfeld, A., Reynolds, L., & Amiri, T. (2017). Exploring the value of inter-professional collaboration between occupational therapy and design: A pilot survey study. *The Open Journal of Occupational Therapy, 5*(3), Article 2.

Wang, D., & MacMillan, T. (2013). The benefits of gardening for older adults: A systematic review of the literature. *Activities, Adaptation & Aging, 37*(2), 153–181.

Wen, C., Albert, C., & Von Haaren, C. (2018). The elderly in green spaces: Exploring requirements and preferences concerning nature-based recreation. *Sustainable Cities and Society, 38*, 582–593.

Whear, R., Coon, J. T., Bethel, A., Abbott, R., Stein, K., & Garside, R. (2014). What is the impact of using outdoor spaces such as gardens on the physical and mental well-being of those with dementia? A systematic review of quantitative and quali-tative evidence. *Journal of the American Medical Directors Association, 15*(10), 697–705.

WHO. (2001). *International classification of functioning, disability and health: ICF*. Geneva: World Health Organization.

WHO. (2015a). *Measuring the age-friendliness of cities: A guide to using core in-dicators*. Geneva: World Health Organization.

WHO. (2015b). *World report on ageing and health*. Geneva: World Health Organization.

Yuan, X.-M., Xie, Q., Zhou, T.-Y., & Wang, Y. (2018). On regional community en-vironment design for seniors based on the managed care (in Chinese). *Architectural Journal, S1*, 7–12.

Zeisel, J. (2006). Observing environmental behavior. In J. Zeisel (Ed.), *Inquiry by design: Environment/behavior/neuroscience in architecture, interiors, landscape, and planning* (pp. 191–226). New York: W.W. Norton & Company.

Zhou, T.-Y., Yuan, X.-M., & Ma, X.-J. (2020). Can an outdoor multisurface terrain enhance the effects of fall prevention exercise in older adults? A randomized con-trolled trial. *International Journal of Environmental Research and Public Health, 17*(19), Article 7023.

8 Healthy ageing and the relationship with the built environment and design

Lina Engelen, Margie Rahmann, and Ellen de Jong

Introduction

Worldwide people are living longer. At present, people live on average 20 years longer than 50 years ago. Globally, the number and proportion of people over 60 years are increasing. By 2050, the world's population aged 60 years and older is expected to total 2 billion, up from 1 billion in 2020 (World Health Organization, 2018). By that time, 1 in 5 older adults will be aged 85 and over. Longevity and global population growth are posing significant economic, social, and environmental challenges for society. Although people are living longer lives than ever before, it is important to consider how wellbeing and high quality of life (QoL) can be retained or even regained.

There are multiple reasons why those in the developed world now live longer, including better control of infectious diseases (e.g., through vaccines), better nutrition and hygiene, and fewer people employed in heavy manual jobs or in toxic environments. While these risk factors have diminished over the last 50 years, mortality and morbidity due to non-communicable diseases that often manifest in middle or older age, like cardiovascular disease, cancer, and dementia, have risen significantly in comparison to 50 years ago (World Health Organization, 2014). As many of these non-communicable diseases are lifestyle related, the opportunity exists to prevent, delay, or manage them to improve health as we age.

Although ageing is a complex process and a consistent definition is difficult to find, most sources describe ageing as an aged-dependent decline of mental and physical function (Flatt, 2012). Loss of function directly correlates with loss of independence. Loss of sight and hearing, muscular decline, and reduction of cognitive functioning may lead to a gradual decrease in physical and mental capacity, an increased risk of disease, and ultimately, death. However, studies have found that with the right support, functional ability can be maintained as we get older (Papa et al., 2017).

Healthy ageing is the focus of the World Health Organization's (WHO) work on ageing between 2015 and 2030 and replaces the previous policy framework, focused on active ageing developed in 2002. The WHO defines healthy ageing as "the process of developing and maintaining the functional

DOI: 10.1201/9781003344711-9

ability that enables wellbeing in older age" (World Health Organization, 2015). To enable this wellbeing (to stay mentally, physically, and socially healthy), active living (integrating physical activity into everyday life), independence, and social interactions need to be supported across the lifespan into old age (Delle Fave et al., 2018). Healthy ageing is most successful with supportive environments and opportunities that enable people to do what is important to them, despite losses in capacity. These environments need to balance basic needs (physiological and safety) (Campbell, 2015) with higher order needs like belonging, dignity, independence, and personal growth, which can promote autonomy, QoL, wellbeing, and slow the decline in function (Maslow, 1943).

QoL and healthy ageing are multidimensional (Cosco et al., 2021), where one can consider QoL as comprised of three factors of wellbeing (physical, social, and mental). To visualise the inter-connectedness of these, we developed the "Balancing pyramid of QoL", a conceptual model, where these factors arranged in a triangular pyramid on top of a balance board act as dynamic forces (see Figure 8.1). When all three forces act in unison, the base is balanced, enabling QoL to be high and healthy ageing to be good.

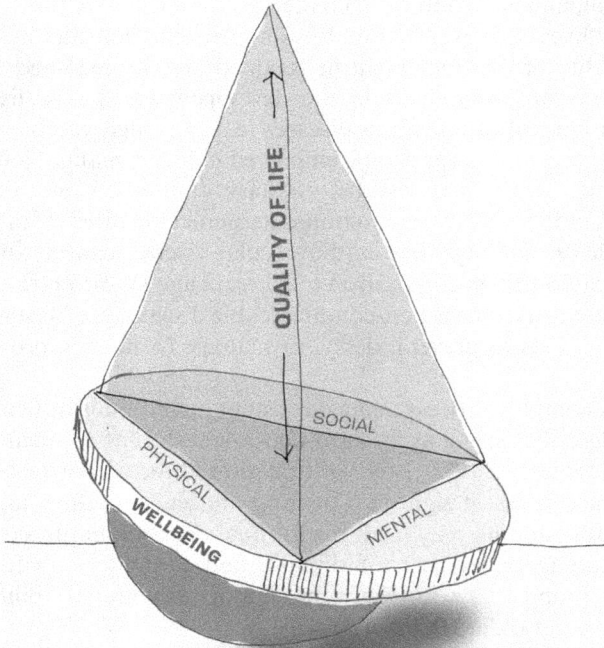

Figure 8.1 The "Balancing pyramid of QoL" conceptual model of the relationship between the triangle of wellbeing in healthy ageing and QoL.

However, if forces are unequal, the balance board becomes askew and QoL is decreased.

The built environment is increasingly recognised as having an impact on health outcomes across an individual's lifespan. For older people with limitations in functional capacity, the design of residential environments is critical (Gitlin et al., 2001). Farage et al. (2012) wrote that "Designing for older adults is inclusive design: it accommodates a range of physical and cognitive abilities and promotes simplicity, flexibility, and ease of use for people of any age". Much research has been conducted around the medical needs of older adults in aged care facilities, however, it has been suggested that there is a significant gap in research evidence between medical and design approaches of the built environment to improving health outcomes for older adults (van Hoof et al., 2013). It is important for a variety of disciplines (architecture and design, policy development, and allied health, among others) to understand the relationship between the built environment and healthy ageing to maximise QoL for older adults.

Given the large and growing proportion of older adults and the potentially considerable role the built environment can play in healthy ageing, this narrative review aims to summarise the current research and draw together an evidence base for how the design of indoor and adjacent environments can support healthy ageing. More specifically, it looks at which aspects of the physical environment, grouped into seven themes, have an impact on the physical, social, and mental wellbeing of older adults (see Figure 8.2). The evidence base is drawn from a variety of disciplines, countries, and cultures. The chapter includes a set of recommendations to inform decision-making for practitioners and researchers, taking a cross-disciplinary approach to provide a diverse set of perspectives and encourage this approach in practice to better support healthy ageing.

Wayfinding and spatial organisation

Wayfinding, or negotiating the spatial arrangement of an environment, is a critical factor in successful physical and mental orientation (Marquardt, 2011). A variety of inputs affect the clarity and success of wayfinding in built environments for older adults, including architectural layout and relationship of spaces (spatial organisation), interior design features and surfaces, signage, and graphic design, as well as operational or service design initiatives. To achieve clarity and success in wayfinding, it is important that spatial organisation be such that "destinations" like the bathroom, shops, or spaces for social interactions are easily located (Elmståhl et al., 1997; Marquardt, 2011). Leung et al. (2019) recommended providing strategically located signage with iconic information using easy-to-understand and remember icons to improve wayfinding and activity (Leung et al., 2019). Lu et al. (2015) found that destinations located along clearly defined paths or corridors contribute to active living in the elderly by being used more often (Lu et al., 2015).

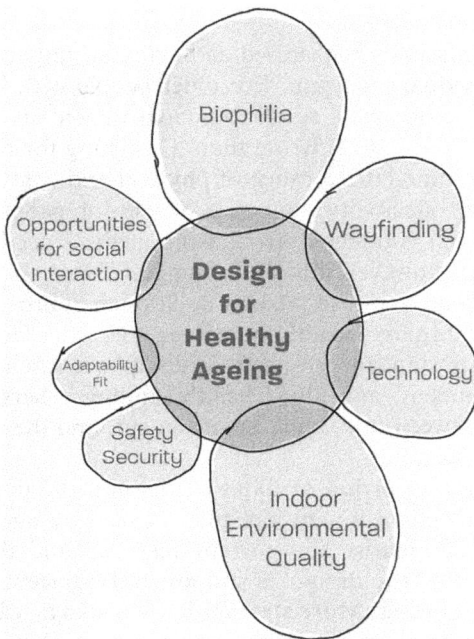

Figure 8.2 Themes related to the overarching review of design for healthy ageing. Strength of evidence is represented by the size of the bubble for each theme.

They found that the degree of indoor "recreational walking" was positively related to the perception of looped corridors and negatively to the number of stories of the building in assisted living facilities. For people living with dementia, on the other hand, environments that provide direct paths with clear sightlines to destinations perform better for orientation than those with changing directions (Marquardt, 2011).

For older adults to achieve successful wayfinding, it is particularly important that the spaces are clearly identifiable by looking different, with, for example, significant changes in materials, textures, and colours. As time passes, the functional abilities of the eye wane, as do the analytical capacities of the central visual system (Salvi et al., 2006). With ageing, contrast sensitivity decreases and the ability to separate colours is diminished. Decreased contrast sensitivity also reduces an older adult's ability to perceive depth, hence strong contrast between architectural elements (like door frames and walls) is an effective design tool for indicating destinations such as bathrooms or social spaces. However, for floor surfaces, contrast should be minimised, as high contrasting patterns or features can be perceived as changes in height, increasing the risks of trips and falls, and anxiety in older adults, especially those living with dementia.

When Lu et al. (2015) looked at "utilitarian walking" for various purposes in 18 residential aged care facilities in Texas, US, they found that the quantity and quality of the space surrounding the mailbox for sitting or waiting were positively related to how often the residents walked to fetch their mail. When there was well-considered space for sitting or waiting, this area was also used for social interactions. By encouraging social interaction and conversation, design features like landscape or artworks in these areas could over time become landmarks for residents, thus assisting successful wayfinding. The researchers found that excessive circulation spaces, repetitive layouts (where differences between areas are indistinguishable to residents), and lack of proximity to communal spaces (for example, common kitchens, laundries, and refuse collection points) all caused disorientation, even for residents with relatively normal levels of cognitive function (Lu et al., 2015). O'Malley et al. (2018) found that when designers engaged directly with the residents (rather than the developer or care provider), the most useful briefing information for input to wayfinding design and spatial planning was obtained. Approaches like human-centred design seek to include "end-users" throughout the design process to better meet their needs in the design outcome.

Henry Brookes Estate, a co-housing development for older single women in Kanahooka, Australia (see Figure 8.3), provides smaller attached single dwellings that surround a shared communal hall with space for larger gatherings.

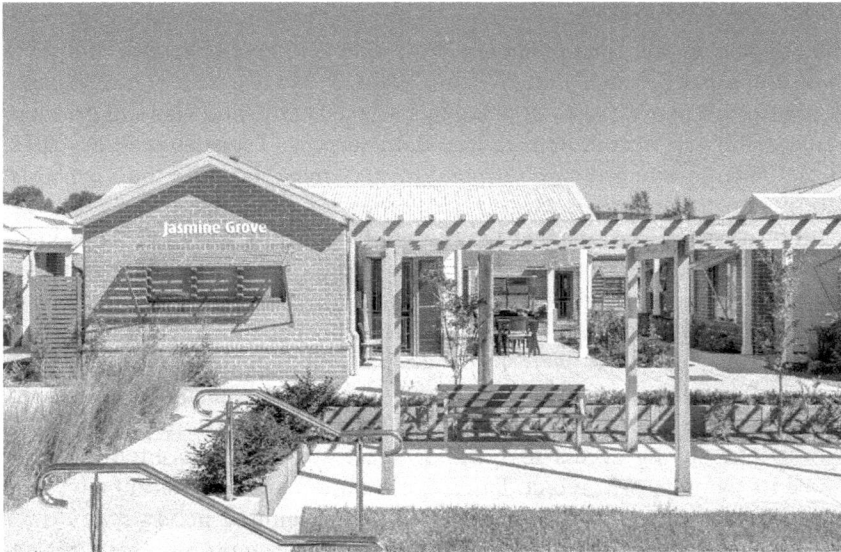

Figure 8.3 Henry Brookes Estate, Kanahooka, Australia. Photo credit: Louise Wellington. IRT Group (developer), Edmiston Jones (architect).

Clear paths and considered seating areas provide opportunities for social connection for residents and their families.

Space, in the sense of sufficient floor area and free space, has been found to be associated with overall QoL, physical health, and social relationships. A study on more than 300 older adults living in private domestic units in Hong Kong highlighted that older adults need enough space to safely move around and be able to welcome social interactions in their home (Leung et al., 2017). In many cities around the world, real estate is becoming increasingly expensive. There is a risk that units affordable to older adults may become smaller, thereby compromising some of these activities. Oswald et al. (2011) also found that apartment size was positively related to QoL in 65–80-year-olds living in the UK. However, they also noted that large apartment sizes were negatively associated with life satisfaction in the 80–94 age group, suggesting that large apartments may diminish life satisfaction in very old age, in part affected by longer walking distances when mobility difficulties become more prevalent.

In summary, there is emerging evidence in the literature that spatial organisation is key to successful wayfinding. Designs based on individuals' needs, understood by direct engagement with older adults, show promise for successful outcomes. This can be enhanced by other interventions such as signage, interior design, contrasts, and decoration. Consideration of how these elements perform together is critical to the successful support of older adults in remaining active, confident, and independent.

Biophilia and green spaces

Humans possess an innate tendency to seek connections with biophilia (nature and other forms of life) (Wilson, 1984). Viewing greenery is associated with physiological indicators of being in a relaxed state, and views of greenery have been shown to promote recovery from surgery (Tsunetsugu et al., 2013; Ulrich, 1984). In an aged care setting, greenery may comprise indoor plants, vegetation in a garden/courtyard, and a view of natural elements outside. The literature reviewed suggests that access to greenery shows great promise in promoting positive mental health among residents of aged care facilities. Positive associations between the presence and use of greenery and the mental wellbeing of aged care residents have been reported in a review by Carver et al. (2020). QoL scores were found to increase and depression scores to decrease after a therapeutic sensory wander garden was installed at an aged care facility in Australia (Edwards et al., 2013). Similarly, Potter et al. (2018) reported that having access to outdoor space was the only environmental variable to significantly predict depressive symptoms in older adults living in residential aged care facilities in the UK, where limited access to outdoor space was associated with higher levels of depressive symptoms. Horticultural therapy (gardening) showed in a systematic review to enhance psychological and physiological health and wellbeing in older adults across a large range of studies (Heród et al., 2022). In a study by Artmann et al. (2017), managers from residential aged care facilities across six European countries were asked to provide insights into the importance of gardens related to residential aged care facilities for the QoL of its residents. The results show that having a usable garden was beneficial to residents' wellbeing by providing opportunities for physical activity, passive recreation, and social interaction. Residents at 14 United States residential aged care facilities were asked to report how they felt after having spent time outdoors at their facility. Three-quarters of the residents reported that they felt slightly better or much better after they had spent time outdoors in gardens or courtyards, while only 3% reported they felt worse (Rodiek, 2006). Residents also reported in interviews that access to outdoor space was restricted in many ways: locked doors, uneven footpaths, steep steps, and needing permission or assistance to go outside. Residents also appreciated the greenery and nature provided in gardens and referred to past times managing and spending time in gardens as positive memories (Potter et al., 2018).

While most studies have looked at gardens and courtyards, a study by Rappe and Topo (2013) found that indoor and outdoor plants contributed to Finnish aged care residents' wellbeing by providing sensory stimulation and a topic of conversation that prompts social interaction. Through nurturing plants, residents reported experiencing positive feelings of self-worth and achievement. A study from the United States associated tree canopy cover around 9186 residential aged care facilities with the percentage of residents suffering from depressive symptoms (Browning et al., 2019). They found that tree canopy cover within 500 metres of the residence was associated with lower depressive symptoms, even when controlling for socio-economic factors, race, gender, air quality, and population density. This suggests that the presence of trees itself plays a significant role and highlights the importance of both nature-based therapy and outdoor landscape greening to improve residents' mental health.

One suggested mechanism that may explain how exposure to greenery can influence mental health is the stress-recovery theory. It posits that positive emotions invoked by spending time in natural settings can reduce physiological responses to stress (Ulrich, 1983). This mechanism seems applicable to residential aged care settings, as residents may have to cope with stressors such as lack of independence and privacy, feelings of social isolation, noise, and institutional regulations (Choi et al., 2008).

In summary, there is good evidence that both visual exposure to greenery (e.g., via a view from a window) and physical exposure to greenery (e.g., gardening, a garden visit, or presence of pot plants) are important in creating an environment that promotes healthy ageing (see Figure 8.4). There were, however, few studies from countries with high-density populations, such as Singapore and Hong Kong, where access to biophilia may be limited and where investigating ways in which nature can be integrated into, around, and on top of buildings in which older adults reside may have a significant effect.

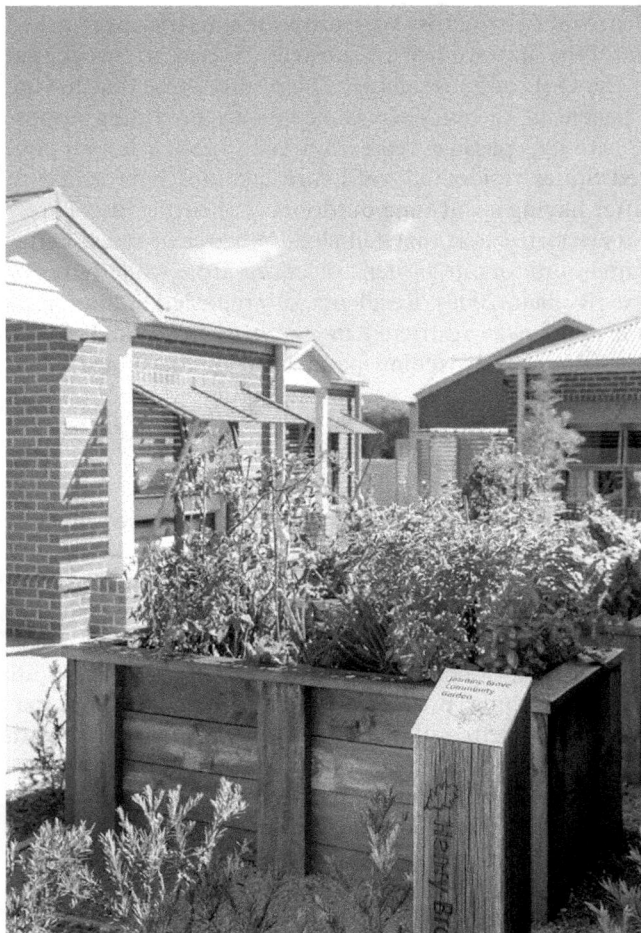

Figure 8.4 The well-tended raised garden beds are shared by residents at Henry Brookes Estate. IRT Group (developer), Edmiston Jones (architect). Photo credit: Louise Wellington.

Technology

Smart technologies and the Internet of Things (IoT) have the potential to play a significant role in enabling older adults to age in place. IoT is a term that relates to the connection of material devices to the internet. Its sensors have the capacity to register changes to the environment and transmit that information over the internet, as well as the potential to store and process information or independently initiate action. According to the IoT paradigm, objects are rendered "smart" – that is, they can be discovered, localised, and acquire, process, and exchange data – which can make them a useful support for healthy ageing and ageing in place.

The literature suggests that the use of new technology in aged care and healthy ageing in place is promising to enable older users to improve their autonomy, engage in daily activities, provide safe conditions, and support the prevention and treatment of older adults. Technology can monitor health, physiological data, daily activities, environmental data, and promote social connections (Rodrigues et al., 2020). IoT devices can also track changes in air quality, carbon monoxide, or temperature, notifying the occupant or caregiver if levels fall outside an acceptable level. The widespread application of this new technology could avoid admission to hospitals or residential aged care facilities, enabling a higher QoL and saving costs for the community (Cesta et al., 2018). In addition to monitoring data, technology can be used to support independence while ageing. One useful implementation is voice-controlled technology, which can be used for adjusting indoor climate and controlling social media and applications. Many smart devices can also "learn" about the users' behaviour and use this information to anticipate changes and register and report cognitive and behavioural anomalies. As such, IoT can assist with the early detection of dementia (Ahamed et al., 2020). Although there has been substantial development of new applications of sensor technology in the home for health purposes, this has mainly been telehealth focused, and there has been less work done on the role of IoT and ageing in place that more broadly considers caregiving and the built environment (Carnemolla, 2018).

Technology is only helpful if the user accepts and uses it. Studies reported a strong need for the technology to be human-centred, with high usability, feasibility, and accessibility (Morato et al., 2021). Cesta et al. (2018) investigated the usefulness and acceptance of using Ambient Assisted Living (AAL) to monitor physiology, social interactions, activity, and environmental factors in three end-user groups in Italy: the user self, the carer, and the health professional. All three groups indicated the key functionalities to include in an AAL system were as follows: facilitated contact with the doctor; monitoring of physiological parameters, such as vital signs at night; reminders to take medicine; falls detection; decline in mobility; and warning of danger in the home environment (gas leaks, etc.). The qualitative data found that the participants had some concerns about continuous monitoring and inappropriate access to the data. In particular, the need to protect data and tailor the data collection to different needs was considered an important aspect of the system. The participants also highlighted that the technical solutions should not replace human contact, but rather should be seen as a means to foster and promote human communication and support. However, Queirós et al. (2015) reported in a systematic review that many research papers are technology-oriented and focus on how technology can be used in the AAL context instead of looking at the users' needs and discussing their implications for practice.

There is also a high potential for exergames, simulations, and virtual reality (VR) to have beneficial outcomes for the health of older adults. In a systematic review of exergame studies, Li et al. (2018) concluded that the interaction of older adults with exergames has promising results regarding the enhancement of social wellbeing, including the increase of positive attitudes and social connection and reduction of loneliness. In a Danish study, residents in a residential aged care facility wore VR goggles while riding stationary bicycles through various virtual landscapes (Bruun-Pedersen et al., 2016). The speed with which the participants biked was reflected in their speed through the landscape. The results suggested that the augmentation increased the level of response for all motivation factors in the study, but predominantly the interest/enjoyment factor. Lee and Park (2020) also pose that it is necessary to expand the scope of VR and augmented reality technology and use them as a means of natural immersion experience linked to the experience of biophilia that is free from spatial and temporal constraints. Hence, the beneficial outcomes of using VR with older adults included more physical activity and increased QoL by getting exposure to biophilia, as well as "getting out" and gaining new experiences.

In summary, new technologies are available for older adults and these are being trialled. Although they seem very promising in supporting healthy ageing, there is at present scarce literature reporting on larger scale implementation and effectiveness in the elderly population. More research on the practical implementation of technology to support healthy ageing and its use in real-world settings is needed (Morato et al., 2021). It is important to understand the extent to which the older population engages with and adopts technology, how this increases with the implementation of user-centred designs, and the affordability of purchasing and using these technologies for older adults. There is also a strong need for digital education and ongoing technology support.

Indoor environmental quality

Indoor environmental conditions are strongly related to health, wellbeing, and overall performance. It is estimated that in developed countries, adults spend 80%–90% of their day indoors (Kembel et al., 2012) and this figure is likely to be higher in older adults. With people spending so much time inside buildings, the issue of indoor environmental quality (IEQ) becomes particularly important. IEQ includes a range of parameters, such as thermal comfort, noise, light, and air quality. In addition to the need to satisfy occupants' comfort requirements, inadequate IEQ can negatively influence the occupants' QoL and health status. According to the Environment Docility hypothesis (Lawton & Simon, 1968), people with lower functional capacity are more sensitive to influence from the environment; hence, older adults with low independence may be particularly sensitive to inadequate indoor environments (Tsuchiya-Ito et al., 2019).

Thermal comfort

As we age, we become less responsive to changes in our thermal environment, leading to a narrowing of the thermal band for performance, health, and comfort (van Hoof et al., 2017). The underlying causes of these changes include reduced ability to detect cold and warm, lower metabolic rate, reduced vascular reactivity, decreased thermoregulatory response, reduced muscle strength, hence reduced work capacity, lower cardiovascular flexibility, and resulting lower cardiac output in older people (Blatteis, 2012; Havenith, 2001; Hoof & Hensen, 2006). These factors have an impact on older adults' thermal sensation and preference.

A number of studies looked at thermal comfort in older adults in various settings. Van Hoof et al. (2017) reported in their review on thermal comfort in the Netherlands that older adults generally prefer a warmer environment than young adults do. They also summarised that to age well in place, older people should be able to control their own thermal environment with their preferred strategies, such as moving around to increase thermogenesis, wearing an extra jumper, or adjusting the indoor temperature and ventilation by opening the window to let in some breeze. This may be possible when ageing at home, but in a residential aged care facility, usually only staff have access to the thermostat, and windows are often locked (Walker et al., 2016). This concept of the physiological, behavioural, and psychological responses of the person and the control opportunities afforded by the design and construction of the building is referred to as adaptive thermal comfort. There are a range of comfort standards available globally, but a review by de Dear et al. (2020) indicated a systematic discrepancy between what is regarded as comfortable among the elderly and that suggested in the current comfort standards.

Weather and thermal conditions impact the activities and health of older adults. Hot summers and cold winters increase the risks of older people contracting pneumonia, heat stroke, dehydration, hypo- and hyperthermia, and the risk of mortality increases (Hajat & Kosatky, 2010). Cheng et al. (2018) found that between 1998 and 2011, heatwaves were associated with an average death increase of 28% in older Australians. However, a study from Japan showed that especially cold temperatures negatively impacted the activities and health of older people (Hayashi et al., 2017). Similarly, a multi-country study reported that temperature-related deaths caused by cold outweighed those caused by heat by more than 17 times (7.29% versus 0.42%) (Gasparrini et al., 2015). Apart from mortality and morbidity due to cold spells and heatwaves, an increase in indoor temperature has been shown to lead to considerable increases in self-reported sleep disturbance and breathing discomfort, where a 5 degree increase in indoor temperature led to a 40% increase in sleep disturbance (van Loenhout et al., 2016). With older adults being more prone to economic vulnerability, they may be more susceptible to suffering energy poverty, which is likely to affect thermal comfort (Porto Valente et al., 2021). Thermal comfort can be achieved through a balanced mix of passive, architectural solutions and active, technological solutions, including smart-home devices for measuring, programming, and controlling functions, which is likely to have beneficial outcomes for healthy ageing.

Indoor air quality

Older adults may be particularly sensitive to indoor air quality. By spending the majority of their time indoors, prolonged exposure to indoor air pollutants may increase deterioration of health more than the damage caused by occasional exposure to outdoor pollutants (Corsi et al., 2012). With ageing also comes a reduced ability to protect our bodies against the intrusion of airborne pathogens. Ageing leads to the deterioration of immune defences and an increased predisposition to respiratory infections (Viegi et al., 2009). Studies in Europe have found that even at low levels, indoor air quality affects respiratory health in older adults living in residential aged care facilities (Bentayeb et al., 2015). Indoor environments can harbour types of microbes not commonly found outdoors, where air temperature and relative humidity, as well as the source of ventilation air, can influence the abundance and transmission of some pathogenic microbes, and hence respiratory issues (Kembel et al., 2012). As these effects can be modulated by ventilation, the importance of effective and clean ventilation systems is highlighted, particularly in spaces where older adults reside. Unfortunately, it is not uncommon that older adults in residential aged care do not have the ability to control when to open or close windows to increase or decrease ventilation.

Light

Light quality and levels have been found to have a range of effects on mental and physical health of the elderly. Gbyl et al. (2017) collected data on socio-demographics, length of stay, and depression severity for patients in an inpatient affective disorders' unit in Denmark over the course of a year. They found that patients in the lighter and sunnier hospital rooms had shorter hospital stay than patients in rooms without sun. Costa et al. (2013) reported that many older adults suffer from disruption of their circadian rhythm, where sleep disorders and depression have been demonstrated to be highly co-prevalent conditions. Bright light has been shown to improve circadian rhythm in people with intact vision living with dementia (Van Someren et al., 1997). Riemersma-van der Lek et al. (2008) conducted a 5-year double-blind, placebo-controlled, randomised study with 189 older adults (most of them with a dementia diagnosis) across 12 residential aged care facilities in the Netherlands. They introduced bright light (1000 lux) during the daytime (9:00–18:00), followed by lower light levels in the evenings in 6 residential aged care facilities from 15 to 40 months.

The 6 control facilities retained the standard light levels of 200–300 lux across the whole day. The residents of the intervention facilities showed slower cognitive decline and less depressive symptoms than residents in the control facilities. Light treatment ameliorated agitated behaviour and resulted in better sleep when combined with melatonin. Leung et al. (2019) found that sufficient lighting levels in eight residential aged care facilities in China were associated with psychological and social health in residents living with dementia. Leung et al. (2020) also found that increased indoor lighting increased positive emotion and reduced sleep disturbances in older adults living with dementia in Hong Kong. Light levels hence have a proven effect on mental health for older adults; however, there is less support for the quality/type of light. A study by Sander et al. (2015) in Denmark found no difference in sleep duration or saliva melatonin levels between older adults being exposed to either blue-enriched or blue-suppressed lighting conditions from morning to midday. However, self-reported sleep quality was higher for women in the blue-enriched condition.

Sound

Acoustics has been found to affect many aspects of human social interactions and performance, such as in schools and workplaces (Engelen et al., 2018; Mealings, 2016); hence, one can presume that acoustics plays a role in well-being for older adults too. There is a range of literature focusing on technical solutions to improve the acoustic performance of aged care facilities (Thomas et al., 2018), with some qualitative feedback evaluation from staff. However, very little research is available on the effects of acoustics on healthy ageing.

In summary, there is strong evidence that thermal comfort, indoor air quality, and light have effects on physical and mental wellbeing, and hence on healthy ageing. The scarce evidence for the role of acoustics and noise does not preclude that noise pollution may play a large part in the physical and mental wellbeing of the elderly. The evidence supports the need for older individuals to be able to control their ambient environment.

Opportunities for social interactions

Most people desire social participation and support, which are strong predictors of health and wellbeing (Global Age-Friendly Cities, 2007). The reviewed literature investigated various topics such as loneliness (Leung et al., 2020), room distance, barrier-free design (Yu et al., 2017), and ageing in place (Mulliner et al., 2020) in relation to social interactions.

Several studies conducted in residential aged care homes found that it is often difficult for elderly residents to move around due to declining mobility. Appropriate distances between rooms of various functions within residential aged care homes allow residents to move independently from their bedroom to bathroom, dining room, and other common areas. Barrier-free design, which is any design to accommodate individuals with physical disabilities, is also important. All this together allows for independent movement, which can encourage the residents to engage in social activities and foster social relationships with other residents (Falk et al., 2009; Kenkmann et al., 2017; Leung et al., 2020).

Leung and their team found that furniture and the placement thereof had significant effects on the sense of loneliness of older adults living with dementia in residential aged care homes in Hong Kong. The participants spent 34% of their time in leisure activities or having meals in communal areas, but only one-third of that time was observed in social interactions. The furniture in those homes was placed far apart and with large tables in straight rows. It was suggested that two to three comfortable chairs around a small table would encourage social interaction. Kenkmann et al. (2017) reported that the arrangement of tables and seats in residential aged care facilities in the UK could determine whether communicating with others was easy to achieve. An abundance of spatial options can help build and sustain relationships as residents have more choices with whom to sit and socialise compared to the limited options offered by more structured environments. Residents commented specifically on positive personal relationships with others that enabled them to feel "at home" in areas with a wide choice of communal spaces (Kenkmann et al., 2017).

Falk et al. (2009) found that improvements to the shared space did not lead to an increase in perceived QoL by residents of aged care facilities in Sweden. In interviews and questionnaires with cognitively alert aged care home residents, they appreciated the changes, but stated it did not change their feelings of community or their habits. In residential aged care facilities, the idea of "home" tends to be mostly felt in residents' individual rooms, where they experience the sense of ownership and control of space normally associated with the notion of home (Kenkmann et al., 2017). The researchers found that some residents preferred to stay in their own room rather than share space with people whose physical or cognitive abilities did not match their own. Watching other residents being fed "publicly", for example, reinforced the institutional nature of their domestic situation in a residential aged care facility.

The "Successful Social Space Attribute Model", introduced by Campbell, identifies that belonging, security, and physical needs are the main factors impacting social interactions (Campbell, 2015). The model sought to compare perspectives on social spaces of people living independently to those living in residential care. This study confirmed that people living in an independent living unit in a retirement community in the United States did not want to relocate when their care needs changed. Active engagement opportunities (i.e., ways to engage with the environment and other people) and "home range" (i.e., residents' daily path of travel and the proximity of the social spaces) were identified as the two main factors in their decision-making. People preferred to keep their existing social connections and wanted to avoid

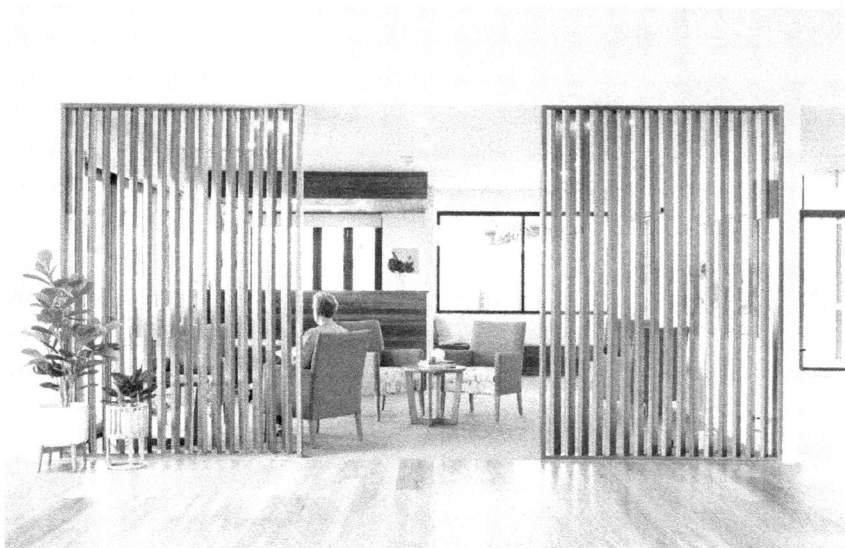

Figure 8.5 A variety of seating areas in the communal spaces at Henry Brookes Estate include smaller more intimate areas with comfortable seating, screened from larger open spaces. Photo credit: Louise Wellington.

losing them. A strong indicator of a well-used social space was the proximity to the person's usual daily route. If the social space was within or close to their usual daily path of travel, it was more likely to be used. The actual distance perceived as within "home range" became shorter as the mobility of the residents declined.

Overall, from the studies reviewed, emerging evidence is available that the built environment has an impact on social interactions in older adults (see Figure 8.5). The way QoL and built environment were measured varied greatly among studies, which makes comparison challenging; however, it is evident that the design of the built environment has a part to play. Healthy behaviours such as increased mobility, walking, and maintaining social interaction can be encouraged by design principles like barrier-free design and proximity by creating inviting small social spaces.

Safety/security

Safety and security are basic needs that are important aspects of our well-being. If our safety needs are not met, our primary behavioural reaction is to "fight or flight". If this state is prolonged, the chronic stress condition can contribute to high blood pressure and mental health issues, such as anxiety, phobia, depression, and addiction (Harvard Medical School, 2020). Three types of safety concerns for older adults have been identified: physical, spatial, and interpersonal (Tong et al., 2016). The research available on safety and security for older adults was limited and general and conducted in Canada and Sweden. We chose to exclude research regarding crime rates in the community and to focus on the safety and security within or around the residence.

Tong et al. (2016) conducted interviews in Canada with community living older adults, who received professional home care support, to understand the feelings of safety of both residents and their home care support workers. Falls at home were the primary safety issue for older adults and their families. Falls can be considered a physical safety concern where reduced physical mobility is a risk factor and a spatial safety concern due to restricted living spaces that have trip hazards. For Canadian home care workers, domestic cleaning tasks were not within their list of funded tasks, and clients had to organise the domestic duties themselves (Tong et al., 2016), resulting in sometimes dirty and messy homes. This increased the safety concerns of both residents and workers.

In Sweden, older adults that had just moved into a residential aged care home were interviewed about their sense of safety and security. Most residents' primary reason for leaving their previous home was due to falls and losing their sense of security in their home. They mentioned that the design of the house and placement of furniture affected their safety. Falling over steps and finding it harder to push wheelchairs or walkers over the carpet were some of the reasons why they choose to move to a perceived safer environment in the aged care facility.

Overall, their feeling of safety and security was the main reason people moved away from their own home in the community. The knowledge of staff being available 24 hours per day, if they needed it provided a great sense of safety for the residents. The residents preferred to continue to do things for themselves, but knowing that someone is there when needed gave them a great sense of security.

In summary, the evidence that was found indicated that older adults' sense of safety and security was linked to the support they had available and their built environment. Knowing people would be there to assist them increased their sense of safety. Having homes adaptable or built to include barrier-free design with wider doorways, minimal steps, easier access, and increased access to home assistance would mean people can continue to live at home longer.

Adaptability/fit

When there is a good "fit" between an older adult's level of function and the environment they inhabit, a higher level of independence can be experienced (Peace & Darton, 2020). With limited research on this theme, frameworks such as "person-environment fit", developed in the field of environmental gerontology, present one avenue for potential future study

(Marquardt, 2011). This model acknowledges the reciprocal effects between the environment and an individual. Although design plays an important role in offering opportunities for healthy ageing in residential settings, without a detailed understanding of the individual's needs, it can inadvertently create barriers.

In reviewing several residential aged care environments in the United Kingdom, Kenkmann et al. (2017) found that enabling the connection of indoors and outdoors achieves optimal results for residents when carefully considered from both a physical and operational perspective and by considering the opportunities for residents to experience leaving and returning to their place of residence, a normal part of daily life for those not living in residential aged care. They found a positive impact on aged care residents' sense of feeling at home, at facilities with an organisational culture that promoted and encouraged independent use of "mediating" spaces. These are semi-public or transition areas that residents can easily and autonomously access and where they can view passers-by, wildlife, or the traffic outside.

Hung et al. (2016) also found that residential aged care facilities in Canada providing home-like environments lead to better functional ability and higher engagement in the residents. Amenities that residents can use under supervision, like a kitchen, for simple tasks such as making a sandwich, enable a greater level of independence of residents. A study by Connell (2002) in a residential aged care centre also looked at the benefits of considering fit. Oral care items were placed on a resident's bedside table in containers with large, high contrast labels rather than in a bathroom cupboard. With this simple and inexpensive adaptation/intervention, the participants were able to engage in more independent oral care, resulting in better oral hygiene.

Jonsson (2013) reports that there is great variety in Sweden in how older adults feel regarding furniture, revealing a diversity of interests, needs, and wishes. Jonsson proposes a model that explains how older people attribute significance to furniture, which consists of four categories: 1) fit usage, 2) fit human body, 3) suit the individual, and 4) fit physical environment. This model highlights the importance of object fit to the user of that object.

In all these studies, a clear and detailed understanding of the needs of the individual was critical to the success of the outcome. The other important factor is the role of the carer and the organisational culture they operate within. Carers must understand how to best employ design interventions or elements and have the time and inclination to facilitate their use by older adults. Living spaces for older adults that are adaptable over time accommodate inevitable changes in an individual's needs and abilities. Van Hoof et al. (2013) found that the success of any modifications made to a dwelling to support an older adult living with dementia while ageing in place, and for how long they remain successful, will depend on the specific needs of the individual in that residence. Similarly, Ahrentzen and Tural (2015) found that some types of accommodation are difficult to adapt to individuals. For example, when designing residential aged care facilities or rental

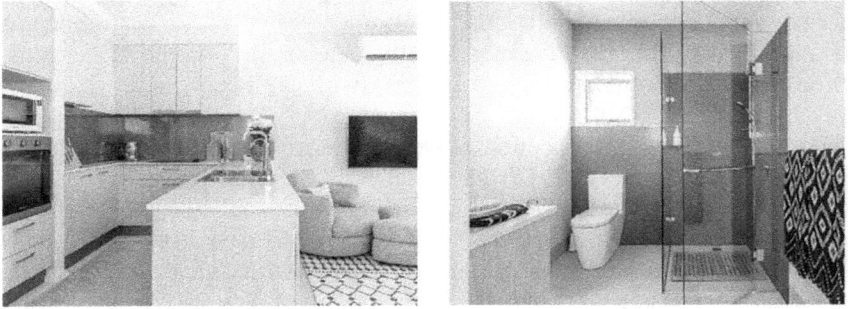

Figure 8.6 The interior design of Henry Brookes Estate accommodates ageing in place by providing kitchens designed with accessible appliances and fittings, adaptable bathrooms, and extra-wide doorways. Photo credit: Louise Wellington.

accommodation where people with different individual needs may occupy the same space at different times, successful individual "fit" can be difficult to achieve. In these cases, designs that are "adaptable" are a better approach to cater for a wider variety of needs (see Figure 8.6).

It is surprising that so little evidence exists for the role of adaptability/fit in improving QoL for older adults, given that these aspects of the built environment have such an intimate psychological relationship with humans, especially the elderly (Marquardt, 2011). It could be that, as this relationship is so subjective and difficult to measure, designing and implementing a research study around these areas is time-consuming and complex. There is some evidence that fit and adaptability are important aspects when creating optimal spaces to support healthy ageing. Consideration of fit at various scales offers a broad range of opportunities for enabling older people to be independent and exercise choice. Their success partly relies on careful consideration of ways to support people's activities of daily living. As needs change during the ageing process or in places where different individuals inhabit the same space at different times, the environment's fit will ideally be adaptable.

Conclusions

This chapter with a cross-disciplinary focus identifies how aspects of indoor and adjacent built environments have an impact on the physical, social, and mental wellbeing of older adults, and hence on healthy ageing. When these aspects of wellbeing are supported equally by the built environment, a high QoL can be experienced as described in the "Balancing pyramid of QoL" model (see Figure 8.1). Design interventions in the built environment have the leverage to adjust this balance, and when carefully considered to maintain harmony between physical, social, and mental wellbeing, they can help support and improve QoL of older adults and healthy ageing. By utilising a cross-disciplinary approach to existing research models such as this, we hope that a more robust and well-balanced evidence base can be formed.

We summarised the reviewed literature into seven key themes. These themes represent different design aspects of the physical environment that can enable "the process of developing and maintaining the functional ability that enables wellbeing in older age", hence healthy ageing.

One very important consideration that emerged was the ability of older adults to maintain agency in their lives, including exerting some level of control over their physical environment. This could range from choosing the furniture in their rooms to controlling temperature and deciding where to have their dinner. Practitioners and researchers ought to closely research the needs and wishes of older people to embrace a holistic view of people and their diverse needs (Jonsson, 2013).

Human-centred and co-design processes give rise to solutions that are not only feasible, meet peoples' needs, and provide good user experiences, but through the process of design, empower these "end-users" to contribute to the solution. When designers immerse themselves in the lived experience and perspectives of the people who will ultimately be using their designs, the outcomes are likely to be more effective. By understanding the physical and psychological needs, motivations, and barriers of those who should enjoy the benefit of design, biases and assumptions can be avoided and design solutions improved. When older adults are included in the design decision-making process, the outcomes can have an even greater impact. In Australia, the final report of the Royal Commission tabled in the federal parliament in 2021 recommended that: "priority [be] given to research and innovation that involves co-design with older people, their families, and the aged care workforce". This will help inform a clear strategy for future adaptability that could improve useability over a longer timeframe.

In practice, the recommendation by the Royal Commission can be difficult to implement – the variety in models of residential care, the number of organisations with diverse business models that deliver care, and the range of cognitive abilities of older adults that require care are but a few impediments to successful co-design. Communication between relevant people (residents, families, carers, health practitioners, designers, builders, and management) with a well-designed engagement process based on the International Association of Public Participation is a successful means by which a smooth co-design process can be facilitated.

Many of these aspects of the built environment are well-understood by design professionals and often legislated in some countries (e.g., lux levels in residential aged care facilities in AS/NZ 1680 (Standards Australia, 2009)). In Australia, the majority of legislation relates more generally to people with disabilities (National Construction Code, (Australian Building Codes Board, 2019) AS 1428) (Standards Australia, 2021) and there are several state-based planning policies that address design for seniors and people with disabilities together (e.g., SEPP Housing for Seniors or People With a Disability) (NSW Government, 2004). There have been calls for a specific Building Code for the design of housing for older people (Paduch, 2008). Certainly, some guidelines do exist (e.g., (Liveable Housing Australia), Specialist Disability Accommodation (SDA) Guidelines) (Liveable Housing Australia, 2019); however, over-reliance on technical specifications or legislative controls can miss opportunities for creating recommendations for functional and operational considerations (van Hoof et al., 2013).

Physical environments that support healthy ageing are dependent on good design, and a range of factors can be considered during planning and design for these environments. Design decisions are often based on cultural tradition, cost, compliance frameworks, and trends instead of scientific evidence. However, as highlighted in this narrative review, there is good evidence available on which to base these decisions. Closing the loop between design intent and operational performance will benefit those living and working in aged care settings and help those designing these settings improve design outcomes. It is also important to maintain focus on the adaptability of our homes in the community, as most older adults have expressed that they would prefer to continue to live relatively independently in the community. As community-dwelling, our older adults increased access to in-home care and barrier-free design in their homes.

Recommendations

Based on the evidence reviewed in this chapter, several recommendations (see Table 8.1) have been produced to support evidence-informed design decisions and to create healthy spaces to support healthy ageing. The recommendations range from simple, low-cost methods that are very straightforward to implement to innovative electronic technology that requires specialist input to design and install, as well as in-depth training for older adults and their carers. Consideration of these recommendations during the early phases of a project (whether a new build or modification), combined with careful interrogation of the specific needs of the older adults, will help close the gap that exists between theory and practice. This will also allow us to create built environments that are more responsive to and supportive of the wellbeing of older adults.

Lessons from the coalface

There is anecdotal evidence that there are discrepancies between design intent and practice and that the loop from bench to bedside (translation of research to implementation and evaluation) is not always closed. This can be seen as a missed opportunity for our older adults, as the research findings may not be used to the best effect in their built environment.

The literature suggests that having looped corridors and relatively close proximity to communal areas is good for effective wayfinding and this is

Table 8.1 Evidence-based recommendations on design for healthy ageing by theme

Theme	Recommendation
Wayfinding	• Physical activity (e.g., walking) in residential aged care settings can be encouraged through designing corridors that lead to a location or utilitarian destination where social interactions can occur. These paths should be designed with a balance of interest (e.g., looped corridors) and clear and simple wayfinding. • Clearly defined paths with signage, inviting space with small seating, encourages social interaction and use of space. • Proximity to communal spaces, avoid repetitive layouts. • Colour and materials contrast to identify different spaces, but not extreme tonal contrast on floor surfaces.
Biophilia	• Ensure a range of biophilic aspects are available to elderly to promote physical and mental health. This includes views, presence of indoor plants, and access to greenery and gardens. Creating a connection to nature can be an easily achievable design modification to a built environment. Even small changes (e.g., caring for indoor plants) can be beneficial. • Physical connection to green spaces needs to be safe, accessible, and user friendly, for example, gardening with raised garden beds.
Technology	• Consider introducing technology based on the user's needs, functionality, and acceptability to monitor health and promote physical activity and social connections.
IEQ[*]	• For optimal health and to support individual variations, it is recommended that older adults are provided with opportunities to control their ambient environment, such as openable windows, ventilation, heating, and light. • For those older adults who are unable to independently control IEQ, other options should be considered (e.g., technological solutions, carer assistance). • It is recommended that light levels are adjusted to provide high light levels during the daytime and low levels during evenings/nights to support mental and sleep health.
Opportunities for social interactions	• Proximity to social spaces is important and ideally should be located on daily activity paths. These spaces for gathering can be small but the key factors are encouraging walking and proximity to daily activities of residents. E.g., "pocket parks" (small open spaces) or sitting areas along corridors of residential developments. They should be safe, well-lit, accessible, and provide appropriate furniture. Maintenance of these spaces is critical to their continued use over time. • Create small-scale "social hubs" to invite social interaction in residential aged care facilities. • Provide opportunities to individualise rooms (e.g., by selecting the furniture, wall decorations, or photographs).

(*Continued*)

Table 8.1 (Continued)

Theme	Recommendation
Safety and security	• Adopt a universal design approach and consider a whole-of-life user experience at the design stage (e.g., Australian Liveable Housing certification system). • Provide enough space in the home to move around freely to reduce trip hazards; this may include accessible storage space.
Adaptability and usability	• Designing buildings for adaptability will allow continued use by a variety of individuals through various life stages (age in place). • Understanding daily tasks of older adults informs better design solutions. For example, ensuring items that support desired behaviours are visible and within easy reach, such as oral care items on bedside table, and understanding storage needs that may change over time. • Adapting existing spaces to allow views to other spaces where activities are occurring (e.g., views to public areas, the outside world (traffic, wildlife)) to feel a greater sense of connection.

Note
* IEQ – Indoor Environmental Quality

sometimes part of the original design. In established facilities, this structural design is not easily changed. Signs, on the other hand, are easier to add later and can be simply changed and updated if required. In a space that is shared by many, some with cognitive decline, the insight into how to maintain and care for their environment might deteriorate and signs may be altered or damaged. If staff who work in these areas do not have a good understanding of the sign's purpose, it is sometimes removed or replaced with another, less effective sign.

Spaces for social interactions are generally integrated into residential aged care settings, but we have experienced them not being used in the most effective way when residents have problems finding them or where staff concerns about supervision may discourage their use.

For example, an accessible kitchen that can be used by residents can improve nutritional outcomes and feelings of autonomy and choice. And placement of private rooms in proximity to shared spaces relevant to the individual's preferences can encourage social interaction and less isolation.

Ideally, the principles of the research findings could be applied in different settings and contexts. For example, research showed that the visibility of and easy access to oral care items increased their use and had beneficial effects on oral hygiene. It is interesting to ponder upon if this same principle would also apply when you, for example, place a bowl of fruit in the communal dining room of a residential facility. Would residents eat more fruit and feel more in control by deciding when they felt the need for a snack and not having to wait for the next set mealtime? Likely so, but would staff agree to have the fruit out in the open when there are residents with swallowing difficulties and a bite of an apple could potentially be fatal for them? Or risk residents with cognitive decline taking all the fruit and hiding it in their wardrobe, only to be found weeks later when the rotting fruit exudes its aroma?

The matter of dignity and choice, which is the first of the Aged Care Quality Standards, is thus raised. We need to consider how we find a balance between providing older people under the care of professionals with dignity and choice and protecting them from potential risks of harm. Risks that are manageable and can provide older adults with opportunities for development and choice should be prioritised. Most care staff have chosen their profession because they care, want to look after people, and want to keep them safe. It is a challenge for staff to re-think safety and allow older adults to take risks while under their care, but a culture shift and enhanced understanding of manageable risks are necessary for well-being. This needs to be recognised, and staff and management need to be trained towards an adaptation that staff are there to support the residents, to allow older adults to control their environment and activities to some degree and not inhibit their preferences to protect the older adults (or the care staff's own security). In many cases, there appears to be a gap in the communication to staff and residents regarding the reasons for change that are based on research findings. Many people have their own opinions and may dismiss research findings if they contradict their own beliefs. Communication is key for these issues, and at present, there might not be enough time and importance placed on that final piece of the puzzle for the research findings to be implemented across a wide range of situations effectively in the long term.

In summary, we have found evidence to support a range of design strategies that support healthy ageing and have provided recommendations based on these. In practice, the benefits of these recommendations will be enhanced and made more successful with a strong emphasis on training and change management of staff and their managers, as well as effective communication with family and carers.

References

Ahamed, F., Shahrestani, S., & Cheung, H. (2020). Internet of things and machine learning for healthy ageing: Identifying the early signs of dementia. *Sensors*, *20*(21), 1–25.

Ahrentzen, S., & Tural, E. (2015). The role of building design and interiors in ageing actively at home. *Building Research & Information*, *43*(5), 582–601.

Artmann, M., Chen, X., Iojă, C., Hof, A., Onose, D., Poniży, L., Lamovšek, A. Z., & Breuste, J. (2017). The role of urban green spaces in care facilities for elderly people across European cities. *Urban Forestry and Urban Greening*, *27*(March), 203–213.

Bentayeb, M., Norback, D., Bednarek, M., Bernard, A., Cai, G., Cerrai, S., Eleftheriou, K. K., Gratziou, C., Holst, G. J., Lavaud, F., Nasilowski, J., Sestini, P., Sarno, G., Sigsgaard, T., Wieslander, G., Zielinski, J., Viegi, G., & Annesi-Maesano, I. (2015). Indoor air quality, ventilation and respiratory health in elderly residents living in nursing homes in Europe. *European Respiratory Journal, 45*(5), 1228–1238.

Blatteis, C. M. (2012). Age-dependent changes in temperature regulation – A mini review. *Gerontology, 58*(4), 2012, 289–295.

Browning, M. H. E. M., Lee, K., & Wolf, K. L. (2019). Tree cover shows an inverse relationship with depressive symptoms in elderly residents living in U.S. nursing homes. *Urban Forestry and Urban Greening, 41*, 23–32.

Bruun-Pedersen, J. R., Serafin, S., & Kofoed, L. B. (2016). Motivating elderly to exercise – Recreational virtual environment for indoor biking. IEEE. 2016 IEEE International Conference on Serious Games and Applications for Health, SeGAH 11–13 May 2016, IEEE.

Campbell, N. (2015). Designing for social needs to support aging in place within continuing care retirement communities. *Journal of Housing and the Built Environment, 30*(4), 645–665.

Carnemolla, P. (2018). Ageing in place and the internet of things – how smart home technologies, the built environment and caregiving intersect. *Visualization in Engineering, 6*(7).

Carver, A., Lorenzon, A., Veitch, J., Macleod, A., & Sugiyama, T. (2020). Is greenery associated with mental health among residents of aged care facilities? A systematic search and narrative review. *Aging and Mental Health, 24*(1), 1–7.

Cesta, A., Cortellessa, G., Fracasso, F., Orlandini, A., & Turno, M. (2018). User needs and preferences on AAL systems that support older adults and their carers. *Journal of Ambient Intelligence and Smart Environments, 10*(1), 49–70.

Cheng, J., Xu, Z., Bambrick, H., Su, H., Tong, S., & Hu, W. (2018). Heatwave and elderly mortality: An evaluation of death burden and health costs considering short-term mortality displacement. *Environment International, 115*, 334–342.

Choi, N. G., Ransom, S., & Wyllie, R. J. (2008). Depression in older nursing home residents: The influence of nursing home environmental stressors, coping, and acceptance of group and individual therapy. *Aging and Mental Health, 12*(5), 536–547.

Connell, B. (2002). Tailoring the environment of oral health care to the needs and abilities of nursing home residents with dementia. *Alzheimer's Care Quarterly, 3*(1), 19–25.

Corsi, R., Kinney, K., & Levin, H. (2012). Editorial microbiomes of built environments: 2011 symposium highlights and workgroup recommendations. *Indoor Air, 22*(3), 171–172.

Cosco, T. D., Howse, K., & Brayne, C. (2021). Healthy ageing, resilience and wellbeing. *Epidemiology and Psychiatric Sciences, 26*, 579–583.

Costa, I. C., Carvalho, H. N., & Fernandes, L. (2013). Aging, circadian rhythms and depressive disorders: A review. *American Journal of Neurodegenerative Diseases, 2*(4), 228–246.

de Dear, R., Xiong, J., Kim, J., & Cao, B. (2020). A review of adaptive thermal comfort research since 1998. *Energy and Buildings, 214*, 109893.

Delle Fave, A., Bassi, M., Boccaletti, E. S., Roncaglione, C., Bernardelli, G., & Mari, D. (2018). Promoting well-being in old age: The psychological benefits of two training programs of adapted physical activity. *Frontiers in Psychology, 9*(MAY), 828.

Edwards, C. A., McDonnell, C., & Merl, H. (2013). An evaluation of a therapeutic garden's influence on the quality of life of aged care residents with dementia. *Dementia, 12*(4), 494–510.

Elmståhl, S., Annerstedt, L., & Åhlund, O. (1997). How should a group living unit for demented elderly be designed to decrease psychiatric symptoms? *Alzheimer Disease and Associated Disorders, 11*(1), 47–52.

Engelen, L., Chau, J., Young, S., Mackey, M., Jeyapalan, D., & Bauman, A. (2018). Is activity-based working impacting health, work performance and perceptions? A systematic review. *Building Research & Information. 47*(4), 468–479.

Falk, H., Wijk, H., & Persson, L. O. (2009). The effects of refurbishment on residents' quality of life and wellbeing in two Swedish residential care facilities. *Health and Place, 15*(3), 717–724.

Farage, M. A., Miller, K. W., Ajayi, F., & Hutchins, D. (2012). Design principles to accommodate older adults. *Global Journal of Health Science, 4*(2), 2–25.

Flatt, T. (2012). A new definition of aging. *Frontiers in Genetics, 3*(AUG), 148.

Gasparrini, A., Guo, Y., & Hashizume, M. (2015). Mortalité attribuable au froid et à la chaleur: Analyse multi-pays. *Environnement, Risques et Sante, 14*(6), 464–465.

Gbyl, K., Østergaard Madsen, H., Dunker Svendsen, S., Petersen, P. M., Hageman, I., Volf, C., & Martiny, K. (2017). Depressed patients hospitalized in southeast-facing rooms are discharged earlier than patients in northwest-facing rooms. *Neuropsychobiology, 74*(4), 193–201.

Gitlin, L. N., Gitlin, N., Mann, W., & Laura, M. T. (2001). Factors associated with home environmental problems among community-living older people. *Disability and Rehabilitation, 23*(17), 777–787.

Global Age-friendly Cities: A Guide (2007). Available at: www.who.int/ageing/enFax: +41 (Accessed: 2 May 2021).

Hajat, S., & Kosatky, T. (2010). Heat-related mortality: A review and exploration of heterogeneity. *Journal of Epidemiology and Community Health*, 753–760.

Harvard Medical School. (2020). *Understanding the stress response - Harvard Health.* Available at: https://www.health.harvard.edu/staying-healthy/understanding-the-stress-response (Accessed: 8 July 2021).

Havenith, G. (2001). Temperature regulation and technology. *Gerontechnology, 1*, 41–49.

Hayashi, Y., Schmidt, S., Malmgren Fänge, A., Hoshi, T., & Ikaga, T. (2017). Lower physical performance in colder seasons and colder houses: Evidence from a field study on older people living in the community. *International Journal of Environmental Research and Public Health, 14*(6), 651.

Heród, A., Szewczyk-Taranek, B., & Pawłowska, B. (2022). Therapeutic horticulture as a potential tool of preventive geriatric medicine improving health, well-being and life quality - A systematic review. *Folia Horticulturae, 34*(1), 85–104.

Hoof, J. V., & Hensen, J. L. M. (2006). Thermal comfort and older adults. *Gerontechnology, 4*(4).

Hung, L., Chaudhury, H., & Rust, T. (2016). The effect of dining room physical environmental renovations on person-centered care practice and residents' dining experiences in long-term care facilities. *Journal of Applied Gerontology, 35*(12), 1279–1301.

Jonsson, O. (2013). *Furniture for Later Life: Design based on older people's experiences of furniture in three housing forms. PhD Thesis, Department of Design Sciences, Faculty of Engineering, Lund University.*

Kembel, S. W., Jones, E., Kline, J., Northcutt, D., Stenson, J., Womack, A. M., Bohannan, B. J., Brown, G. Z., & Green, J. L. (2012). Architectural design influences the diversity and structure of the built environment microbiome. *The ISME Journal, 6,* 1469–1479.

Kenkmann, A., Poland, F., Burns, D., Hyde, P., & Killett, A. (2017). Negotiating and valuing spaces: The discourse of space and "home" in care homes. *Health and Place, 43,* 8–16.

Lawton, M., & Simon, B. (1968). The ecology of social relationships in housing for the elderly. *Gerontologist, 8,* 108–115.

Lee, E. J., & Park, S. J. (2020). A Framework of Smart-Home Service for Elderly's Biophilic Experience. Sustainability, *12*(20), 8572.

Lester, P. (2013). *Visual communications: Images with messages.* Wadsworth.

Leung, M. Y., Famakin, I., & Kwok, T. (2017). Relationships between indoor facilities management components and elderly people's quality of life: A study of private domestic buildings. *Habitat International, 66,* 13–23.

Leung, M. Y., Wang, C., & Chan, I. Y. S. (2019). A qualitative and quantitative investigation of effects of indoor built environment for people with dementia in care and attention homes. *Building and Environment, 157,* 89–100.

Leung, M. Y., Wang, C., & Wei, X. (2020). Structural model for the relationships between indoor built environment and behaviors of residents with dementia in care and attention homes. *Building and Environment, 169.*

Li, J., Erdt, M., Chen, L., Cao, Y., Lee, S.-Q., & Theng, Y.-L. (2018). The social effects of exergames on older adults: Systematic review and metric analysis. *Journal of Medical Internet Research,* e10486.

Liveable Housing Australia. (2019). *Design guidelines.* Available at: https://livablehousingaustralia.org.au/design-guidelines/ (Accessed: 5 September 2021).

Lu, Z., Rodiek, S., Shepley, M. M., & Tassinary, L. G. (2015). Environmental influences on indoor walking behaviours of assisted living residents. *Building Research & Information, 43*(5), 602–615.

Marquardt, G. (2011). Wayfinding for people with dementia: A review of the role of architectural design. *Health Environments Research and Design Journal, 4*(2), 75–90.

Maslow's Hierarchy of Needs | Simply Psychology (1943). Available at: https://www.simplypsychology.org/maslow.html#gsc.tab=0 (Accessed: 2 May 2021).

Mealings, K. (2016). Classroom acoustic conditions: Understanding what is suitable through a review of national and international standards, recommendations, and live classroom measurements. 2nd Australasian Acoustical Societies Conference, pp. 1047–1056. ACOUSTICS 2016, *2*(November), 1047–1056.

Morato, J., Sanchez-Cuadrado, S., Iglesias, A., Campillo, A., & Fernández-Panadero, C. (2021). Sustainable technologies for older adults. In *Sustainability, 13*(15), 8465.

Mulliner, E., Riley, M., & Maliene, V. (2020). Older people's preferences for housing and environment characteristics. *Sustainability, 12*(14).

NSW Government. (2004). *State Environmental Planning Policy (Housing for Seniors or People with a Disability) 2004 - NSW Legislation.* Available at: https://legislation.nsw.gov.au/view/html/inforce/current/epi-2004-0143 (Accessed: 5 September 2021).

O'Malley, M., Innes, A., Muir, S., Wiener, J., *et al.* (2018). "All the corridors are the same": A qualitative study of the orientation experiences and design preferences of UK older adults living in a communal retirement development. *Ageing and Society, 38*(9), 1791–1816.

Oswald, F., Jopp, D., Rott, C., & Wahl, H.-W. (2011). Is aging in place a resource for or risk to life satisfaction? *Gerontologist*, *51*(2), 238–250.

Paduch, M. (2008). 'Designing Housing for Older People: The need for a Design Code'. Thesis, University of New South Wales Faculty of the Built Environment Bachelor of Planning.

Papa, E. V., Dong, X., & Hassan, M. (2017). Skeletal muscle function deficits in the elderly: Current perspectives on resistance training. *Journal of Nature and Science*, *3*(1). Available at: (Accessed: 2 May 2021). http://www.ncbi.nlm.nih.gov/pubmed/28191501.

Peace, S., & Darton, R. (2020). Reflections on cross-cultural comparison of the impact of housing modification/adaptation for supporting older people at home: A discussion. *Journal of Ageing and Environment*, *34*(2), 210–231.

Porto Valente, C., Morris, A., & Wilkinson, S. J. (2021). Energy poverty, housing and health: The lived experience of older low-income Australians. *Building Research & Information*, *50*(1-2), 6–18.

Potter, R., Sheehan, B., Cain, R., Griffin, J., & Jennings, P. A. (2018). The impact of the physical environment on depressive symptoms of older residents living in care homes: A mixed methods study. *The Gerontologist*, *58*(3), 438–447.

Queirós, A., Silva, A., Alvarelhão, J., Rocha, N. P., & Teixeira, A. (2015). Usability, accessibility and ambient-assisted living: A systematic literature review. *Universal Access in the Information Society*, *14*(1), 57–66.

Rappe, E., & Topo, P. (2013). Contact with outdoor greenery can support competence among people with dementia. *Outdoor Environments for People with Dementia*, Journal of Housing For the Elderly, *21*(3–4), 229–248.

Riemersma-van Der Lek, R. F. *et al.* (2008). Effect of bright light and melatonin on cognitive and noncognitive function in elderly residents of group care facilities: A randomized controlled trial. *JAMA - Journal of the American Medical Association*, *299*(22), 2642–2655.

Rodiek, S. (2006). A missing link: Can enhanced outdoor space improve seniors housing? *Seniors Housing and Care Journal*, *14*(1), 3–19.

Rodrigues, M. J., Postolache, O., & Cercas, F. (2020). Physiological and behavior monitoring systems for smart healthcare environments: A review. *Sensors*, *20*(8), 1–26.

Salvi, S. M., Akhtar, S., & Currie, Z. (2006). Ageing changes in the eye. *Postgraduate Medical Journal*, 581–587.

Sander, B., Markvart, J., Kessel, L., Argyraki, A., & Johnsen, K. (2015). Can sleep quality and wellbeing be improved by changing the indoor lighting in the homes of healthy, elderly citizens? *Chronobiology International*, *32*(8), 1049–1060.

Standards Australia. (2009). *Code of practice for interior lighting and the visual environment, AS1680*. Available at: https://www.standards.org.au/standards-catalogue/sa-snz/building/lg-001/as-slash-nzs–1680-dot-0-colon-2009.

Standards Australia. (2021). *Design for access and mobility*. Available at: https://www.standards.org.au/standards-catalogue/sa-snz/building/me-064/as–1428-dot-1-colon-2021.

Thomas, P., Aletta, F., Filipan, K., vander Mynsbrugge, T., de Geetere, L., & Dijckmans, A. (2018). Noise environments in nursing homes: An overview of the literature and a case study in Flanders with quantitative and qualitative methods. *Applied Acoustics*, *159*, 107103.

Tong, C. E., Sims-Gould, J., & Martin-Matthews, A. (2016). Types and patterns of safety concerns in home care: Client and family caregiver perspectives. *International Journal for Quality in Health Care*, *28*(2), 214–220.

Tsuchiya-Ito, R., Slaug, B., & Ishibashi, T. (2019). The physical housing environment and subjective well-being among older people using long-term care services in Japan. *Journal of Housing For the Elderly*, *33*(4), 413–432.

Tsunetsugu, Y., Lee, J., Park, B.-J., Tyrväinen, L., Kagawa, T., & Miyazaki, Y. (2013). Physiological and psychological effects of viewing urban forest landscapes assessed by multiple measurements. *Landscape and Urban Planning*, *113*, 90–93.

Ulrich, R. S. (1983). Aesthetic and affective response to natural environment. In I. Altman & J. Wohlwill (Eds.), *Human behavior and environment*. (6th ed., pp. 85–125). Plenum Press.

Ulrich, R. S. (1984). View through a window may influence recovery from surgery. *Science*, *224*(4647), 420–421.

van Hoof, J., Blom, M. M., Post, H. N. A., & Bastein, W. L. (2013). Designing a "think-along dwelling" for people with dementia: A co-creation project between health care and the building services sector. *Journal of Housing for the Elderly*, *27*(3), 299–332.

van Hoof, J., Schellen, L., Soebarto, V., Wong, J. K. W., & Kazak, J. K. (2017). Ten questions concerning thermal comfort and ageing. *Building and Environment*, *120*, 123–133.

van Loenhout, J. A. F., le Grand, A., Duijm, F., Greven, F., Vink, N. M., Hoek, G., & Zuurbier, M. (2016). The effect of high indoor temperatures on self-perceived health of elderly persons, *Environmental Research*, *146*, 27–34.

Van Someren, E. J., Kessler, A., Mirmiran, M., & Swaab, D. F. (1997). Indirect bright light improves circadian rest-activity rhythm disturbances in demented patients. *Biological Psychiatry*, *41*(9), 955–963.

Viegi, G. *et al.* (2009). The epidemiological link between ageing and respiratory diseases. *Respiratory Diseases in the Elderly*, (July), 1–17. European Respiratory Society.

Walker, G., Brown, S., & Neven, L. (2016). Thermal comfort in care homes: Vulnerability, responsibility and thermal care. *Building Research & Information*, *44*(2), 135–146.

Wilson, E. O. (1984). *Biophilia*. Harvard University Press.

World Health Organization. (2014). *Global status report on noncommunicable diseases 2014*. World Health Organization. Global status report on noncommunicable diseases 2010. 2011.

World Health Organization. (2015). *World report on ageing and health*. Available at: https://apps.who.int/iris/handle/10665/186463 (Accessed: 2 May 2021).

World Health Organization. (2018). *Aging and health*. Available at: https://www.who.int/news-room/fact-sheets/detail/ageing-and-health (Accessed: 2 May 2021).

Yu, J., Ma, G., & Jiang, X. (2017). Impact of the built environment and care services within rural nursing homes in China on quality of life for elderly residents. *Engineering, Construction and Architectural Management*, *24*(6), 1170–1183.

9   Energy poverty, poor housing, and the wellbeing of older Australians

Caroline Valente, Sara Wilkinson, and Alan Morris

Introduction

The Russian invasion of Ukraine has thrust energy poverty (EP) into the news. It has massively increased the cost of energy globally and the extent of EP (Nelson & Gilmore, 2022; Tollefson, 2022). Even prior to the war in Ukraine, the International Energy Agency (IEA) estimated that around 2 billion people globally experienced EP. EP is not confined to less developed countries. The IEA estimated that in the European Union, between 50 and 125 million people are energy-poor (ENPOR, 2022). Post the Russian invasion of Ukraine, it is expected that rising energy prices and supply disruptions have pushed millions more people into EP (Benton et al., 2022).

Although what it means to be in EP is contested, it can be broadly defined as a household's inability to secure or afford an acceptable level of energy services (electricity, gas, and other fuel sources) in the home (Bouzarovski & Petrova, 2015; Culver, 2017; Simcock et al., 2018). In Australia, the setting for this chapter, EP is a major issue for many low-income households (Chai et al., 2021; Churchill & Smyth, 2021; KPMG, 2017; Wilkinson et al., 2021). According to a Brotherhood of St. Laurence study (Bryant et al., 2022), over the period 2006–2020, 18–23% of households in Australia experienced EP to some extent. A recent survey based on a representative sample of 1,000 people found that electricity remains the primary cost of living concern for Australian households. It was ranked above private health, mortgages, and food and groceries (ACOSS et al., 2018). Another study in 2016 estimated that low-income households (defined as households in the bottom 40% of Australia's income distribution) spent 12.4% of their weekly income on utility bills and fuel, whereas high-income households spent 2.9% (Cornwell et al., 2016). During the COVID-19 pandemic, household energy debt increased by 21% to $AU124 million between March and November 2020 (Curtis, 2020). A report from the Australian Energy Regulator concluded that 178,901 residential customers were repaying energy debt in the quarter ending March 2022 and the average debt was $AU1,060 (AER, 2022b). Furthermore, in June 2022, after the Russian invasion of Ukraine, the average debt of customers on hardship programmes was around 30–40% higher than pre-pandemic levels (AER, 2022a).

DOI: 10.1201/9781003344711-10

A particularly vulnerable group are older people (over 65 years of age) who are reliant solely on the government Age Pension for their income. The maximum government Age Pension in November 2021 for a person living by themselves was $513 a week. The Melbourne Institute's well-recognised poverty line for a single person (not in the workforce) in December 2020 was $500 a week, including housing (The Melbourne Institute, 2022). According to the annual Household, Income and Labour Dynamics Survey survey, poverty rates among older single people and older couples have been consistently higher than any other household type (Wilkins et al., 2020). An Australian study estimated more than one-third of households identified as energy-poor have a reference person aged 65 years or older (Azpitarte et al., 2015). The 2021 Census established that in mid-2021, 4,317,634 people, 16.8% of Australia's population, were aged 65 years and over (ABS, 2022).

Research on EP and older people has historically focused on patterns of mortality and morbidity (Rudge & Gilchrist, 2005; Wilkinson et al., 2004). More recently, studies have focused on older people's lived experience of EP and their coping mechanisms (Chard & Walker, 2016; Willand et al., 2017). This study aims to expand our knowledge of the impacts of EP on older Australians who are solely or primarily reliant on government benefits for their income. Drawing on 23 in-depth, semi-structured interviews with older Australians in Sydney and Melbourne, we examine how EP impacts on their everyday lives, health, and wellbeing.

Housing, older people, and EP in Australia

In Australia, there is a strong preference among older people to age in their own home (Judd et al., 2014). A consequence is that many older Australians are living in old homes that are not energy efficient (Porto Valente et al., 2020; Romanach et al., 2017). In Australia, the Nationwide House Energy Rating Scheme assessments are the most common way to meet the minimum energy efficiency requirements of the National Construction Code. Ratings range from zero to ten stars (Department of Industry, Science, Energy and Resources, 2021). A zero-star rating means that the building envelope does little to reduce the discomfort caused by hot or cold temperatures. The Australian Housing Conditions Dataset, which is based on a sample of 4,501 households, including 1,999 households with a household head aged 65 or over, found that 78% of homes of older Australians were 25 years old or more. Minimum energy efficiency standards for residential property were only mandated in the Building Code of Australia in 2006. This is significant, as studies indicate that much of the housing stock built before 2006 has a star rating of two or less (Berry & Marker, 2015; Sustainability Victoria, 2014; Willand et al., 2019). The poor energy efficiency of homes is potentially a serious issue, especially for older people reliant on the government Age

Pension. The homes concerned are difficult to heat or cool adequately and a challenge for older people who are less tolerant of extreme temperatures (van Hoof et al., 2017).

The lack of thermal comfort represents a health risk for older people (Dear & McMichael, 2011; Howden-Chapman et al., 2012). The risk has been accentuated by climate change. In 2018/19, New South Wales, the state where Sydney is located, experienced the hottest summer on record – 3.41 degrees Celsius above average (Climate Council, 2020). On 4 January 2020, Penrith, in outer Sydney, recorded the hottest day ever in the Sydney region – 48.9 degrees Celsius (Australian Government, 2021). The average maximum daytime summer temperature in Sydney is 26 degrees. Melbourne in Victoria is located on the southern end of the country. On 31 January 2020, Laverton, in Melbourne's outer suburbs, recorded a temperature of 44.1 degrees Celsius. The average summer temperature in Melbourne is 26 degrees Celsius. In terms of climate zones, Sydney is in Zone 5 Warm Temperate, and Melbourne is in Zone 6 Mild Temperate (ABCB, 2019). As such, Melbourne buildings typically require heating for longer periods of the year than Sydney. Both zones can experience periods of extreme heat. In buildings with poor thermal design and performance, extreme heat makes the dwelling very uncomfortable. Mechanical cooling is required to make the environment tolerable. This adds to energy costs. One response is to cut down on energy use and endeavour to cope with the consequences of high indoortemperatures (Sherriff et al., 2019; Thomson et al., 2019). Australian air conditioning providers recommend a standard air conditioner's temperature be set to 25–27 degrees for cooling in summer (Canstar Blue, 2019). Clearly, to achieve temperatures in the comfortable 25–27 degrees Celsius range, home occupiers would need to use air conditioning extensively.

Within the older cohort, there is also a significant gender factor with respect to EP. Although EP is generally presented as gender-neutral, its impact is often uneven (O'Neill et al., 2006; Robinson, 2019). In Australia, like many other advanced economies, older women are more likely to suffer from entrenched poverty and experience EP as a result (Robinson, 2019; Wilkins et al., 2020).

The impacts of EP

EP has a range of impacts, and older people, especially if they have health issues and limited income, are particularly vulnerable. The most concerning impacts are food insecurity, inability to purchase essential items, poor health due to thermal discomfort, and social exclusion. The definition of food security, agreed to at the World Food Summit in 1996, refers to "a situation that exists when all people, at all times, have physical, social, and economic access to sufficient, safe, and nutritional food that meets their dietary needs and food preferences for an active and healthy life" (World Food Summit, 1996). There is increasing evidence that in advanced economies, money spent on energy bills is contributing to food insecurity (Hernández, 2016; Kearns et al., 2019). After paying their energy bills, some people do not have the ability to purchase an adequate supply of nutritious food (Tuttle & Beatty, 2017). In Australia, this is especially the case for those older private renters who are reliant on government benefits for their income. High accommodation costs, in combination with energy costs, place them in a particularly vulnerable position (Morris, 2016). Besides food, their high energy costs can also result in an inability to purchase other essentials such as prescription medicines (Nord & Kantor, 2006; Porto Valente et al., 2021).

A comparative study conducted by Thomson et al. (2017) found that in most European countries, the energy-poor population is statistically more likely to report poorer physical and mental health than the non-energy-poor population. To avoid high energy bills and avoid or lessen EP, many low-income households reduce their energy use (Judson et al., 2019; Roberts & Henwood, 2019). This can result in thermal discomfort and impact the health of the household (Hernández & Siegel, 2019). The relationship between excess winter deaths, low thermal efficiency of housing, and low indoor temperature during cold weather is well-established (Anderson et al., 2012; Day & Hitchings, 2011; Hamza & Gilroy, 2011).

Heatwaves and an inability to cool the home adequately are also major health risks. It has been argued that in Australia, in the last couple of decades, wildfires and heatwaves have been responsible for over 60% of deaths related to natural hazards (Borchers Arriagada et al., 2020). People experiencing EP are more prone to suffer during heatwaves, as they cannot afford the cooling required to feel comfortable at home (Nicholls & Strengers, 2018; Nicholls et al., 2017). In both Melbourne and Sydney, cooling is required from November to the end of February. Physical fragility increases with advancing age and reduces people's ability to keep cool or warm and maintain their health during extreme temperature events (Steffen et al., 2014). For older people who may be frail, maintaining thermal comfort is a major challenge.

Social isolation is another possible outcome of EP. If a person's expenditure on energy consumes a substantial proportion of their disposable income, it makes it difficult for them to partake in social activities (Chester, 2013; COTA, 2018). They simply do not have the requisite funds (Morris, 2012). Also, some households may not have visitors because their home is thermally uncomfortable or they fear it will increase their energy use (Kearns et al., 2019; Middlemiss et al., 2019).

EP and capabilities

Amartya Sen (1997) and Martha Nussbaum (2000) developed the capability perspective to analyse social inequality, wellbeing, and poverty. This approach is particularly useful in expanding on the analysis of the impacts of EP on households' wellbeing. The capabilities approach addresses the question of what social justice, freedom, and development require (Nussbaum, 2003, 2011; Sen, 1992, 1993). A key question posed is *what are people actually able to do and to be?* (Nussbaun, 2011). Three linked concepts, functionings, capabilities, and resources are used to address this question.

Functionings represent the various things that a person manages to do or be in leading a life; the capability of a person reflects the alternative combinations of functionings they can achieve and from which they can choose (Sen, 1993). As Sen (1993, 1997) describes, some capabilities are very elementary, such as escaping morbidity and mortality, being adequately nourished, being in good health, and/or being well sheltered. Others may be more complex, but still widely valued, such as being happy, achieving self-respect, being socially integrated, or appearing in public without shame. Nussbaum (2000, pp. 70–71) developed a list of ten central capabilities (as depicted in Table 9.1) as "universal values" that must be seen as a "foundation for basic political principles that should underwrite constitutional guarantees".

The freedom to lead different types of lives and achieve different functionings is intrinsic to a person's capability set, and that will depend on a variety of factors, including their income, personal characteristics, social arrangements, and the environment (Sen, 1993, 1997). The concept of resources as "instrumentally valuable means to intrinsically valuable human ends" is then applied (Kelleher, 2015, p. 8). For Nussbaum (2003), individuals will inherently need different levels of resources to achieve similar levels of capability to function.

Whilst the capabilities approach places particular importance on the diverse and differing abilities of people to convert their resources into actual functionings, there is no doubt that the lack of access to different forms of resources, monetary or not, will deprive individuals from achieving certain capabilities.

Day et al. (2016) conceptualised energy use and, therefore, EP, through the capabilities' perspective. They argued that such a broader understanding of the ways in which energy use is connected to socio-economic development, wellbeing, and quality of life can provide a useful theoretical framework for comprehending the wider impacts of EP. They argue that there are basic and secondary capabilities (Smith & Seward, 2009) within the energy use needs. Whilst a basic capability might be "being in good health", several secondary capabilities related to energy services would be needed to achieve this, including being able to keep adequately warm or cool (heating or cooling services), being able to take a shower (hot water service), and being able to acquire and cook nutritious meals (refrigeration and cooking services). All these energy services require an energy supply (and finally an energy source). The links between the energy source and basic capabilities are illustrated in Figure 9.1.

EP, in this sense, can be understood under the corrosive disadvantage concept (Wolff & de-Shalit, 2007), as the energy-poor restrict their energy

Table 9.1 Nussbaum's list of central human capabilities

Central capability	Brief description
Life	Being able to live to the end of a human life of normal length; not dying prematurely or before one's life is so reduced as to be not worth living.
Bodily health	Being able to have good health, including reproductive health; to be adequately nourished; to have adequate shelter.
Bodily integrity	Being able to move freely from place to place, and having one's bodily boundaries treated as sovereign.
Senses, imagination, and thought	Being able to use the senses to imagine, think, and reason – and to do these things in a "truly human" way, a way informed and cultivated by an adequate education, including, but by no means limited to, literacy and basic mathematical and scientific training. [...] Being able to search for the ultimate meaning of life in one's own way. Being able to have pleasurable experiences and avoid non-necessary pain.
Emotions	Being able to have attachments to things and people outside ourselves; to love those who love and care for us, to grieve in their absence; in general, to love, to grieve, to experience longing, gratitude, and justified anger. Not having one's emotional development blighted by overwhelming fear and anxiety, or by traumatic events of abuse or neglect.
Practical reason	Being able to form a conception of the good and to engage in critical reflection about the planning of one's life.
Affiliation	Being able to live with and toward others, to recognise and show concern for other human beings, to engage in various forms of social interaction; [...] having the social bases of self-respect and non-humiliation; being able to be treated as a dignified being whose worth is equal to that of others.
Other species	Being able to live with concern for and in relation to animals, plants, and the world of nature.
Play	Being able to laugh, play, and enjoy recreational activities.
Control over one's environment	Political, as in being able to participate effectively in political choices that govern one's life; and material, as in being able to hold property (both land and movable goods) and having the right to seek employment on an equal basis with others.

Source: Adapted from Nussbaum (2000, pp. 78–80).

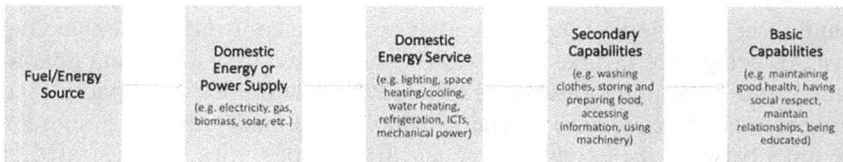

Figure 9.1 The relationship between energy, services, and capabilities.

Source: Adapted from Day et al. (2016).

consumption to situations of compromised secondary capabilities that largely affect basic ones (Day et al., 2016). The inability to achieve those capabilities influence an individual's wellbeing and self-esteem (Baudaux et al., 2019; Longhurst & Hargreaves, 2019; VCOSS, 2018). As a result, there has been increasing agitation that universal access to a minimum level of energy services be considered a human right based on the capabilities approach (Frigo et al., 2021; Sovacool & Dworkin, 2014).

Besides analysing the impacts of EP (Middlemiss et al., 2019; Willand & Horne, 2018), the capabilities approach has been applied more recently to explore other energy issues. For example, Lee et al. (2021) and Willand et al. (2021) used the capabilities approach to evaluate current EP relief policies and strategies. They found that compensation measures associated with financial assistance are ineffective in solving the problem in the long term; empowerment measures related to increasing households' capabilities and energy efficiency measures, conversely, can create long-lasting improvement. To corroborate that, Chipango (2021, p. 447) emphasises that some basic capabilities are required for households to take full advantage of their energy services: "what matters most is not only the provision of the energy services, but the person's capabilities to promote their ends". Therefore, it is suggested that the lack of certain capabilities (which are mostly related to economic and cultural capital) can also influence the experience of EP.

In light of the capabilities approach (Sen, 1999), in this research, we examine how EP undermines older Australians' capacity, opportunities, and freedoms to lead a decent and pleasant life. Evidence is given as to how EP impacts many of the central capabilities outlined by Nussbaum (2003).

Methodology

An inductive approach using semi-structured in-depth interviews was adopted to obtain an understanding of how older Australians use energy and are impacted by EP. The interview guide was designed around six main topics – background and housing characteristics; use of energy at home and strategies to reduce energy consumption; the impacts of the home on energy usage; difficulties in paying the energy bill; impacts of the energy costs; and awareness of energy hardship programmes and assistance.

Recruitment was severely disrupted by the COVID-19 pandemic, as social distancing and self-isolating measures meant community centres were closed and offline advertising was not possible. In response, contact was made with relevant organisations that advocate for older Australians and/or provide assistance with energy hardship. The organisations approached to provide support included the Combined Pensioners and Superannuants Association, the Public Interest Advisory Centre, the NSW Council of Social Services, and the Council on the Ageing. They all agreed to advertise the study through their networks and publications. In addition, a couple of older people who had participated in an earlier separate study by one of the authors were contacted and agreed to participate.

The sensitivity of the interviews meant that interviewees were given every chance to stop the interview at any point. It was made clear that they did not have to answer a question if they felt it was too challenging. The information sheet that was given to interviewees provided details as to where counselling could be obtained if required. Ethics approval for the study was granted by the ethics secretariat of the university. Informed consent was obtained from all interviewees.

In total, 23 low-income older Australians were interviewed (see Table 9.2) of whom 17 were solely or primarily reliant on the government Age Pension for their income. The focus was on older Australians; however, there were five outliers, of which three were in their fifties and two in their early sixties. Of the five outliers, two were reliant on their own minimal savings, one on the government unemployment benefit, and two on the Disability Support Pension (a government benefit) for their income. We decided to include these interviewees due to them being in a very similar situation to the interviewees on the Age Pension with respect to income and frailty. Noteworthy, is that 18 of the 23 interviewees were female.

To analyse the data, we conducted a thematic analysis of the interviews. The process started with transcribing verbatim the audio recordings into text and isolating relevant themes. The transcripts were then loaded into NVivo. NVivo facilitated the organisation of the transcripts into themes. For this chapter, we focused on the following themes: EP's impact on food insecurity, consumption of essential consumer items, medical expenses, capacity to maintain thermal comfort, and social exclusion.

Findings and discussion

EP and food insecurity

As indicated, there is evidence from previous research (Hernández & Siegel, 2019; O'Neill et al., 2006) that EP has the potential to contribute to food insecurity. A nutritious diet is a key capability for bodily health and essential for human development. The interviews indicated that, for several interviewees, prioritising paying their energy bill meant that they compromised on their food consumption. Sonia (74 years old, private renter) was in a particularly difficult position. Not only was she totally reliant on the government Age Pension for her income, but she was also a private renter. This meant that, unlike older social housing tenants, whose rent is set at a maximum of 25% of their income, Sonia had to pay a market rent. In Sydney, at the end of 2019, the median weekly rent was $525 for houses and $510 for apartments. In contrast, the rent for social housing tenants, calculated at 25% of income, was around $119. After paying her rent (she had somehow managed to find an apartment for $290 a week) and energy bill, approximately $50 a week, Sonia had little money left over for food:

Table 9.2 Profile of interviewees*

Pseudonym	Location in Sydney	Gender	Age	Household composition	Main income source	Source of energy	Housing tenure
Bill	Inner ring	M	70	Single	Age pension	Electricity	Social housing
Gloria	Inner ring	F	70	Single	Age pension	Electricity	Social housing
Charles	Inner ring	M	70	Couple	Age pension	Electricity and gas	Social housing
Lauren	Middle ring	F	87	Single	Age pension	Electricity and gas	Homeowner
Iris	Inner ring	F	77	Single	Age pension	Electricity	Affordable rent
Mary	Middle ring	F	70+	Single	Age pension	Electricity and gas	Homeowner
Megan	Inner ring	F	93	Single	Savings	Electricity and gas	Homeowner
Adam	Middle ring	M	63	Family with child	Wages and salaries	Electricity and gas	Homeowner
Sonia	Outer ring	F	74	Single	Age pension	Electricity	Private renter
Anna	Not fixed	F	51	Single	Disability pension	Electricity and gas	Private renter
Amelia	Inner ring	F	70	Single	Age pension	Electricity and gas	Social housing
Phoebe	Middle ring	F	71	Single	Age pension	Electricity and gas	Homeowner
Samantha	Inner ring	F	77	Single	Age pension	Electricity	Social housing
Janine	Inner ring	F	64	Single	Savings	Electricity and gas	Social housing
Denise	Outer ring	F	77	Single	Age pension	Electricity	Social housing
Chloe	Outer ring	F	70	Single	Age pension	Electricity	Affordable rent
Marisa	Outer ring	F	70	Single	Age pension	Electricity	Affordable rent
Rose	Outer ring	F	65	Single	Age pension	Electricity	Affordable rent
Daniel	Outer ring	M	53	Single	Disability pension	Electricity	Social housing
Violet	Melbourne	F	67	Single	Age pension	Electricity and gas	Social housing
Jessica	Melbourne	F	65	Single	Age pension	Electricity and gas	Social housing
Jasmine	Melbourne	F	53	Single	Unemployment benefit	Electricity	Social housing
Anthony	Outer ring	M	69	Single	Savings	Electricity	Homeowner

Notes
* All the names used are pseudonyms.

And [I had] to agree for a payment plan for that one [overdue bill]. But my payment plan [for electricity] has always been self-organised at $50 a fortnight. But it did leave me with not that much left over [for] food and stuff. It was a regular drain on my income … It effects the amount I'll have left to eat with. And I know that my electricity bill is manageable if I don't eat too much.

Despite being a social housing tenant, Jessica (65 years old) was also struggling to eat adequately. Her energy bills accounted for about 10% of her disposable income. When asked whether her energy costs had an impact on her ability to purchase essential items, Jessica lamented that she was forced to buy "cheaper food".

I have to admit, you buy cheaper things for food, the cheaper quality, rather than the better quality because it's cheaper. You can buy that [the cheaper food] rather than the dear stuff because you can get more.

Violet (67 years old, social housing tenant) also felt that her high energy bills were compromising her health. Like Jessica, she was unable to buy enough nutritional food:

You can't shop properly and then your health goes down the plug, you know. If you go to shops, you see the chips and the lollies and that. They are cheaper and the people are buying those because they can't afford to buy broccoli … So you know, what do you do first? You feed yourself, put the heater on and hope that it's [the energy bill] not going to be too high. It's very, very hard … Sometimes I just, you don't know what to do first. So, I opt to pay my bills and pay my rent first and whatever is left over, then I see where I am and how I am, and what I can afford I buy, and what I can't afford doesn't get bought. That's all there is to it.

Jasmine (53 years old, social housing tenant) was reliant on the government unemployment benefit for her income. The unemployment benefit, the official government name is Jobseeker, is much lower than the Age Pension; in November 2022, it was $376 a week for people 60 and over. Jasmine was struggling to pay her energy bill; she owed her electricity provider close to $500 and was forced to rely on charities for most of her food requirements:

I go to food banks and then I might go to three or four food banks … A lot of the stuff from the food banks are mainly out of date and they are just rubbish … And I try and save that way. It's a lot of work to kind of go like that and then you get confused [as to] which ones you've been to …

Jasmine felt that the food she got from the food banks contributed to her gaining weight, which in turn worsened her mental health and ultimately the amount of time she spent alone at home, further increasing her energy costs. Her situation illustrates how it is possible for EP to contribute to food insecurity, unhealthy eating, and depression.

> I live on bread and baked beans, or spaghetti, or something like that ... All it does is make you put on more weight. It makes you more depressed and then you stay home more, and you use more heater or cooling because you don't want to go out ... You don't get no meat or nothing. You just get like tins of baked beans and some frozen stuff sometimes and out of date food. I mean, I shouldn't be ungrateful, but I just throw it out. It's disgusting, you know. You just get so angry, you know if I am eating food that is out of date by a month of something, you know what I mean ... terrible.

There is the possibility that the out-of-date food was still edible, but Jasmine was not prepared to risk it.

EP and the capacity to purchase essential items

High energy bills contributed to other essentials being out of reach. Being able to purchase clothing, hygiene products, and other necessities enhances one's sense of dignity and self-image, which reflects Nussbaum's central capability of affiliation, as in "having the social bases of self-respect" (see Table 9.1). Jasmine restricted her use of basic items like shampoo and deodorant:

> Oh no, I can't just buy what I want. No, it does stop you from buying certain things. No, I can't do that. You know, like, a lot of personal hygiene stuff. You can't just go and get [them]. Like, say a body wash. I'd buy a body wash, but I might not buy shampoo. So I use the body wash to wash my hair instead ... And If I don't go out, I don't use deodorant ...

Violet spoke about how her high energy bill contributed to her not being able to purchase basic clothing items.

> It [her energy bill] prevents you [from buying essentials] because it [the bill] goes so high, you can't afford to eat properly, can't afford to go buy underwear or can't buy a blouse. You can't afford to get any of those things. There is not enough money in the budget ... I don't have a bra ... I can't afford to buy one. There is no money in the budget for that.

Daniel (53 years old, social housing tenant) also found it difficult to purchase clothes:

I mean a couple of extra dollars a fortnight probably won't matter too much to anyone, but yeah, I mean over a year or something, it may be $100 total or something and that can be used for other things. It might be to, you know, buy some clothes or to buy a new pair of sneakers or something like that. It's better for the older person who is on a limited income, you know, if they can use that money for those sorts of things, instead of paying for the electricity.

As elaborated in the following text, the inability to purchase basic items probably contributed to depression and social exclusion (Baudaux et al., 2019).

EP and the capacity to cover medical expenses

In some cases, the limited disposable income of interviewees meant they could not obtain the proper medical care or medication they required. This had an impact on their capacity to maintain bodily health. Medicare in Australia covers most medical costs, but there are important omissions. For example, most dental treatments, physiotherapy, podiatry, glasses, and contact lens are not covered or coverage is limited. Also, many specialists do not bulk bill, which means that patients must pay "the gap". The gap refers to what they pay for their treatment and what they get back from government (Medicare). If a specialist bulk bills, there is no gap, and the treatment is essentially free. Daniel had been referred to medical specialists but could not afford to see them. He felt that his energy bills were a factor:

Like I have some specialist referrals that I haven't been able to afford to go [to] … because of the cost of those … If I had solar power and had an almost zero electricity cost, then I could certainly use that money towards the medical bills, yeah.

At the time of the interview, Amelia (70 years old, social housing tenant) had recently seen an ophthalmologist. This expenditure meant that she was now worried that she would be unable to pay her energy bill: "if I have an unusual expense, for example, I had to go to an eye specialist recently, and that was an unusual expense. And so, if I have unusual expenses, it puts me behind [on the energy bill]".

Not being able to afford the gap in specialist consultations because of EP gives greater urgency to Sherriff et al.'s (2020) argument that there is a need for an innovative and integrated approach to identifying and assisting people whose health is compromised directly or indirectly by EP. Rose (65 years old, social housing tenant) knew she needed an MRI (MRIs are not covered by Medicare) as soon as possible but could not afford the procedure. She was worried that if she went for an MRI she would not be able to pay her energy bill and other bills.

I am a bit scared at the moment because I should be getting an MRI this year, but I don't have the money to pay for that, you know what I'm saying. What [if] another bill comes and I realise that, you know, that's not enough?

When asked if her energy bills affected her quality of life, Lauren, an 87 years old homeowner, mentioned that despite being a homeowner and thus having low housing costs, she had had to cut back on the physiotherapy sessions she required:

Ah, look, I have the physio bills, for example, that are not covered [by Medicare], so well I have to pay for them. They [the government's scheme] give you five treatments a year ... but [for my condition] it adds up to 24 [sessions] a year, so I pay for 19 that are not covered [by Medicare]. But what I've been doing is, instead of going twice a month, I go only once a month.

The health conditions of some interviewees required treatments that increased energy usage. However, they restricted their treatments due to concerns that their energy bill would increase significantly (Snell et al., 2015; Willand et al., 2019). Charles, a 70 years old, social housing tenant, did not use his CPAP machine to treat his sleep apnoea "as much as I need it", because he was worried about the energy costs.

Concern about energy usage and cost did not only impact physical health. Research has shown a relationship between EP and poor mental health (Marmot Review Team, 2011; Thomson et al., 2017). Reducing energy consumption to the very basic energy needs and cutting expenditure on essentials in some cases evoked constant stress, anxiety, and depression, which significantly affected interviewees' capabilities. Jasmine mentioned she had had suicidal thoughts because of her vulnerable situation, which included late payments of energy bills:

It makes me feel, you know ... how depressed it makes me feel. I tried to suicide twice. It's just so, so embarrassing. Do you know what it's like to line up? [Jasmine is referring to charities where food is handed out and people have to queue]. You know my back hurts, my knee hurts. You have just got to line up for food. It's so, so embarrassing, and you just feel like you're being judged.

Rose passed up events which involved her having to spend money. This caused significant distress:

If there is another birthday coming up and it's like, you know, that's a stress on my part, because then I won't go to that party, because you know, I don't have a gift. So, it impacts my, you know, the way that I look at myself, you know. So yeah, psychologically it affects me.

'for Samantha, (77 years old, social housing tenant)', high hot water costs associated with the inefficient electric storage system she had at home meant she decided not to use the bath for the polymyalgia rheumatica pain management treatment anymore:

> The way my body feels like … I don't use hot water anymore for pain treatment. In the other house I had a big old-fashioned bath and because I had instantaneous [gas hot] water supply, I would have a big hot bath and that would reduce the pain level by 50%. But I don't do that here because of the [inefficient] hot water system that I've got. Those sorts of little decisions I've sorted out since I've been here. So that does add to that level of anxiety.

Not only did she have to endure persistent body pain and stiffness, but her anxiety levels were also very high. Hence, the central capabilities of bodily health and emotions were severely compromised. As Nussbaum (2000, p. 79) argues, no one should have their life "blighted by overwhelming fear and anxiety". Besides worrying about reducing their energy consumption to reduce costs, interviewees also feared potentially unaffordable bills – despite all efforts – and felt anxious and stressed as the next meter reading approached.

EP and the ability to maintain thermal comfort

Physical and mental health might be compromised by thermal discomfort (Ormandy & Ezratty, 2012; WHO, 2018). Particularly for older people, who are more likely to have other comorbidities such as heart disease and high blood pressure, it is harder to cope with temperature extremes (Day & Hitchings, 2011; Gronlund et al., 2016; van Hoof et al., 2017). In the context of climate change, this may become more serious, putting more pressure on the public health infrastructure. Usually, the focus is on winter temperatures (Daniel et al., 2019), but in cities such as Sydney and Melbourne, the impact of extreme summer temperatures is more pertinent. Melbourne typically experiences 30 days over 30 degrees Celsius per annum, whereas Sydney Central Business District typically experiences 18 days over 30 degrees Celsius per annum. In 2021 in Penrith, western Sydney, there were 67 days with temperatures over 30 degrees Celsius, 19 days over 35 degrees Celsius, and 4 days over 40 degrees Celsius (Bureau of Meteorology, 2021).

Many of the older women interviewed complained about the difficulty of coping with both the cold and the heat. Research has found that women are more sensitive to extreme temperatures (Clancy et al., 2017). On hot summer days, the poor energy efficiency of their homes was a major factor contributing to thermal discomfort. Several of our interviewees did not have an air conditioner or, alternatively, could not afford to run the one they had. Despite needing to be cool for health reasons, Adam (63 years old, home-owner), who was unemployed at the time of the interview and had serious health issues, did not have the financial resources to replace his old, inefficient air conditioner:

> But we don't use the air conditioner because it's too old and inefficient for our purpose. But I really do need it. I really desperately need the air conditioner because of my recent operation ... I have a heart condition, so I get very tired and hot easily because of my inability to cope with the hotter weather and humid[ity] ... The hotter weather, especially this summer, it's been very energy sapping, very tiring for me ... When I'm just trying to do little things, housework or do a little bit of gardening ... I can't get any relief at home.

Violet described how she was overcome on a particularly hot day:

> Like I can't stay here [in her house] in the summer. It's just too hot. I can't breathe in here. One day a friend came over here and I was passed out almost on the couch and she grabbed me and took me outside and took me to her place to cool down. Put me on the couch ... got me a cold towel on my head to revive me again. She was ready to call the ambulance. That's how bad it was.

Like Violet, Janine (64 years old, social housing tenant) was adamant that the building envelope of her social housing apartment meant it was difficult to cope with hot summer days:

> It definitely does affect my health during the summer months because I'm just totally exhausted, you know, and the perspiration [is] just pouring off me. I've never felt anything like where I've moved to now. It's just, it's, it's the worst I've ever, ever felt. And unless you're here and experience [it], it's very hard for anyone to realise how bad it really is. So that has affected, that does affect me, too. It's too hot. Even if you hop under the shower, a cool shower, and you step out of it, there is just too much heat, you know. You're just hot again, so there's no point in doing that. I'd do anything to try and keep cool, but it's ... virtually impossible. It's because of the building.

Anna (51 years old, private renter, reliant on the government Disability Support Pension for her income) blamed her unhealthy eating and weight gain during an extremely hot summer on not being able to afford an air conditioner:

Because of the unusual heat, I found the only way I could keep cool was with ice cream and cold fizzy drinks. Normally I never put drinks in the fridge, but I had to then. I'd just lost 15 kilograms and was insistent I would keep it off - but even I can't deal with 47degree centigrade heat unaided. Instead, I put on 20 kilograms. If I'd had air con to use, I'd be 25 kilograms lighter than I am now. Air con is high on the too expensive to use list.

Some of the interviewees found the winter cold difficult to deal with. In Sydney, the average day temperature in mid-winter is 17 degrees Celsius and the average night temperature is 8 degrees Celsius. Melbourne is colder. The average day temperature in mid-winter is 14 degrees Celsius and the at night the average is 7 degrees Celsius. Winter was a major problem for Sonia. Her apartment was extremely cold, and she could only afford to run a small heater:

So, I was living with the most atrocious carpet ... Very thin, threadbare. I could feel the stone underneath. Very cold. It was extremely cold in there. The first winter, I nearly froze to death. So, I think I've had that little heater on a lot. But even so, $600 [her energy bill] was a lot. So, I think I was being overcharged ... They [the energy company] were really gouging money from me.

Lauren found it easier to deal with the winter cold than the summer heat:

But, you know, my philosophy is that the cold is easier to fix, because you put something warmer on and that's it. But in summer it's worse, because how do you combat the heat? It's very difficult. To me, summer is more [uncomfortable].

Recent research on the nexus between housing and wellbeing drawing on the capabilities approach argues that this relationship is highly subjective and complex, with many social and cultural factors contributing to diverse experiences (Harris & Mckee, 2021; Irving, 2021). Nevertheless, adequate housing conditions are essential to the exercise of key functionings. The findings above indicate that EP plays an important role in how households experience their home and how this affects their health, wellbeing, and capabilities. Key capabilities associated with emotions (mental health), bodily health and integrity, and control over one's (home) environment are potentially impaired by EP.

EP and social isolation

In this section, we underline what Middlemiss et al. (2019) found in their research: being energy-poor can lessen opportunities to socialise and intensify a sense of feeling socially excluded. Furthermore, a key capability, affiliation, as in the ability to engage in various forms of social interaction and having the social bases of self-respect and non-humiliation, is diminished (Nussbaum, 2000). Interviewees noted that they avoided going out as they needed to "budget for every cent". A persistent question was whether the money spent on social activities could be better spent on food, paying for energy, and other essentials. Outings with friends or family that involved any expenditure were avoided and often evoked anxiety and embarrassment (Longhurst & Hargreaves, 2019; Morris, 2016). Sonia explained how her energy costs and rent had had a dramatic impact on her social life:

> I have no social life. I can't afford it ... There is one neighbour who was very friendly, and she would ask me out for coffee. Often, I would have to say, "No, I can't afford to." That's very embarrassing. It really cuts down your social life completely. You can't even afford to go out for a bit of lunch and a coffee.

Even though Mary (70 years old) is a homeowner, she is constantly worried about her financial situation and found it difficult to tell her friends about her situation:

> If some friend[s] call me and they say, "Oh, we [would] like to go for a lunch together", and I have to think, "If I go out, I have to spend the money, you know, and pay [for] the food ... Maybe later they want to have coffee and have a cake." How much money spent, huh? And I say, "Sorry, today I can't." I don't say, "I don't have enough money".

Connon (2018) in her case study of four communities in the UK found a similar pattern. The people she interviewed tended to hide their EP situation and become isolated. Violet was unable to join her friends for a restaurant meal or accompany them to the cinema:

> I tell you what, unless my friend pays for a meal if I want to go out with them, I can't afford it. I just can't afford it. There is just no way. It's too much. I'd like to go to a restaurant with my friends every once in a while. I like to go out and see what's happening, but I can't. I can't even go to the movies, you know. I can't afford the movies. It's just not in the budget.

Another common anxiety was having visitors or family stay and the higher energy costs that accompanied their stay. Samantha had her nephew living with her for a few months, but was relieved when he left:

> When my nephew came to live [here with me], the electricity bill doubled, just with one young man in the house ... So that's something that I have

learned. And I decided … [to avoid guests] because I've exhausted my finances.

Denise (77 years old, social housing tenant) lives alone and would normally shower every second day to reduce her hot water use. However, when somebody stayed over, she felt compelled to shower every day:

And because I live on my own, I can be dirty for as long as I like. I'm not a dirty person, don't get me wrong, but I don't have to have two showers a day, let's put it that way. [But] if I have a friend stay, of course I shower in the afternoon as distinct from the morning so that he can have the morning shower … It's only then [when I have a guest staying] I have a shower a day. The shower gets used on a daily basis, but if it's only me, it's every two days. So, I suspect that I might actually save a bit on that, I don't know.

Jessica could not contemplate socialising when she was a private renter. When interviewed she was living in social housing and her situation had improved because of her lower housing costs. When she was a private tenant, after paying the rent and energy bill, she had very little money left and would prefer to spend it on food rather than outings:

I hardly bought anything then [when she was a private tenant] because I couldn't afford it, yeah … I never went out for a meal, I never went shopping for clothes. Not even a coffee because to me going out for a coffee, I could get something else with it. I could get a packet of Weetabix or something, if that makes sense.

For some interviewees, spending a good part of their income on energy had an impact on their internet usage. They either limited its use, turned off the modem to reduce electricity costs, or could not pay for a good service. During the COVID-19 pandemic and the resultant lockdown, Rose maintained social contact using her phone and Zoom, but was concerned that ultimately she would need to purchase a better plan:

So even though I am at home [during the COVID-19 pandemic], it's the internet [costs] and all that, because now instead of going out and not using the internet to be able to interact, now I have to use Zoom, which means I have to have, I have to think about - okay two or three months later - I have to sign up for a better internet data connection, NBN or something like that. At the moment I [can still] use my phone because I have [data] credits still available. When that runs out, I have to [get a new plan], and that is going to be a major expense and I am telling you, at the moment I keep postponing it, because I know it's going to be really tight.

Reducing the opportunity for social connection because of EP can create a cycle of EP problems. For older low-income households, mostly for those who lack computer literacy or have poor access to internet services, social connections can play an important part in alleviating EP, as they provide an opportunity to receive trustworthy information and advice from friends and family regarding their energy bills. Face-to-face conversations were, in many cases, their only way to learn about energy-related subjects.

EP, housing conditions, and the wellbeing of older Australians

The interviews reflected the complex interaction of variables which impacted whether a person experiences EP or not. It is apparent that a relatively simple method and succinct overview of housing, health, and EP are needed for stakeholders, particularly policymakers. After analysing the interview data, we propose the following conceptualisation of the relationship between housing, health, and EP (see Figure 9.2) as a means of determining where people are on the EP continuum. The variables found in the literature and the interviews were housing conditions which fluctuate from good to poor in respect of thermal performance and running costs. The impact of the housing conditions varied depending on the health of the occupants which are categorised broadly into those with good or poor health.

	Poor health		Good health	
Good housing conditions	Health condition affecting energy use to the extent of aggravating energy poverty and vice-versa; i.e. particular health needs are not being met (and limited income factor possibly)	Health condition may be affecting energy use but not to the extent of putting household in energy poverty (likely not low income situation)	Energy poverty situation likely to be mainly related to limited income and poor energy literacy skills	Best (and rarest) possible combination but not likely among low income older households
Poor housing conditions	Poor health and housing conditions aggravating energy poverty | Energy poverty and housing conditions compromising health	Poor health and housing conditions affecting energy use but not to the extent of putting household in energy poverty (likely not low income situation, but susceptible to boiling frog effect)	Poor housing conditions might be aggravating energy poverty situation, but not to the extent of compromising health (likely to be a household with strong adaptive behaviour and susceptible to boiling frog effect)	Poor housing conditions not affecting health nor putting household in energy poverty | DYI retrofits likely to improve overall comfort but not urgent
	In energy poverty	Not in energy poverty	In energy poverty	Not in energy poverty

Figure 9.2 Relationships between housing conditions, health, and EP among older Australians.

Source: The authors.

The colours/tones in the figure indicate the severity of the situation. The worst possible combination, bottom left (in red), refers to an older low-income person in poor health living in inadequate housing (i.e., a home that is not energy efficient and/or needing major repairs/maintenance) and suffering from EP. On the other side of the continuum, top right (in green), is the best combination – an older person in good health, living in an energy-efficient house, and not experiencing EP. This is followed by the bottom right (light green) combination of bad housing conditions not affecting health or pushing the person into EP. This situation is not likely to pertain to low-income older households but is possibly the situation of older households with adequate income. The top left (dark orange) combination refers to a person whose housing conditions are good, but whose health might affect their energy use. As discussed, health issues can contribute to EP due to increased energy consumption and can also be aggravated by EP.

The two central lower combinations (light orange beige) describe the situation of most older Australians. They mostly live in homes with poor energy efficiency that may influence their energy consumption patterns. However, income and health play an important role in determining whether they will experience EP. Older Australians in these two lower combinations are susceptible to Handy's (2012) "boiling frog" effect. The boiling frog effect refers to a situation where a person does not realise that they may slide into EP. Gradual changes go unnoticed. In the case of older low-income Australians not yet in EP, minor "unnoticed" changes in energy costs or a decline in their health status might rapidly push them into EP. The individuals already experiencing it may have strong resilient and adaptive (and conditioned) behaviours, but if conditions due to climate change get worse, EP will likely affect their health.

The upper central combinations (in yellow) describe two less severe cases. The first one refers to a situation where an older household member has a health condition that may affect their energy usage, but, because their housing conditions and income are adequate, this does not result in EP. The other combination (central, yellow) describes an older household whose occupants have no health issues and reside in a good home with respect to energy efficiency, but still experience EP. This is most likely due to low income and low energy literacy. In this case, providing this household with assistance and the opportunity to obtain a fair energy deal could lessen or even resolve their EP.

Conclusions

The findings reinforce previous research on the impacts of EP on older people (Day & Hitchings, 2011; O'Neill et al., 2006; Waitt et al., 2016; Willand et al., (2017). The interviews showed that, for low-income older Australians, EP is a central issue impacting the quality of their lives. The thermal discomfort they experience at home, particularly in summer, is an issue that needs to be addressed in the context of climate change and rising temperatures. Those older pensioners struggling with long-term health conditions that affect the way they experience their home and use energy are often in situations where their health is impaired by EP. The interviews showed how health issues can either be a significant cause of EP due to the need for increased energy use or can be aggravated by EP when medication and medical treatment are difficult to afford.

The interviews also demonstrated the detrimental effects of EP on the capabilities of older low-income Australians and corroborated previous studies (Melin et al., 2021; Middlemiss et al., 2019; Willand & Horne, 2018). The findings revealed the impacts of EP on mental and physical health and on the capacity of interviewees to consume essentials such as food, clothing, hygiene products, prescriptions, and engage in recreational activities. Worrying about energy bills, cutting other expenses, and, ultimately, compromising their quality of life made interviewees anxious, stressed, and, in some cases, depressed. High levels of anxiety, stress, and depression caused by high energy costs undermined their capacity to lead a joyful life. The thermal discomfort they experienced in their energy-inefficient homes during summer and winter and the compromises on medical treatments that either required extra energy use or money they did not have, further affected physical health. The vicious cycle of social isolation and EP impacted their capacity to retain social ties with family, friends, and support networks.

Basic capabilities are then severely affected. Energy-poor older households lack the opportunities, resources, and freedom to achieve valuable functionings, some as basic as being able to have a balanced and nutritious diet. This research provided evidence that Nussbaum's (2000) list of central capabilities associated with being able to have good health and bodily integrity, being able to socialise and enjoy recreational activities, being able to live and not be overwhelmed by anxiety and fear, and being able to control one's environment are often unachievable for energy-poor older Australians.

A further contribution of this study is the conceptualisation of how health, housing, and EP correlate. Previous research on the impact of energy-efficient features and EP helps us understand this relationship, and this study provided more information on how older Australians experience extreme temperatures, an emerging research topic (Judson et al., 2019; Willand et al., 2015, 2019). Figure 9.2 illustrates the different combinations of EP, poor housing conditions, and poor health, suggesting where older pensioners might be situated and opening discussion for targeted solutions to alleviate EP.

The overall cost of EP to society and individuals may be far higher than what recent statistics indicate. Also, the health impacts are probably underestimated. Currently, the measurement of EP is inadequate. In Australia, it is measured by a few questions related to financial strain, inability to heat the home properly, and paying energy bills on time (ABS, 2012;

Baker et al., 2019; Wilkins et al., 2020). There is a need for more comprehensive and refined survey instruments and a wider use of qualitative methods to capture the extent of EP and its various impacts.

The findings suggest that policymakers need to rethink the way EP is managed. This is especially so considering the substantial increase in energy costs post the energy crisis precipitated by Russia's invasion of Ukraine. The expectation that older low-income households should just weather EP on their own with no active intervention from government places the individuals concerned in vulnerable situations. The opportunities for older pensioners to learn about and engage with the energy market should be increased. This may help lessen the power and knowledge imbalance between energy retailers and consumers.

Acknowledgements

The authors would like to thank all interviewees for their time and for sharing their stories about their lived experience of energy poverty.

References

ABCB (2019). *Climate Zone Map Australia.* Australian Building Codes Board. https://www.abcb.gov.au/resource/map/climate-zone-map-australia

ABS (2012). *Household energy consumption survey, Australia: Summary of results.* Australian Bureau of Statistics. http://www.abs.gov.au/ausstats/abs@.nsf/Lookup/bySubject/4670.0~2012~Main Features~Summary of Findings~13

ABS (2022). *2021 Australia, census all persons quickstats.* Australian Bureau of Statistics.

ACOSS, PCA, & EEC (2018). *Energy bills & energy efficiency.* Australian Council of Social Services, Property Council of Australia and Energy Efficiency Council.

AER (2022a). *AER starts a journey towards energy equity.* Australian Energy Regulator.

AER (2022b). *Quarterly retail performance report Q3 2021–2022.*

Anderson, W., White, V., & Finney, A. (2012). Coping with low incomes and cold homes. *Energy Policy, 49,* 40–52.

Australian Government (2021). *Reduce your energy bills.* Department of Industry, Science, Energy and Resources. https://www.energy.gov.au/households/household-guides/reduce-energy-bills

Azpitarte, F., Johnson, V., & Sullivan, D. (2015). *Fuel poverty, household income and energy spending: An empirical analysis for Australia using HILDA data.* The Brotherhood of St Laurence: Fitzroy.

Baker, E., Beer, A., Zillante, G., London, K., Bentley, R., Hulse, K., Pawson, H., Randolph, B., Stone, W., & Rajagopalan, P. (2019). *The Australian housing conditions dataset.* ADA Dataverse.

Baudaux, A., Coene, J., Delbeke, B., Bartiaux, F., Sibeni, A., Fournier, F., Oosterlynck, S., & Lahaye, W. (2019). Living in energy poverty: A qualitative approach. In B. Françoise (Ed.), *Generation and gender energy deprivation: Realities and social policies* (pp. 43–72). Brussels: BELSPO.

Benton, T. G., Froggatt, A., & Wellesley, L. (2022). *The Ukraine war and threats to food and energy security: Cascading risks from rising prices and supply disruptions,* Research Paper, London: Royal Institute of International Affairs.

Berry, S., & Marker, T. (2015). Residential energy efficiency standards in Australia: Where to next? *Energy Efficiency, 8*(5), 963–974.

Borchers Arriagada, N., Bowman, D. M. J. S., Palmer, A. J., & Johnston, F. H. (2020). Climate change, wildfires, heatwaves and health impacts in Australia. In R. Akhtar (Ed.), *Extreme weather events and human health: International case studies* (pp. 99–116). Springer International Publishing.

Bouzarovski, S., & Petrova, S. (2015). A global perspective on domestic energy deprivation: Overcoming the energy poverty-fuel poverty binary. *Energy Research and Social Science, 10*, 31–40.

Bryant, D., Porter, E., Rama, I., & Sullivan, D. (2022). *Power pain: An investigation of energy stress in Australia,* Brotherhood of St. Laurence, Fitzroy, Victoria. (https://library.bsl.org.au/bsljspui/bitstream/1/13115/1/Bryant_etal_Power_pain_energy_stress_in_Australia_2022.pdf).

Bureau of Meteorology (2021). Climate statistics for Australian locations. In *Statistics.*

Canstar Blue (2019). *Electricity Costs Per kWh | QLD, SA, VIC, NSW Rates – Canstar Blue.* https://www.canstarblue.com.au/electricity/electricity-costs-kwh/

Chai, A., Ratnasiri, S., & Wagner, L. (2021). The impact of rising energy prices on energy poverty in Queensland: A microsimulation exercise. *Economic Analysis and Policy, 71*, 57–72.

Chard, R., & Walker, G. (2016). Living with fuel poverty in older age: Coping strategies and their problematic implications. *Energy Research and Social Science, 18*, 62–70.

Chester, L. (2013). *The impacts and consequences for low-income Australian households of rising energy prices.* Department of Political Economy, Faculty of Arts and Social Sciences, The University of Sydney: Sydney.

Chipango, E. F. (2021). Beyond utilitarian economics: A capability approach to energy poverty and social suffering. *Journal of Human Development and Capabilities, 22*(3), 446–467.

Churchill, S. A., & Smyth, R. (2021). Energy poverty and health: Panel data evidence from Australia. *Energy Economics, 97*(105219), 11.

Clancy, J., Daskalova, V., Feenstra, M., Franceschelli, N., & Sanz, M. (2017). *Gender perspective on access to energy in the EU.* Brussels: Study for the FEMM Committee. European Parliament Policy Department for Citizens' Rights and Constitutional Affairs.

Climate Council (2020). *Hottest of the hot: Extreme heat in Australia.* https://www.climatecouncil.org.au/resources/hottest-of-the-hot-extreme-heat-in-australia/

Connon, I. L. C. (2018). Transcending the triad: Political distrust, local cultural norms and reconceptualising the drivers of domestic energy poverty in the UK. In N. Simcock, H. Thomson, S. Petrova & S. Bouzarovski (Eds.), *Energy poverty and vulnerability: A global perspective* (1st ed., pp. 46–60). Routledge.

Cornwell, A., Hejazi Amin, M., Houghton, T., Jefferson, T., Newman, P., & Rowley, S. (2016). *Energy poverty in Western Australia: A comparative analysis of drivers and effects.* Perth: Bankwest Curtin Economics Centre. http://bcec.edu.au/assets/bcec-energy-poverty-in-western-australia.pdf

COTA (2018). *State of the (Older) Nation 2018.* Canberra: Council on the Ageing Australia.

Culver, L. C. (2017). *Energy poverty: What you measure matters*. Pre-symposium white paper for: Reducing Energy Poverty with Natural Gas: Changing Political, Business, and Technology Paradigms. Stanford University.

Curtis, K. (2020, December 9). Powerful debts on energy bills are tipping Australians "off a cliff". *The Sydney Morning Herald*.

Daniel, L., Baker, E., Beer, A., & Pham, N. T. A. (2021). Cold housing: Evidence, risk and vulnerability. *36*(1), 110–130.

Day, R., & Hitchings, R. (2011). "Only old ladies would do that": Age stigma and older people's strategies for dealing with winter cold. *Health and Place*, *17*(4), 885–894.

Day, R., Walker, G., & Simcock, N. (2016). Conceptualising energy use and energy poverty using a capabilities framework. *Energy Policy*, *93*, 255–264.

Dear, K. B. G., & McMichael, A. J. (2011). The health impacts of cold homes and fuel poverty. *British Medical Journal*, *342*, 1–2.

DEE (2019). *Nationwide house energy rating scheme*. Department of the Environment and Energy. http://www.nathers.gov.au/

Department of Industry, Science, Energy and Resources (2021). *Nationwide House Energy Rating Scheme (NatHERS)*. https://www.nathers.gov.au/

ENPOR (2022). *Energy poverty*. https://www.enpor.eu/energy-poverty/

Frigo, G., Baumann, M., & Hillerbrand, R. (2021). Energy and the good life: Capabilities as the foundation of the right to access energy services. *Journal of Human Development and Capabilities*, *22*(2), 218–248.

Gronlund, C. J., Zanobetti, A., Wellenius, G. A., Schwartz, J. D., & O'Neill, M. S. (2016). Vulnerability to renal, heat and respiratory hospitalizations during extreme heat among U.S. elderly. *Climatic Change*, *136*(3–4), 631–645.

Hamza, N., & Gilroy, R. (2011). The challenge to UK energy policy: An ageing population perspective on energy saving measures and consumption. *Energy Policy*, *39*(2), 782–789.

Handy, C. (2012). *The age of unreason*. Random House.

Harris, J., & Mckee, K. (2021). *Health and wellbeing in the UK private rented sector | Enhancing capabilities*. Glasgow: UK Collaborative Centre for Housing Evidence (CaCHE).

Hernández, D. (2016). Understanding 'energy insecurity' and why it matters to health. *Social Science and Medicine*, *167*(October), 1–10.

Hernández, D., & Siegel, E. (2019). Energy insecurity and its ill health effects: A community perspective on the energy-health nexus in New York City. *Energy Research and Social Science*, *47*(July 2018), 78–83.

Howden-Chapman, P., Viggers, H., Chapman, R., O'Sullivan, K., Telfar Barnard, L., & Lloyd, B. (2012). Tackling cold housing and fuel poverty in New Zealand: A review of policies, research, and health impacts. *Energy Policy*, *49*, 134–142.

Irving, A. (2021). Exploring the relationship between housing conditions and capabilities: A qualitative case study of private hostel residents. *Housing Studies*.

Judd, B., Liu, E., Easthope, H., Davy, L., & Bridge, C. (2014). *Downsizing amongst older Australians*. AHURI Final Report No. 214. Melbourne: Australian Housing and Urban Research Institute.

Judson, E., Zirakbash, F., Nygaard, A., & Spinney, A. (2019). *Renewable energy retrofitting and energy poverty in low-income households*. Hawthorn: Research report prepared by the Centre for Urban Transitions for United Housing Cooperative.

Kearns, A., Whitley, E., & Curl, A. (2019). Occupant behaviour as a fourth driver of fuel poverty (aka warmth & energy deprivation). *Energy Policy*, *129*(March), 1143–1155.

Kelleher, J. P. (2015). Capabilities versus resources. *Journal of Moral Philosophy*, *12*(2), 151–171.

KPMG (2017). *The rise of energy poverty in Australia* (Issue Census Insight Series). KPMG International Limited.

Lee, J., Kim, H., & Byrne, J. (2021). Operationalising capability thinking in the assessment of energy poverty relief policies: Moving from compensation-based to empowerment-focused policy strategies. *Journal of Human Development and Capabilities*, *22*(2), 292–315.

Longhurst, N., & Hargreaves, T. (2019). Emotions and fuel poverty: The lived experience of social housing tenants in the United Kingdom. *Energy Research and Social Science*, *56*(June), 101207.

Marmot Review Team (2011). *The health impacts of cold homes and fuel poverty*. London: Friends of the Earth & the Marmot Review Team - University College London.

Melin, A., Day, R., & Jenkins, K. E. H. (2021). Energy justice and the capability approach—Introduction to the special issue. *Journal of Human Development and Capabilities*, *22*(2), 185–196.

Middlemiss, L., Ambrosio-Albalá, P., Emmel, N., Gillard, R., Gilbertson, J., Hargreaves, T., Mullen, C., Ryan, T., Snell, C., & Tod, A. (2019). Energy poverty and social relations: A capabilities approach. *Energy Research and Social Science*, *55*(September 2018), 227–235.

Morris, A. (2012). Older social and private renters, the neighbourhood, and social connections and activity. *Urban Policy and Research*, *30*(1), 43–58.

Morris, A. (2016). *The Australian dream: Housing experiences of older Australians*. CSIRO Publishing.

Nelson, T., & Gilmore, J. (2022, March 21). Energy bills are spiking after the Russian invasion. We should have doubled-down on renewables years ago. *The Conversation*.

Nicholls, L., & Strengers, Y. (2018). Heatwaves, cooling and young children at home: Integrating energy and health objectives. *Energy Research and Social Science*, *39*(February 2017), 1–9.

Nicholls, L., McCann, H., Strengers, Y., & Bosomworth, K. (2017). *Electricity pricing, heatwaves and household vulnerability in Australia*. Melbourne: Centre for Urban Research, RMIT University.

Nord, M., & Kantor, L. S. (2006). Seasonal variation in food insecurity is associated with heating and cooling costs among low-income elderly Americans. *The Journal of Nutrition*, *136*(11), 2939–2944.

Nussbaum, M. (2000). *Women and human development: The capabilities approach*. Cambridge University Press.

Nussbaum, M. (2003). Capabilities as fundamental entitlements: Sen and social justice. *Feminist Economics*, *9*(2–3), 33–59.

Nassbaum, M. C. (2011). *Creating capabilities: The human development approach*. Harvard University Press.

O'Neill, T., Jinks, C., & Squire, A. (2006). Heating is more important than food. *Journal of Housing for the Elderly*, *20*(3), 95–108.

Ormandy, D., & Ezratty, V. (2012). Health and thermal comfort: From WHO guidance to housing strategies. *Energy Policy, 49*, 116–121.

Porto Valente, C., Morris, A., & Wilkinson, S. J. (2021). Energy poverty, housing and health: the lived experience of older low-income Australians. *Building Research & Information, 50*(1-2), 6–18.

Porto Valente, C., Wilkinson, S., & Morris, A. (2020). Age pensioners' homes: current state and adaptation for climate change. *Proceeding of the 26thAnnual of the Pacific Rim Real Estate Society (PRRES)*, Canberra, Australia, 19–22 January 2020.

Roberts, E., & Henwood, K. (2019). "It's an old house and that's how it works": Living sufficiently well in inefficient homes. *Housing, Theory and Society*, 1–20.

Robinson, C. (2019). Energy poverty and gender in England: A spatial perspective. *Geoforum, 104*(May), 222–233.

Romanach, L., Hall, N., & Meikle, S. (2017). Energy consumption in an ageing population: Exploring energy use and behaviour of low-income older Australians. *Energy Procedia, 121*, 246–253.

Rudge, J., & Gilchrist, R. (2005). Excess winter morbidity among older people at risk of cold homes: A population-based study in a London borough. *Journal of Public Health, 27*(4), 353–358.

Sen, A. (1992). *Inequality reexamined*. Clarendon Press.

Sen, A. (1993). Capability and well-being. In M. Nussbaum & A. Sen (Eds.), *The quality of life*. Oxford University Press.

Sen, A. (1997). From income inequality to economic inequality. *Southern Economic Journal, 64*(2), 383–401.

Sen, A. (1999). *Development as freedom*. Oxford University Press.

Sherriff, G., Lawler, C., Martin, P., Butler, D., Probin, M., & Brown, P. (2020). *Reshaping health services and fuel poverty in the Outer Hebrides*. Final report of the Gluasad Còmhla project. Salford: SHUSU, University of Salford.

Sherriff, G., Moore, T., Berry, S., Ambrose, A., Goodchild, B., & Maye-Banbury, A. (2019). Coping with extremes, creating comfort: User experiences of 'low-energy' homes in Australia. *Energy Research and Social Science, 51*(July 2018), 44–54.

Simcock, N., Thomson, H., Petrova, S., & Bouzarovski, S. (2018). Conclusions. In N. Simcock, H. Thomson, S. Petrova & S. Bouzarovski (Eds.), *Energy poverty and vulnerability: A global perspective* (pp. 249–256). Routledge.

Smith, M. L., & Seward, C. (2009). The relational ontology of Amartya Sen's capability approach: Incorporating social and individual causes. *Journal of Human Development and Capabilities, 10*(2), 213–235.

Snell, C., Bevan, M., & Thomson, H. (2015). Justice, fuel poverty and disabled people in England. *Energy Research and Social Science, 10*, 123–132.

Sovacool, B. K., & Dworkin, M. H. (2014). *Global energy justice*. Cambridge University Press.

Steffen, W., Hughes, L., & Perkins, S. (2014). *Heatwaves: Hotter, longer, more often*. Climate Council of Australia Ltd.

Sustainability Victoria (2014). *Victorian Households Energy Report*.

The Melbourne Institute (2022). *Poverty Lines: Australia*.

Thomson, H., Simcock, N., Bouzarovski, S., & Petrova, S. (2019). Energy poverty and indoor cooling: An overlooked issue in Europe. *Energy and Buildings, 196*, 21–29.

Thomson, H., Snell, C., & Bouzarovski, S. (2017). Health, well-being and energy poverty in Europe: A comparative study of 32 European countries. *International Journal of Environmental Research and Public Health*, *14*(6).

Tollefson, J. (2022). What the war in Ukraine means for energy, climate and food. *Nature*, *604*(7905), 232–233.

Tuttle, C. J., & Beatty, T. K. M. (2017). *The effects of energy price shocks on household food security in low-income households* (Issue ERR-233). U.S. Department of Agriculture, Economic Research Service.

van Hoof, J., Schellen, L., Soebarto, V., Wong, J. K. W., & Kazak, J. K. (2017). Ten questions concerning thermal comfort and ageing. *Building and Environment*, *120*, 123–133.

VCOSS (2018). *Battling on persistent energy hardship*. Melbourne: Victorian Council of Social Service.

Waitt, G., Roggeveen, K., Gordon, R., Butler, K., & Cooper, P. (2016). Tyrannies of thrift: Governmentality and older, low-income people's energy efficiency narratives in the Illawarra, Australia. *Energy Policy*, *90*, 37–45.

WHO (2018). *WHO housing and health guidelines*. World Health Organisation.

Wilkins, R., Botha, F., Vera-Toscano, E., & Wooden, M. (2020). *The household, income and labour dynamics in Australia survey: Selected findings from waves 1 to 18* (p. 171). Melbourne Institute: Applied Economic & Social Research, University of Melbourne.

Wilkinson, P., Pattenden, S., Armstrong, B., Fletcher, A., Kovats, R. S., Mangtani, P., & McMichael, A. J. (2004). Vulnerability to winter mortality in elderly people in Britain: Population based study. *British Medical Journal*, *329*(7467), 647–651.

Wilkinson, S., Valente, C. P., & Morris, A. (2021, January 25). "I can't save money for potential emergencies": COVID lockdowns drove older Australians into energy poverty. *The Conversation*, https://theconversation.com/i-cant-save-money-for-potential-emergencies-covid-lockdowns-drove-older-australians-into-energy-poverty-153096.

Willand, N., & Horne, R. (2018). "They are grinding us into the ground" – The lived experience of (in)energy justice amongst low-income older households. *Applied Energy*, *226*, 61–70.

Willand, N., Maller, C., & Ridley, I. (2017). "It's not too bad" - The lived experience of energy saving practices of low-income older and frail people. *Energy Procedia*, *121*, 166–173.

Willand, N., Middha, B., & Walker, G. (2021). Using the capability approach to evaluate energy vulnerability policies and initiatives in Victoria, Australia. *Local Environment*, 1–19.

Willand, N., Ridley, I., & Maller, C. (2015). Towards explaining the health impacts of residential energy efficiency interventions - A realist review. Part 1: Pathways. *Social Science and Medicine*, *133*, 191–201.

Willand, N., Sharrock, D., & Long, D. (2019). *Integrating energy efficiency & hardship improvements into the care at home system*. Report for publication: RMIT University.

Wolff, J., & de-Shalit, A. (2007). Disadvantage. In *Oxford political theory*. Oxford University Press.

World Food Summit (1996). *Report of the World Food Summit*.

Conclusion

It is never an easy task attempting to conclude an edited book, especially one that contains a wide range of topics and building types. However, reflecting on the content of the chapters, it is possible to tentatively suggest some areas for further investigation that appear to be pertinent. The themes and issues that emerge have revealed unique insights into how our buildings influence our wellbeing and how building users may attempt to influence their internal environments. Of course, the limitations of a book format means that the chapters can only cover some of the many aspects concerning health and wellbeing and not all building types. We have been able to address a range of physical and mental abilities, a wide age range, and a variety of building typologies. There was, however, insufficient space to include educational buildings, such as schools and universities, and hence the younger members of society. We have not been able to dedicate space to building materials and how they influence the internal environment and affect our health and wellbeing. Nor have we had space to address the policy issues relating to, for example, housing and healthcare provision. These are areas that will continue to feature in articles published in *Building Research & Information*, which may form the focus for forthcoming books in this series.

Despite the omissions, the overall message in this book is encouraging and positive. Health and wellbeing relate to physiological and psychological issues as much as it does the physical building fabric. The contributors to this book have engaged with a wide variety of research methods to achieve their aims and objectives, from which readers can take inspiration and direction. Methods include monitoring and shadowing, interviews and longitudinal research. The takeaway is the importance of time in research programmes to better understand the complex interactions between people and buildings. Collectively, the chapters have demonstrated a need for a better understanding of how buildings affect our comfort, health, and wellbeing. Assembling the contributors and contributions to this book has been rewarding in terms of making new acquaintances and rekindling established ones. It has also resulted in a better understanding of some of the issues at play. The chapters have primarily addressed the indoor environment, with one focusing on the external space adjacent the building.

DOI: 10.1201/9781003344711-11

The building types have included offices, homes, and healthcare facilities. The building users have included staff, patients, and residents.

The link to building design is dealt with directly and indirectly in this book, with the chapters raising different aspects for further consideration. What is evident is the need to better understand the needs, and hence the characteristics, of building users. The book content also does help to reinforce the value of good design as a determinant of comfort, health, and wellbeing; something that we must continue to cherish and promote. Building designers are usually faced with uncertainty about the characteristics of the people using their buildings. To be able to deal with that uncertainty assumptions about users' general needs and requirements, physical size, age range, and mobility are required. Indeed, a feature of design guides is the use of average sizes and typical space requirements and characteristics. As witnessed in this book, such assumptions may be misleading as nothing is particularly typical or average about the individuals featured in these chapters. Different users have, not surprisingly, different expectations and requirements of buildings. Understanding the wide range of user needs and abilities, both physical and mental, is one step towards designing a more inclusive and accessible built environment that supports and stimulates a healthy existence. This needs to be addressed with an awareness of the prevailing local, national, and global social and economic situation. For example, at the time of compiling this book, there is intense interest in the cost of the fuel used to heat, cool and power our buildings. For many businesses and individuals, the cost is such that difficult decisions must be made that will undoubtably impact the comfort, health, and wellbeing of many building users. Decisions need to be made within the context of our climate emergency.

We return to the aim of this book, which is to act as a primer for further research into the link between our buildings and our health and wellbeing. That has been achieved in these chapters, which offer a variety of perspectives from a multitude of users, building types, and geographical locations. Underlying much of the content is the importance of design and how building inhabitants use, perceive, and adjust their internal and immediate external environments. This is related to our perception of comfort. Comfort with our physical and sensory built environs, the stimuli we need for an active life, and the support required to enable us to control and adapt our milieu. Although we have not included articles that are specific to thermal comfort and adaptive thermal comfort, some of the chapters have implicit links to that body of literature. Similarly, there are parallels with the literature on inclusive design and useability. These are topics that will, no doubt, feature in future investigations.

Index

accessibility 176
acoustics 126, 205
active living 195
activity-friendly 164
adaptability 196, 208
adaption 44, 92
adaption strategies 88, 94
adequacy of: healthcare environment 122; housing 239; impatient facilities 122
aesthetics, of offices 20
age-friendly 166
ageing 164, 193
air pollutants 60
air purifiers 60, 63
air quality sensors 69
Alzheimer's disease 170
analytical methods 119, 172
anthropometric factors 41
architecture 195
Australia 197, 221

barriers, to mobility 146
bedrooms 72
behavioural adaption 89, 96
behavioural health environments 111
behavioural, observations 172
behavioural rules 21
Belgium 91
biophilic design 10, 196, 198, 213
building design 10, 142, 159, 249
building use 103
built environment, design of 193, 210

capability, of people 226
carbon dioxide (CO_2) 80
care facility 164, 168
case study 10, 91, 164, 187

changes (in perception) 18
characteristics, of participants 170, 229
Chile 33
China 164
coherence, sense of 6, 16
cold climates 61
comfort 36, 77, 90, 96
comfortable walking environments 177
context 10, 21, 64
control of one's environment 20, 38, 77, 92, 99
convenience sample 64
cost of energy 224
courtyards use of 182, 199
COVID-19 25, 45, 63, 159, 227, 238
crossover study 70
cross-disciplinary 210
cross-sectional 49

data analysis (procedure) 14, 43, 94, 147, 172
data collection procedure 12
deductive coding 14
dementia 144, 176, 193, 204
dementia-friendly 166
demographics 12, 65, 118, 171
design 155, 193
design characteristics 112
design of outdoor environment 166
design practice 104
design research 111, 155
design tool 113
designers 25, 104
designing 34, 133, 195
diabetes 170
disabilities 164, 206
dissatisfaction 79, 98
distance, as a barrier 141

distance travelled 148, 156
diversity, of people 102, 182

economic reality 82
effectiveness: of air purifiers 78; of
    environmental qualities 121; of
    healthcare settings 112
employees 5
energy efficiency standards 222
energy poverty 221
environmental: evaluation 185; model
    164; qualities 111, 121
essential items, purchase of 231
eudaimonic wellbeing 37, 100
evaluations, staff and patient 122
evidence-based design 111, 213
exercise 179
experience of distance and barriers 153
explorative research 100, 187

facility managers 25
features, environmental 111
Finland 60
food insecurity 228
framework 8, 118
functioning, of people 164, 225

gardening spaces 176, 199
Germany 142
goodness of fit 52
green spaces 198

health 7, 61, 90, 165, 171
health and wellbeing agenda 5
health: outcomes 195; promoting 7; risk
    223; status 102
healthcare 89
healthcare buildings (settings) 10, 113,
    140, 145
healthy: ageing 193, 196; employees 5;
    office 5
heatwaves 224
heating season 61
hedonic wellbeing 100
home air purifiers 63
homes 60, 221
hospital 88; staff 91; ward 91
housing conditions 239
housing, for older people 222
human centred design 103, 201

impact 80, 149, 223
importance and effectiveness 125

independence, of patients 139, 149
individual preferences 22
indoor air quality 60, 70, 204
indoor environmental comfort 88
indoor environmental quality (IEQ) 88,
    196, 202
IEQ indicators 89, 95
IEQ parameters 89, 95
indoor temperatures 74
indoor thermal environment 31
inpatients 118
Internet of things (IoT) 200
interviews 12, 70, 92, 168, 171, 227

landscape architecture 184
L=light, quality of 204
limitations *see* research limitations
logistic regression model 71

manageability 9
materials, interior 132
mean temperature 75
meaningfulness 9
medical: expenses 232; needs 195
mental health environments 111
method(s) 10, 41, 64, 91, 113, 142, 167,
    195, 227
mixing, of people 182
mixed methods 91
mobility, of patients 139, 141, 149, 167
monitoring 68

narrative review 195
natural environments 174
nature 9, 166
needs, environmental 185
Netherlands, The 60
normality (of work) 45

observation (method of) 12, 147, 172
occupant behaviour 60, 64, 77
office: context 7; environment 22, 31, 33;
    occupants 31; temperature 39
older adults 164, 195, 221, 239
organisational influence 21
outdoor activities 184
outdoor friendly environments 164, 184

Parkinson's disease 170
particulate matter 61
patient experiences 92, 95
patient mobility 145
patient needs 140

patients 88, 111
path analysis 52
parameters 46, 76
perceived: comfort 97; control 92
perception of: indoor air quality 62, 76;
     thermal environment 35
personalisation 23
perspectives, of staff and patients 126
physical activity 166
physiology 42
physiological: adaption 89, 96; factors 41
Pittsburgh Sleep quality Index (PSQI) 70
place attachment 9
pollutant levels 70
poor quality housing 221
portable air filters 60
practical implications 25
productivity 31, 44; gains 40;
     measurement 41
psychological adaption 89

qualitative analysis 94
quantitative data 35
quality of life 102, 139, 193, 225
questions 116
questionnaires 35, 92, 171

random sampling 92
recruitment, of participants 144, 168
rehabilitation: centres 139; environments
     140; of older people 166
relationships, with buildings 193
relative humidity 62
research design 15
research limitations 24, 80, 100, 130,
     158, 187
research method *see* method(s)
retrospective questionnaire 36
rooms, configuration of 132
routes 146

safe environments 177, 196, 207
safety, of staff and patients 132
salutogenesis 6
security 196, 207
self-esteem 227
self-perception 44
sensors 68, 92
sensory 167
sensory stimuli 174
shadowing, of patients 145

sleep 62
sleep quality 70, 82, 166
smart technologies 200
social: atmosphere 19; cohesion 186;
     interactions 9, 23, 32, 166, 196,
     205; isolation 236
spaces: for gathering 182; outside 179
spatial arrangement 34, 142, 195
spatial distance 139
staff 111, 118, 171
statistical analysis 71, 120, 150
stimuli 64
stroke 139
structural equation models 48
summer: indoor air quality 76;
     temperatures 36
survey tool 112, 114
surveys 142, 168
Sweden 10

task-related 22
thematic analysis 228
theoretical framework 102
theoretical model 165
therapeutic gardens 167
thermal: behaviour 32; conditions 62;
     comfort 33, 39, 62, 203, 223, 234;
     environment 35; stimuli 62
thermoregulation 32
time log 146
transcription 15, 94, 172

United Kingdom (UK) 60
United States of America (USA) 111

ventilation 40, 60, 91, 204

walker (aid) 144
walking 196
walking routes 178
wards 140
wayfinding 8, 141, 195
wellbeing 37, 81, 90, 100, 193, 221, 239
wheelchair 144
winter indoor air quality 76
winter temperatures 36
work culture 32
workspace personalisation 16
World Health Organisation 6, 60, 71, 90,
     102, 164, 193

For Product Safety Concerns and Information please contact our EU
representative GPSR@taylorandfrancis.com
Taylor & Francis Verlag GmbH, Kaufingerstraße 24, 80331 München, Germany

www.ingramcontent.com/pod-product-compliance
Lightning Source LLC
Chambersburg PA
CBHW060248220326
41598CB00027B/4023

9 781032 383750